THE TROUBLED ADOLESCENT
as He Emerges on Psychological Tests

THE TROUBLED ADOLESCENT

as He Emerges on Psychological Tests

ERNEST A. HIRSCH, Ph.D.

INTERNATIONAL UNIVERSITIES PRESS, INC.

New York   New York

To the adolescents whom I examined or in whose psychological examinations I had a part, I dedicate this volume.

Topeka, January 1970

Contents

Preface   1

1. Introduction   3

2. The Intellectually Limited Adolescent   16
   - CLINICAL SUMMARY: Claire 17
   - THE PSYCHOLOGIST'S DESCRIPTION 19
   - WECHSLER INTELLIGENCE SCALE FOR CHILDREN . . . 20
     - INFORMATION 22
     - COMPREHENSION 24
     - ARITHMETIC 26
     - DIGIT SPAN 26
     - SIMILARITIES 26
     - PICTURE COMPLETION 28
     - PICTURE ARRANGEMENT 28
     - BLOCK DESIGN 33
     - OBJECT ASSEMBLY 34
     - VOCABULARY 35
     - CODING B 36
   - THE BENDER GESTALT TEST 38
   - THE DRAW A PERSON TEST 38
   - RORSCHACH TEST 42
   - CHILDREN'S APPERCEPTION TEST 49
   - SENTENCE COMPLETION TEST II 55
   - THE PSYCHOLOGIST'S REPORT 59
   - DISCUSSION 62
   - CLINICAL SUMMARY: Stan 64
   - THE PSYCHOLOGIST'S DESCRIPTION 65

WECHSLER INTELLIGENCE SCALE FOR CHILDREN . . . 66
   INFORMATION 66
   COMPREHENSION 68
   DIGIT SPAN 70
   ARITHMETIC 70
   SIMILARITIES 71
   PICTURE COMPLETION 72
   PICTURE ARRANGEMENT 72
   BLOCK DESIGN 72
   OBJECT ASSEMBLY 72
   VOCABULARY 73
   CODING B 74
THE TACTUAL FORM TEST 74
THE BENDER GESTALT TEST 76
RORSCHACH TEST 79
THEMATIC APPERCEPTION TEST 86
THE PSYCHOLOGIST'S REPORT 88
CLINICAL SUMMARY: George 92
THE PSYCHOLOGIST'S DESCRIPTION 93
WECHSLER INTELLIGENCE SCALE FOR CHILDREN . . . 94
   INFORMATION 96
   COMPREHENSION 98
   ARITHMETIC 101
   DIGIT SPAN 102
   SIMILARITIES 102
   PICTURE COMPLETION 104
   PICTURE ARRANGEMENT 106
   BLOCK DESIGN 108
   OBJECT ASSEMBLY 109
   CODING B 110
   VOCABULARY 110
STANFORD-BINET SCALE, FORM L 112
EXAMINING FOR APHASIA 113
   AGNOSIAS 113
   APHASIAS 114
THE BENDER GESTALT TEST 116
THE DRAW A PERSON TEST 120
RORSCHACH TEST 122
CHILDREN'S APPERCEPTION TEST 123
THE PSYCHOLOGIST'S REPORT 129

Discussion 133
Conclusion 133

3. The Adolescent with Central Neurological Impairment 136
 Clinical Summary: Ken 137
 The Psychologist's Description 139
 The Wechsler-Bellevue Scale 139
  INFORMATION 140
  COMPREHENSION 142
  DIGIT SPAN 143
  ARITHMETIC 144
  SIMILARITIES 145
  PICTURE COMPLETION 146
  PICTURE ARRANGEMENT 147
  BLOCK DESIGN 148
  OBJECT ASSEMBLY 149
  DIGIT SYMBOL 150
  VOCABULARY 150
 Story Recall 152
 The BRL Sorting Test 152
 The Story Completion Test 157
 The Bender Gestalt Test 159
 Rorschach Test 161
 Thematic Apperception Test 169
 Sentence Completion Test II 174
 Word Association Test 177
 The Psychologist's Report 185
 Discussion 189
 Clinical Summary: Hal 190
 The Psychologist's Description 191
 The Wechsler-Bellevue Scale 192
  INFORMATION 193
  COMPREHENSION 195
  DIGIT SPAN 197
  ARITHMETIC 197
  SIMILARITIES 198
  PICTURE COMPLETION 199
  PICTURE ARRANGEMENT 199
  BLOCK DESIGN 200
  OBJECT ASSEMBLY 200

DIGIT SYMBOL 200

VOCABULARY 200

STORY RECALL 201

THE BRL SORTING TEST 201

THE BENDER GESTALT TEST 204

THE TACTUAL FORM TEST 209

THE DRAW A PERSON TEST 209

RORSCHACH TEST 211

THEMATIC APPERCEPTION TEST, WORD ASSOCIATION
TEST AND SENTENCE COMPLETION TEST 216

THE PSYCHOLOGIST'S REPORT 217

DISCUSSION 219

CONCLUSION 220

4. The Disorganized Adolescent   221

CLINICAL SUMMARY: Al 221

THE PSYCHOLOGIST'S DESCRIPTION 223

THE WECHSLER-BELLEVUE SCALE 224

INFORMATION 225

COMPREHENSION 227

DIGIT SPAN 229

ARITHMETIC 230

SIMILARITIES 231

PICTURE COMPLETION 232

PICTURE ARRANGEMENT 234

BLOCK DESIGN 235

OBJECT ASSEMBLY 236

DIGIT SYMBOL 236

VOCABULARY 236

THE BENDER GESTALT TEST 238

THE DRAW A PERSON TEST 240

RORSCHACH TEST 242

THEMATIC APPERCEPTION TEST 249

SENTENCE COMPLETION TEST II 251

WORD ASSOCIATION TEST 253

THE PSYCHOLOGIST'S REPORT 256

DISCUSSION 260

CLINICAL SUMMARY: Bill 261

THE PSYCHOLOGIST'S DESCRIPTION 262

THE WECHSLER-BELLEVUE SCALE 263

INFORMATION 263
COMPREHENSION 266
DIGIT SPAN 267
ARITHMETIC 268
SIMILARITIES 268
PICTURE COMPLETION 269
PICTURE ARRANGEMENT 270
BLOCK DESIGN 272
OBJECT ASSEMBLY 272
DIGIT SYMBOL 272
VOCABULARY 273
THE DRAW A PERSON TEST 276
RORSCHACH TEST 278
THEMATIC APPERCEPTION TEST 290
SENTENCE COMPLETION TEST II 296
THE PSYCHOLOGIST'S REPORT 297
DISCUSSION 301
CONCLUSION 301

5. The Doubt-Ridden Adolescent   304
CLINICAL SUMMARY: Paul 305
THE PSYCHOLOGIST'S DESCRIPTION 306
THE WECHSLER-BELLEVUE SCALE 307
INFORMATION 308
COMPREHENSION 311
DIGIT SPAN 313
ARITHMETIC 314
SIMILARITIES 314
PICTURE COMPLETION 316
PICTURE ARRANGEMENT 317
BLOCK DESIGN 320
OBJECT ASSEMBLY 322
DIGIT SYMBOL 322
VOCABULARY 322
THE BENDER GESTALT TEST 327
THE DRAW A PERSON TEST 333
RORSCHACH TEST 337
THEMATIC APPERCEPTION TEST 353
THE PSYCHOLOGIST'S REPORT 354
DISCUSSION 359

CLINICAL SUMMARY: Wes 360
THE PSYCHOLOGIST'S DESCRIPTION 362
THE WECHSLER-BELLEVUE SCALE 362
  INFORMATION 363
  COMPREHENSION 366
  DIGIT SPAN 368
  ARITHMETIC 368
  SIMILARITIES 371
  PICTURE COMPLETION 372
  PICTURE ARRANGEMENT 372
  BLOCK DESIGN 373
  OBJECT ASSEMBLY 373
  DIGIT SYMBOL 373
  VOCABULARY 374
STORY RECALL 377
THE BENDER GESTALT TEST 377
THE DRAW A PERSON TEST 381
THE BRL SORTING TEST 384
THE STORY COMPLETION TEST 389
RORSCHACH TEST 389
THEMATIC APPERCEPTION TEST 398
WORD ASSOCIATION TEST 401
SENTENCE COMPLETION TEST II 410
THE PSYCHOLOGIST'S REPORT 415
DISCUSSION 420
CONCLUSION 420

6. The Nonreflective Adolescent   422
CLINICAL SUMMARY: Joan 423
THE PSYCHOLOGIST'S DESCRIPTION 424
THE WECHSLER-BELLEVUE SCALE 425
  INFORMATION 426
  COMPREHENSION 428
  DIGIT SPAN 429
  ARITHMETIC 430
  SIMILARITIES 431
  PICTURE COMPLETION 432
  PICTURE ARRANGEMENT 432
  BLOCK DESIGN 433
  OBJECT ASSEMBLY 435

DIGIT SYMBOL 435
VOCABULARY 436
STORY RECALL 438
THE BRL SORTING TEST 438
THE BENDER GESTALT TEST 440
THE DRAW A PERSON TEST 442
RORSCHACH TEST 443
THE STORY COMPLETION TEST 445
THEMATIC APPERCEPTION TEST 445
SENTENCE COMPLETION TEST II 451
WORD ASSOCIATION TEST 454
THE PSYCHOLOGIST'S REPORT 461
DISCUSSION 464
CLINICAL SUMMARY: Helen 465
THE PSYCHOLOGIST'S DESCRIPTION 467
THE WECHSLER-BELLEVUE SCALE 468
INFORMATION 470
COMPREHENSION 472
ARITHMETIC 474
SIMILARITIES 475
PICTURE COMPLETION 476
PICTURE ARRANGEMENT 478
BLOCK DESIGN 480
OBJECT ASSEMBLY 481
DIGIT SYMBOL 482
VOCABULARY 482
THE BRL SORTING TEST 484
THE BENDER GESTALT TEST 488
THE DRAW A PERSON TEST 492
RORSCHACH TEST 495
THEMATIC APPERCEPTION TEST 503
SENTENCE COMPLETION TEST II 509
THE PSYCHOLOGIST'S REPORT 513
DISCUSSION 517
CONCLUSION 518

7. The "Delinquent" Adolescent 519
CLINICAL SUMMARY: Don 520
THE PSYCHOLOGIST'S DESCRIPTION 522

THE WECHSLER-BELLEVUE SCALE 523

  INFORMATION 524

  COMPREHENSION 526

  SIMILARITIES 526

  PICTURE COMPLETION 527

  PICTURE ARRANGEMENT 528

  BLOCK DESIGN 529

  OBJECT ASSEMBLY 529

  VOCABULARY 530

THE BRL SORTING TEST 533

THE BENDER GESTALT TEST 535

THE DRAW A PERSON TEST 537

RORSCHACH TEST 539

THEMATIC APPERCEPTION TEST 552

SENTENCE COMPLETION TEST II 555

THE PSYCHOLOGIST'S REPORT 560

DISCUSSION 564

CLINICAL SUMMARY: Chuck 565

THE PSYCHOLOGIST'S DESCRIPTION 566

THE WECHSLER-BELLEVUE SCALE 567

  INFORMATION 568

  COMPREHENSION 570

  ARITHMETIC 571

  SIMILARITIES 573

  PICTURE COMPLETION 575

  PICTURE ARRANGEMENT 575

  BLOCK DESIGN 576

  OBJECT ASSEMBLY 576

  DIGIT SYMBOL 577

STORY RECALL 577

THE BRL SORTING TEST 578

THE BENDER GESTALT TEST 578

RORSCHACH TEST 580

THEMATIC APPERCEPTION TEST 592

WORD ASSOCIATION TEST 598

SENTENCE COMPLETION TEST II 598

THE PSYCHOLOGIST'S REPORT 602

DISCUSSION 606

CLINICAL SUMMARY: Jack 607

THE PSYCHOLOGIST'S DESCRIPTION 608

THE WECHSLER-BELLEVUE SCALE 609

   INFORMATION 610

   COMPREHENSION 613

   DIGIT SPAN 614

   ARITHMETIC 615

   SIMILARITIES 616

STORY RECALL 618

THE BRL SORTING TEST 619

RORSCHACH TEST 619

THEMATIC APPERCEPTION TEST 626

SENTENCE COMPLETION TEST II 628

WORD ASSOCIATION TEST 633

THE PSYCHOLOGIST'S REPORT 633

DISCUSSION 637

CONCLUSION 638

8. Final Thoughts   639

Bibliography   644

Preface

The contents of this book are intended as a series of one-sided supervisory sessions which deal with the test performances of various psychologically troubled adolescents. The book does not refer to studies which corroborate any points of view. Instead, clinical judgments are based on experience with the psychological examinations of children, adolescents and adults. For this reason, the judgments expressed may well be open to critical evaluation by persons whose opinions, based on *their* experiences and theoretical preferences, differ. These pages are intended for student clinicians who wish to come in contact with inferences based on adolescents' test behavior and for colleagues who wish to compare their methods and inferences with those of a fellow clinician. It is not a book that concerns itself with teaching how to administer psychological tests. It is assumed that the reader is familiar with this skill, or that it is irrelevant to him, and that he wishes to relate psychological constructs to the behavior which these types of procedure lay bare. Or he may simply want to come in contact with material produced by adolescents.

The Menninger Foundation offers an exciting experience to anyone interested in working with colleagues and teachers in order to be of psychological help to those who need it. The atmosphere which has been created by the Menninger family stimulates a dedication, first to the process of understanding, and then to doing something constructive with it. The same atmosphere has encouraged the writing of this book, which concerns itself with the young person on the threshold of adulthood. For the opportunity to participate in an institution with such a pervading intellectual and helping tone, I am more than grateful.

1

I also wish to express gratitude to the persons who broke the ground for this kind of psychological study: to David Rapaport and Roy Schafer, whose books were invaluable, both in my graduate studies and until a time when I was able more effectively to walk on my own.

Many thanks are due my clinical teachers: Dorothy Fuller, Cotter Hirschberg, Walter Kass, Arthur Mandelbaum, Martin Mayman (whose idea it was to write this book), Rudolf Ekstein, and the many others whose clinical sensitivities and capacities for infecting others with their abilities and enthusiasms did so much to help develop my own and their other students' clinical skills.

Heartfelt thanks are due my colleagues and students, who participated in setting up an environment which stimulated thought, encouraged discussion, and refined conceptualization.

My warm feelings of gratitude go, of course, to the troubled adolescents whose protocols appear in this book, and from whom (and from other adolescents, as well as from children and adults) I learned so very much.

I thank Gardner Murphy, who read each of this book's chapters while it was still in an inchoate stage, and who made his gentle and helpful comments from a somewhat different frame of reference than the clinical. My grateful thanks to the others who read various of these chapters, whose thoughtful comments I found extremely useful: Sydney Smith, Howard Shevrin, Walter Kass, Gary Goldenberg and Cotter Hirschberg.

To Linda Davis who typed and retyped (and typed again) the manuscript of the book, my very special gratitude.

1

Introduction

Who is meant by "the adolescent"? Who should be included in this category?

A distinction between "adolescence" and "puberty," the former referring to psychological, the latter to physiological, characteristics which appear during a certain period of development, somewhat clarifies the problem. But it does not help enough. For example, is the young person who is neither in the midst (or even at the apparent edge) of the psychological ferment of adolescence, and who has also not yet shown the physical signs of change which come with puberty, not "really" an adolescent, even though he is fourteen years old? Particularly if such a young person is a "late developer," he may be experiencing major unhappiness about not undergoing the same physical and psychological changes as his peers. Since a concern with development is intimately associated with the adolescent process, such a child certainly has a place in a book which deals with psychological problems especially associated with this period.

The question about whom to include in the book was solved arbitrarily. It was decided to include any child whose age fell vaguely within the range of the teen-ager—"vaguely," because not rarely one meets a preteen-ager who tries to deal with many of the issues commonly associated with adolescence.

The adolescents who appear in these pages are limited to the middle and lower age ranges, to the young persons trying to deal with the beginning or middle phases of the adolescent period. Older adolescents, working to resolve the last stages of this period, were not examined at The Menninger Foundation's Children's Service and were therefore not included here. This omission, as will be seen, represents only one of the book's sampling deficiencies.

The primarily upper middle-class composition of the adolescents who appear in these pages also results in a somewhat distorted picture. The unbalanced sample leaves out the very large group of adolescents which more typically comes to the attention of local diagnostic and treatment centers. It is the author's conviction, however, that much can be learned even from this economically, socially and culturally special group. Adolescence presents similar psychological problems to all young people, regardless of class or caste. Adolescent rebellion takes place regardless of a family's economic status; so does the wish to remain in childhood; so does the wish to leap into adulthood without going through adolescence; so do most other attempted efficient and less efficient adolescent solutions. In other words, differences between social classes seem to involve not so much differences in the basic nature of problems to be solved, nor even in the major ways to solve them, but rather in the *specific contents* of these problems and their solutions. An adolescent of relatively low socioeconomic status may speak a different language from one who comes from a group of higher socioeconomic status; he may take part in activities which differ in content from those of his economically more well-off fellows; he may have different life ambitions. But the basic directions his conflicts take will emerge in much the same way—i.e., with his parents, his school, his peers and, of course, inwardly, with his new impulses, with his controls and with his many different strivings.

This volume is incomplete in other respects as well. Obviously not every kind of disturbed adolescent, with every kind of inefficient life solution, could be included. Case presentations are limited in number, not only because of lack of room but also because this work is not intended as an encyclopedia of adolescent disorders. The intention is, rather, to illustrate some major ways adolescents attempt to solve problems accompanying their development into adulthood. Obviously not all such efforts can be demonstrated. Only enough types of solution in enough types of adolescents can be shown to give the reader the additional understanding that will help him to deal more effectively with the young people who are experiencing this aspect of their maturation.

The author has in mind two kinds of reader whose understanding of adolescents might be furthered by a book of this kind:

1. The graduate student, who is familiar with some techniques of psychological testing and who wishes to see how these techniques can be concretized, specifically with adolescent test reactions.

2. The other group for whom this book is intended consists of psychological journeymen and masters who may find value in comparing their inferences and testing methods with those of another psychologist who works with adolescents. In some matters these readers will agree, in others they will disagree, but it is hoped that discussion and thought will be stimulated in either case.

Verbatim recordings of portions of the psychological test batteries of some adolescents who were seen at the Menninger Clinic for a ten-day examination, as well as the author's discussions of selected aspects of their test protocols, comprise the major part of this book.

The author's theoretical points of view are consonant with those expressed in psychoanalytic ego psychology and in what has more recently been referred to as humanistic psychology. He makes little effort to examine psychological phenomena from other possible vantage points (e.g., learning theory, neobehavioristic theory), with which he is on much less familiar ground. Some readers may well feel that the author's inferences are made too intuitively, so that they lack the experimental underpinnings that will eventually serve as an acceptable foundation for a valid clinical psychology. But the aim of this volume is modest: namely, to offer, for the examination of clinicians and others interested in adolescents, the convictions, thoughts, occasionally even the guesses, of one clinical psychologist who has worked intensively with young people, and who wants to share his understanding.

There are many ways one can get to know a child, an adolescent or an adult. How the other person eventually emerges partially depends on (1) the person who tries to describe him, (2) the methods he uses to arrive at his description and, (3) at least to some extent, the ways the person being described wishes to present himself. An adolescent may at various times be described by his teacher, parent, sweetheart, psychiatrist, friend, or probation officer. Methods for evaluation may include a Scout leader's report, a police blotter, a clinical interview, a friend's sketch, a history teacher's description, a younger sibling's complaints, and many others. The adolescent may wish to appear exactly the same as his peers, as much better than they, as overwhelmed by problems he cannot handle, as "cool," or "hip," or "hep," as not understood by those who count, as picked on, as tougher than most, and so on. Depending on the person doing the describing, on the method used for evaluation, and on the impression the person described wishes to make, the personality picture which emerges may be somewhat (occasionally quite extraordinarily) different from what it would be under other circumstances.

This book attempts to describe various adolescents through their performance on psychological tests. No claim is made that psychological tests represent a *via regia, the* way through which other persons can be fully known. Psychological tests cannot present the entire way a person "really" is, any more than can any other *single* procedure. Nevertheless, as part of a more comprehensive examination, psychological test results help significantly toward the construction of reasonably exhaustive, reasonably three-dimensional portrayals of a number of more or less representative adolescents.

To gain a relatively thorough understanding of these adolescents during their ten-day stay at the Children's Service of the Menninger Foundation, and to deal as much as possible with the built-in limitations of all examinational procedure, certain steps were taken:

1. To help overcome the distortions almost certain to appear whenever a single individual examines another, the adolescent and his parents were studied by a team.[1] The adolescent alone was seen by at least four different persons, representing not only four different professions, but also four separate personal, points of view. Although the members of this examining group were rather homogeneously (i.e., clinically) oriented, they nevertheless seemed to represent a sufficient variety of observational viewpoints so that the adolescents emerged in a sufficient breadth of dimension to permit the team to make useful recommendations.

2. To attenuate the distortions which would probably follow were information obtained by using only one method, various ways for gathering data were employed. The adolescent was physically examined, psychiatrically interviewed, neurologically evaluated, his parents were asked to present their views, and he was given x-ray, EEG and other laboratory examinations. Psychological testing, therefore, represented simply a portion of the entire investigation; it was made part of the other findings, so that a heterogeneous but still unified (and presumably fairly valid) picture of the adolescent could finally be constructed.

To assure that the psychologist would obtain as complete a pic-

---

[1] The team consisted of a psychiatrist, psychologist, social worker, neurologist, laboratory technicians and whatever other persons (e.g., ophthalmologist, speech pathologist, orthopedist) seemed required for consultation.

ture of the adolescent as possible, the psychological testing procedures used were also diversified. So that a high degree of descriptive differentiation could be achieved, a battery of tests (tapping different levels of awareness, different aptitudes, different qualities of conflict and conflict solution, etc.) was given each adolescent. Occasionally (e.g., when a question of intellectual ability was involved) different tests with similar purposes were used. Thus, a WISC and a Stanford-Binet might both be administered when mental limitation was suspected or observed. The psychologist would then be able to offer a more diversified opinion to the persons who could help the parents reach a decision about their child. While a "basic" test battery was always used, flexible modifications (i.e., substitutions, additions, omissions) were made whenever such changes seemed called for.

3. In order to deal optimally with the adolescent's mask, his need to present himself in a certain, ordinarily not spontaneous, way to an examining adult, the examiner invariably paid particular attention to trying to establish a trusting, nondefensive rapport. Once the adolescent felt relatively comfortable in the testing situation, it was felt, he would be able to relax enough to shed the psychological armor which always makes it so much more difficult for the examiner to see important, but too frequently disguised or covered up, personality facets.

The establishment of a relationship of trust with an adolescent is often a good deal more complicated than might at first appear. Young persons tend to raise their defensive guard whenever they consider their autonomy threatened, either by *too little psychological distance* between themselves and an adult, or by *too much*.

As for the danger of insufficient psychological distance, an examiner should probably avoid attempting to be just another adolescent. This particular effort to establish rapport is almost certain to fail. The adolescent mistrusts and secretly (sometimes not so secretly) ridicules the adult who rejects adulthood, who tries to talk the adolescent's language, and who attempts to adopt the adolescent's interests and attitudes. An adult simply cannot be a genuine adolescent, and for that reason he can never be accepted as one by adolescents. The adolescent, who usually feels that the adult ought to act his age, is uncomfortable in dealing with a pseudo adolescent. While the adolescent may characteristically rail against grownups, he also knows, somewhere, how much he needs to have them around. He realizes that he requires the adult, not only for physical and emotional support, not only as teacher and guide; he "knows" that he requires him in order to be able to crystallize an identity, through *incorporation-identification* on the one hand, and through *opposition-resistance* on the other. Without adults around to catalyze identificatory processes, the adolescent would be hard put to make his transition into adulthood successfully. Therefore, it not only embarrasses him to come in contact with an adult who acts a much younger role—it frightens him to see his adult model, whom he wishes both to copy and to resist, abdicate his duties as an identification standard. From the point of view of the clinical team trying to arrive at valid conclusions about the adolescent being examined, the adult who empathizes completely with (i.e., who "becomes") the adolescent can hardly function as an objective evaluator.

To avoid creating too much psychological distance, the examiner has to be wary of being the judgmental, condescending, moralistic adult whom many adolescents consider their natural enemy and to whom they are unable to reveal themselves. The examiner who wishes to gain an adolescent's confidence reaches his aim most effectively by imparting his sincere wish to learn about the adolescent, about his interests, activities, conflicts and fears (the last of which are usually directly stated only with great reluctance, if at all). The adult should certainly avoid conveying the attitude that the adolescent's values are rather ridiculous and his behavior immature. The psychologist should be willing to recognize that "even" an adolescent can sometimes fill gaps in an adult's knowledge.

The psychologist should be able to laugh with an adolescent. There is little that destroys affective barriers more effectively than shared humor—provided the adolescent first introduces the humor as a coin of interchange. The examiner must take care to avoid using his humor as a weapon (e.g., as a way to make the adolescent feel less adequate). Nor can humor be permitted to get out of hand, so far as the adolescent's aggressions are concerned. Nothing falls quite so flat as humor introduced to an adolescent who is not amused by it, who is threatened by it, or who becomes fearful and disorganized because of the destructive use to which he himself puts it. Humor, in other words, although it can be extremely helpful when used judiciously, needs to be utilized in a highly selective fashion—much better to omit humor altogether than to employ it poorly.

Such procedural caveats lead to a general rule which the examiner is probably wise to follow: usually wait for the adolescent to take interpersonal initiative. The examiner does well to avoid taking the relationship lead with an adolescent; he is wise to maintain initiative only with the mechanics of the tests themselves. The examinational relationship works most effectively when the examiner volunteers little more than his generally friendly, interested attitude, while, for the rest, he remains pleasantly businesslike and *reacts to* whatever tone the adolescent sets. More active efforts to create a relaxed examinational situation had best come from the adolescent—and they usually do, though not always. The psychologist ought to respond fully to the adolescent's wish to draw nearer, but he is rarely well advised to do more than respond. Each adolescent, as is true of any person, has his own level of tolerance of friendliness; if he is shown more warmth than he can comfortably handle, he becomes preoccupied, in one way or another, with fending off the other person's approach. Although many examiners leave interpersonal initiative not only to adolescents, but to children and adults as well, it seems particularly important to leave first moves in the hands of these young people who are so exquisitely sensitive to, and preoccupied with, problems of independence.

A major reason that trusting rapport is frequently difficult to establish with an adolescent is that he is often taken to a clinic involuntarily or against his will. Because the solutions adolescents try do not work well for themselves, their family, their community, or any combination of these, their parents often *bring* them to be examined. A psychiatric clinic represents, of course, only one of the available places where it is hoped adolescents' ineffective solutions will be remedied. Other times adolescents are brought to court, or sent to a military academy, or encouraged to go on an extended trip. In such ways, other persons try to help either the troubled youngsters or themselves.

Adolescents are very often reluctant to take the initiative in asking for psychological help, since by seeking help they appear to be admitting an inability to run their lives adequately. A great number of, if not most, adolescents react to the problems they create for themselves and their environment by projecting blame—in that way they are able to remain much less aware of their own participation in ineffectual solutions. Since the fault, after all, is "out there," it is rare to find an adolescent who spontaneously expresses a wish for psychological help for himself.

The presentations of the test protocols that follow are intended to serve several purposes. The primary one is to draw attention to the major tasks which the adolescent must undertake in order to deal with his inevitable, imminent transition into adulthood. The special character of this period of development has been described in a most useful fashion by A. Freud (1958), Blos (1962) and Erikson (1956). The reader familiar with the concepts of these theorists will easily identify them as they are implicitly touched on by the author. All three analysts stress how critical a developmental time adolescence is. They point out that adolescence is a time during which early dependencies should be discarded and replaced by more adult relationships; a time when resolutions should be made to enable the young person to become increasingly willing to enter adulthood, to become independent, to reach decisions about who he wants to be and what he wants to do with his future; a time when dormant impulses appear with new violence and must be dealt with.

Not only does this book try to demonstrate how these tasks are *general* to all adolescents (i.e., how the nature of the tasks tends to override individual reactions, so that the process of adolescence faces a diversity of young persons with the *same* growth phenomena); the book also tries to demonstrate the variety of *individual* ways the members of this heterogeneous young group try out in order to deal with a childhood that is already gone and an adulthood that has not yet arrived. In order to demonstrate this diversity of solution, these pages contain the test batteries of a rather wide range of young people. Cases range from adolescents whose difficulties seem produced almost entirely by "organic" features, to ones whose behavior patterns seem to result fairly exclusively from "functional" influences.

The book begins with the protocols of some young people who are intellectually "retarded"; it goes on to present a few who suffer from "organic dysfunction"; then it presents several "schizophrenic" adolescents (in whom the degree of "organic involvement" remains uncertain). It continues with test batteries of adolescents who are usually designated "neurotic" (i.e., "obsessive" and "hysterical"), and ends with several "characterologically" disturbed or "delinquent" adolescents.

The book also stresses the heterogeneities so obvious in the psychic organizations of young people, who, in spite of their frequently significant diversities, have often been squeezed into diagnostic categories which imply a spurious equivalence. Thus, for example, one can see major differences in how "even" the mildly retarded adolescent, each with his unique personality organization, deals with the important life decisions that assume a special quality because of his limitations.

The diversity of personality organizations cannot be overemphasized. It should become apparent that an enormous oversimplification is involved when one speaks of "the" adolescent, even "the" retarded or "the" delinquent one. Comments regarding each person's uniqueness represent, of course, barely more than clinical truisms, since, starting with their earliest training, psychologists are enjoined to respect the individuality of each person. And yet, there exists a difficult-to-resist inclination to speak and think about individuals (particularly adolescents) categorically. Categorization can, of course, lead to exceedingly important understanding, so long as differences are not ignored. In part, this book will emphasize the *variety* of adolescents, the contrasting solutions they try out, and the vastly different appearance they present, even though they may have been given identical diagnostic labels.

As soon as one touches on the diagnosis of adolescent disorders, one unavoidably raises questions about diagnosis in general. The protocols that follow will touch on issues that seem pertinent to present-day diagnostic considerations, similar to a number of points raised by Menninger, Mayman and Pruyser (1963). The diagnosis of childhood disorders involves innumerable problems; the diagnosis of adolescent disorders seems barely less complex. As the adolescent test protocols are presented, certain diagnostic issues are raised and discussed. Such lengthy and involved deliberations seem important to clarify diagnostic thoughts with which the psychologist must wrestle as he works with poorly organized adolescents.

The emphasis on uniqueness, and the wish to demonstrate the differences that exist among adolescents, reflect adult values much more than adolescent ones. Uniqueness, so highly valued by many adults, is not at all highly valued by the majority of adolescents. Frequently, in fact, a difference from adolescent peers can be the source of intense unhappiness, and often a major reason for a clinical examination stems from the adolescent's need to act "like the others," to meet the standards of some adolescent ideal. Problems involving uniqueness and sameness are of special significance among so-called "delinquent" adolescents, since the need to be "the same" not infrequently leads to behavior which ends with the adolescent's colliding with the law.

Another purpose of the book is to illustrate the special issues the psychologist must come to grips with in order to reach valid diagnostic conclusions about adolescents. Not only do adolescents have to solve typical problems which crop up during the six to seven years (sometimes more, sometimes less) that set the boundaries of adolescence; the clinician also has to grapple with characteristic and unique diagnostic considerations. The clinical psychologist working with adolescents probably finds that he thinks about them more as he would about adults than as he would about younger children. Especially in cognitive functioning, the adolescent is able to perform in much the way he will later on, when he has reached full maturity. Such capacities as memory, concept formation, motoric skill, perceptual accuracy and so on, will probably not undergo much further significant change. But there the resemblance with adults ends.

Emotional factors are another story altogether. Perhaps the clinician's chief concern in working with adolescents is in estimating how severely deviant, how disorganized, is the behavior he witnesses. It is often said, although it may not seem very helpful to hear it, that it is "normal" for the adolescent to act in "abnormal" ways. Even though this statement sounds paradoxical, there is a good deal of truth to it. Unfortunately, as clinicians working with adolescents, we often cannot be certain of our diagnostic conclusions, so that we find ourselves unable to assert unequivocally that a certain adolescent's behavior goes beyond the bounds of what might "normally" be expected during this period. Often, we find ourselves relying on little more than a "feeling" as we try to determine at what place the behavior steps over the frontiers of whatever we think of as adequate affective, cognitive and behavioral organization. This state of affairs reflects our ignorance about adolescence. We will have to be content with this approach, however, until a time when we know much more about the process involved in the transformation from the fulmination of adolescence into the greater stability of adulthood. Adolescence is a time when aspects of personality are still falling into place, when the young person is actively trying to find suitable (for him) ways of living, i.e., when he is investigating various life solutions for himself. Since psychological upheaval is usually par for this period, it is the clinician's task to determine when the furor is too extreme. The clinician who works with adolescents must avoid two extremes of error in this regard: using the adult as his absolute prototype, the psychologist may overreact to a fairly peripheral and transitory piece of somewhat extraordinary behavior by considering the adolescent in whom it appears "deeply disturbed"; or the psychologist may take the opposite position, i.e., that adolescence has nothing in common with other life periods, so that any behavior, no matter how peculiar, is shrugged away as "only adolescent."

Illustrations of the author's inferences, and of ways he seeks to translate them into a comprehensive clinical summary, constitute a further reason for presenting a book of this sort. Much clinical inference is done without ever being made explicit; the process of inference often takes place immediately and rather intuitively particularly once the clinician has had the opportunity to study a good number of cases. While much inference is of this almost instantaneous nature, the effort is made here to show where and how hypotheses originate and what their various clinical implications might be. The attempt is made to say in some (sometimes perhaps in too obvious) detail what is often taken for granted, what for many clinicians may have become second nature. Every clinician arrives at his clinical deductions in his own way, and the author as clinician makes inferences in ways which may seem invalid to others. But the author does not mean to imply that his are the only possible inferences; rather, he wishes to present inferential processes of a sort that have worked for him. Many readers may find it difficult to accept either the content of the inferences, or the ways the author goes about making them, or both. It is largely because of basic differences of this kind that we must agree that clinical psychology still lacks and is still groping toward a sturdy, easily communicable, scientific foundation. Until such a dependable basis is achieved, differences of theoretical approach are both necessary and desirable.

In the cases that follow, the reader will participate in the actual testing of adolescents as it takes place in one clinic. The author has tried to furnish verbatim accounts of what these young people say, of what they do, and of what the examiner says and does in response. The reader will note that the examiner tries to walk a fine line between, on the one hand, adhering to the letter of standardization and, on the other, momentarily disregarding the letter of standardization in order to pursue leads that promise increased understanding. If the illustrated testing technique seems to lack a certain type of rigor, it can nevertheless be noted that the method has a rigor of its own. Some of the examiner's questions which at first may seem "irrelevant" turn out not to be so after all. The ground rules for using the testing method illustrated here are to modify standardized instructions as little as possible and then *only* for purposes of increasing the examiner's understanding of the person's test response. To that end, the examiner asks only those questions which will more fully clarify the meanings of answers given or not given. Concrete results (e.g., I.Q. scores) of examinations conducted in this way can obviously not be interpreted as having meanings identical to ones derived from different procedures.[2]

Some further comments about how the material that makes up this book was collected: the adolescents whose test batteries follow were all examined by the author, serving as a member of the usual clinical team, a number of years ago. The psychiatrist and psychologist saw each child, and the social worker the parents. The adolescent was also given neurological, physical and laboratory examinations. As already indicated, whenever it seemed important to do so, further (e.g., visual, hearing) examinations were given. All the examiners presented their findings at a final conference, where a case synthesis was made.

The psychologist based his contribution to the final conference on the sorts of test protocols that follow. At this final meeting, attended by the team members and by other professional persons, differences were resolved, points of view were related to each other, a dynamic formulation was made, and a plan of action was agreed upon. What follows in this volume, therefore, rather than reflecting *final* formulations of cases, represents semifinal (or quarter-final) résumés of the ways one team member understood the adolescents he examined. While, for the reasons mentioned previously, the clinical team could not pretend to say what the adolescent was "really" like, the conclusions it reached at each final conference, as the result of its pooling of information, resulted in a rather complex, rather valid portrait of the adolescent being considered.

How about the validity of the tests used in the examination batteries presented in this volume? As will be seen, many of the tests are used rather differently from the way in which they were originally intended. Rather than being interested in "the I.Q.," for

[2] The testing approach used in these pages is discussed by Rapaport, Gill and Schafer in their *Diagnostic Psychological Testing* (1945-1946). It is illustrated by Schafer in *The Clinical Application of Psychological Tests* (1948).

instance, the author is interested in the way the individual presents himself stylistically, characterologically, defensively and so forth. The "tests," rather than testing in the established sense, serve as relatively stable ways (stable from individual to individual) through which people express themselves. The examiner, using his awareness of the way people behave, tries to make clinical sense of their test responses. The tests, in other words, serve as a kind of structured clinical interview. The examiner is interested not so much in the validity of the *examinations* as he is in his *own* validity—that is, how well he is able to understand and productively use the responses. Thus, the author is less concerned with the degree to which "the I.Q." score is accurate, and more concerned to find out, for example, what personal characteristics the individual uses to deal with tasks, what kind of blockages and emotional detours occur while he works them, what are the significances to the individual of dealing with the test problems, what sorts of interactions go on between the person taking and the one giving the test, and so on. Validity in the usual sense, therefore, plays only the smallest role in the way that psychological examinations are used here.

2

The Intellectually Limited
Adolescent

This chapter contains portions of the psychological tests of adolescents who lack the cognitive equipment that would permit them adequately to manage the problems brought into focus by changing stages of their development. Young people who, because they are "mentally retarded," lack the organizing tools necessary for dealing effectively with the psychological and physiological features of adolescence, will be presented.

One cannot speak of a "typical retarded" person, just as one cannot speak of a "typical" adolescent, or child, or adult of any sort. Retarded adolescents usually differ significantly from one another. They differ in the degree to which they accept their more limited abilities; in the degree to which they deny recognition of their limitations; in the degree to which they suffer as a result of comparisons they make with intellectually more able age mates; in the degree to which some cognitive functions are differentially affected, and in the degree to which they get along with their peers and with adults. Significant differences exist, too, in the amount of security such children feel within themselves—how helpless they feel because they know less and can do less. Do they live in fear of their environment and of their impulses because they consider themselves to have insufficient capacity to handle either? Retarded adolescents differ, of course, in the extent of their total impairments. They differ in the etiology of their retardation. Most of all, they differ in the organization of their personality—in the nature of their motivations and of their defensive styles and structures.

But these differences hold for all retarded persons—children, adolescents and adults. What is unique about the retarded adolescent? His uniqueness lies in facing the special, very major task of entering adulthood, leaving behind early dependencies, and becoming self-sufficient.

A retarded adolescent naturally cannot make a truly major break with his past the way young people with nonimpaired cognitive functioning can. But some retarded adolescents can take much firmer steps in that direction than others.

This chapter contains test records of three adolescents who have made three types of solution to their cognitive disability and to the change demanded by adolescence. The first adolescent, Claire, is of borderline intelligence. She wishes to avoid recognizing that her abilities are limited, and she tries to ignore her inability to do many things as well as others her age can do them. She feels insecure at home and in school and tries to handle this insecurity by remaining a little girl who does not intend to grow up. Claire remains young and passive; she deals with others' wishes by quietly resisting them, by spoiling their plans and by remaining immovable.

The second adolescent, Stan, differs from Claire because his retardation is complicated by an occasional tendency to abrogate reality. Rather than needing to deny his inability (and thereby implicitly recognizing it, as Claire does), he tends to ignore it. By not taking cognizance of his retardation, he avoids needing to correct for it.

The third adolescent, George, is more severely retarded than the other two, but he permits himself to recognize his limitations. He can accept them better than either Claire or Stan can. Although his intellectual difficulties create major problems as he needs to deal with the many intricacies of adolescence, he will probably be able to enter adulthood a good deal more successfully than either Claire or Stan.

Following is Claire's record. The brief résumé of her clinical history which begins immediately below is prepared from the examining psychiatrist's summary. This summary, in turn, is based on information gained from examinations by the psychiatrist, caseworker, neurologist, internist, speech pathologist, laboratory staff and psychologist.

CLINICAL SUMMARY: Claire

Claire is thirteen years old and an only child.

During the pregnancy with Claire, her parents were concerned because the mother is Rh negative and the father Rh positive, but no complications developed. There was a thirty-one-hour labor and a "new" anesthetic was used. Claire was born tongue-tied and underwent immediate minor surgery for this condition. She had "colic" as an infant, crying for hours at a time. She first sat up at six-and-a-half months and did not walk until sixteen-and-a-half months. She spoke simple words, however, before one year of age. Toilet training was begun at the age of four months and completed by the age of six months, though it had to be repeated later. She showed chronic constipation during infancy. She was enuretic until five-and-a-half years and continued to wet the bed occasionally until the age of ten years. She was described as a quiet, reserved, uncommunicative and sometimes negativistic child from an early age, and she showed little interest in toys or other activities.

At eleven months of age, she was hospitalized for five days for a fever of undetermined origin and for refusal to eat. She recovered promptly with intravenous feedings and penicillin. From an early age she showed what doctors thought was muscle weakness, and she had callouses on her feet as a result of foot deformities for which special shoes were prescribed. She suffered many injuries as a result of falls, including a chipped left elbow at the age of four-and-a-half, a fracture of both bones of the right forearm at the age of seven, a severe sprain (requiring five weeks of hip-to-ankle cast) of the left lower extremity in the fifth grade, a chipped tooth in the sixth grade and several cut lips and fractured teeth within the last year.

Complaints about Claire's behavior came from the school system through the years, but any suggestion that she might be retarded was always met with vigorous opposition from her parents. When she began kindergarten, the school nurse, for reasons unknown, wondered if she might have a brain tumor. This suggestion led to an examination by a neurologist who found no evidence of a tumor, but who thought that Claire was retarded in both motor and mental functioning.

In the fifth grade she was not promoted, but her extreme reaction to this situation resulted in her not being returned to the fifth grade. When she began junior high school, her school adjustment worsened, and this worsening led to the present examination.

At present, although Claire's school attendance has been perfect, she is often late to school and tardy to class. She wanders around the school aimlessly, leaves her possessions behind, almost always forgets her homework, provokes teasing by other children and often stands and stares at people in the hallway. Her schoolwork, which has progressively deteriorated, is of failing quality, and she is maintained in school only through the special consideration given her by her teachers.

Little is known about Claire's adjustment at home, although it is known that she has frequently locked herself in the bathroom and has talked to herself for long periods of time. She has had fantasies about being a member of an imaginary family.

Physical and Neurological Examinations: Physical findings include a shortness of the trunk of the body compared to the length of the legs, a mild upper-dorsal scoliosis to the left and increased elevation of the left shoulder, scapula and breast. Both ears stand out and their markings are primitively differentiated. Neurological examination shows a generalized hypotonia, a marked hyperextensibility at the elbows, knees, and toes and a limitation of supination in the right forearm. The gait is awkward, with a clumsy rotation of the hips and some unsteadiness. A mild disarthria is intermittently present.

The EEG shows bilateral positive spike dysrhythmia, predominantly six per second, seen alternately on the left and right in the temporal areas, especially during drowsiness and light sleep.

THE PSYCHOLOGIST'S DESCRIPTION

Claire's somewhat odd appearance is accentuated by a prominently missing front tooth. She is awkward, particularly as she walks and goes up and down stairs. Her gait is so stiff that she gives the appearance of wearing leg braces.

Her general manner is that of a child much younger than thirteen. At times she is passive, trusting and naïve; at others she is stubborn and petulant. Often she attempts to play on my sympathy. As I administer the test, she often looks reproachful and helpless, hoping to stop my questions. At other times she tries at least to slow me down by twisting her face into a seductive grimace, which turns into a petulant one when I continue as before. At these times she seems truly forlorn. Her efforts to ingratiate herself, meant sincerely enough, seem to be a parody of a friendly, social approach.

A need to cling to me is particularly evident at the end of each test session. Sometimes she can not leave the office until I also leave and close the door behind both of us. At the end of each interview she usually finds something of interest which prolongs the termination of our meeting.

Together with her passive clinging, Claire's tendency to be resistive and obdurate can be seen. Fairly often she does not answer a question; instead, she makes herself appear engrossed in another activity; or she simply smiles. Sometimes she claims not to know an answer when she obviously does. Throughout, she protects herself against the possibility of humiliating failure. She avoids vulnerability by not attempting the things she might do poorly.

The degree to which Claire depends on others for cues about how to act in a social situation is seen by the ways she parrots my comments. Sometimes she appropriates them *in toto*. I mention, for example, that there is much ice on the ground; a few seconds later Claire says, "Boy, there certainly is a lot of ice on the ground." In such a way, she depends on others to discover what to think and how to organize her thinking into words.

Claire is engaged in a constant power struggle: with her parents, teachers, with other adults and with her contemporaries. She feels under great pressure to obey, to produce, to bow under, and much of her behavior has the aim of resisting demands which she cannot or does not want to meet.

WECHSLER INTELLIGENCE SCALE FOR CHILDREN[1]

[A glance at Claire's WISC Scattergram reveals her mild intellectual disability. Her Verbal and Performance capacities are about equally developed and place her intellectual ability in the Borderline range.

[As one studies her subtest performances more closely, one sees that Claire's abilities range from a weighted score of 4 on Comprehension and Coding to one of 10 on Arithmetic. The age equivalents range for these performances is from about seven to eight years (Comprehension and Coding) to approximately fourteen years (Arithmetic). In other words, on the Arithmetic subtest, Claire functions as well as, or better than, one might expect of any person her age, while on Comprehension and Coding she functions only

---

[1] Wechsler (1949). The Rapaport method (Rapaport et al., 1945-1946) of administering, scoring and interpreting the Wechsler-Bellevue, Adult Form, has been adapted for use with the WISC.

slightly better than one would expect of someone half her age. One suspects that numbers, possibly because they are so impersonal, may offer Claire a special haven of safety and therefore a special opportunity for excellence of performance.]

Name:	Claire		Age:	13-1

	RS	WTS	0 1 2 3 4 5 6 7 8 9 10 11 12 13 14 15 16 17 18 19 20
COMPR.	8	4	
INFOR.	12-13	6	
DIG.	9	8	
ARITH.	12	10	
SIMIL.	10	8	
VOCAB.	26	5	
P. A.	26	8	
P. C.	10	7	
B. D.	19-27	8-9	×
O. A.	18	6	
CODE	26	4	

TOT. VERB.	33
TOT. PERF.	33-34
TOT. SCALE	66-67

VERBAL I.Q.[2]: 79 LEVEL: Borderline

PERFORMANCE I.Q.: 76-78 LEVEL: Borderline

TOTAL I.Q.: 75-76 LEVEL: Borderline

This Scattergram points to an important issue: the I.Q. figure may conceal at the same time that it reveals. Still, the I.Q. should not be abandoned or ignored, as some suggest, because it does not tell the whole story. It was never meant to do that. What the I.Q. does tell is extremely valuable, but this one measure certainly does not give the much more complete information (e.g., concerning cognitive style) which is needed for a more thorough understanding of the person undergoing psychological examination. Particularly with the retarded, it is necessary to look first at the quantitative, and then at the qualitative, features which make up this global (I.Q.) index.

[2] In accordance with the Rapaport scoring of the Wechsler-Bellevue, the Digit Span subtest score is omitted in the computation of the I.Q.

INFORMATION

No.	Question	Response and Comments	Score
1.	How many ears have you?	(She says nothing. I repeat the question. She gives me a long, puzzled look.) . . . . (I repeat the question.) . . . . Thirteen. ("Are you sure?") Two. [These responses give us a good deal of information. We see Claire's hesitation in complying, and we see her efforts to appear helpless and very ignorant. She first gives a somewhat ridiculously incorrect answer; once I challenge it, she emerges with the correct one. One can see that Claire tries to push me away by telling me something obviously incorrect, perhaps hoping unrealistically that I will give up asking further questions. Claire apparently needs to appear more limited than she really is. With a little firmness she momentarily gives up this position. One wonders, too, whether her negativism might be in response to an insult she feels about my asking her such a very easy question—as though I expected only so little of her.]	1
2.	What do you call this finger? (Show thumb.)	Thumb. (She leans over to look at my writing.) [She is trying to establish an intimate and young relationship, or, particularly considering her high Arithmetic subtest score, she is being hyper-alert.]	1
3.	How many legs does a dog have?	Four.	1
4.	From what animal do we get milk?	Ah . . cow.	1
5.	What must you do to make water boil?	You make it . . you put it over heat.	1
6.	In what kind of a store do we buy sugar?	Groshery store. [Claire shows the type of speech immaturity commonly found among retarded children.]	1
7.	How many pennies make a nickel?	. . . . Five, I believe.	1
8.	How many days in a week?	. . . . Uh, seven, I believe. [The "I believe" in this and the last answer suggests Claire is no longer certain of her ground. She is trying her best, however, and for the moment has given up needing to demonstrate less ability than she has. Perhaps as she finds the going harder, she considers the questions worthy of her best efforts.]	1

No.	Question	Response and Comments	Score
9.	Who discovered America?	. . . . . Columbus? [As the questions are becoming harder, Claire's uncertainty increases.]	1
10.	How many things make a dozen?	Twelve.	1
11.	What are the four seasons of the year?	Uh . . well, first there's . . ah . . another one is winter . . and autumn . . spring and fall. ("What comes after spring?") Winter, doesn't it? Summer!! [Facts that a thirteen-year-old should know are not easily at hand. "Another one is" suggests the unavailability of the concept, or word, "summer."]	1
12.	What is the color of rubies?	Red . . a real deep red. [After the preceding near failure, Claire seems happy to know a correct response again and volunteers additional information.]	1
13.	Where does the sun set?	I believe in the east? [Claire has apparently reached the limits of her available information. She receives credit for only one more answer.]	0
14.	What does the stomach do?	That I don't know. ("Can you think of anything it might do?") No. (She says this very definitely.)	0
15.	Why does oil float on water?	(She shakes her head and makes it apparent that she has no idea.)	0
16.	Who wrote Romeo and Juliet?	. . . . That's . . I don't know that one either. I'm sorry, but I just don't know it. [Claire's "I'm sorry" suggests that taking these tests is a favor to me; because she does not know, she hurts me. The phrase probably also reflects distress about the gaps in her knowledge.]	0
17.	What is celebrated on the Fourth of July?	Ah . . . . . . tsk . . . . . (She looks embarrassed) Firecracker day, isn't it? Fireworks day. ("Why do we have fireworks?") I don't know. [Young and retarded children know the Fourth of July primarily as a day on which to explode firecrackers. They have little idea why firecrackers are set off. This "concrete" response exemplifies a sensory-motor type of conception.]	0
18.	What does C.O.D. mean?	Don't know.	0
19.	How tall is the average American man?	I'd say he's about six feet, 2 inches.	0
20.	Where is Chile?	I don't know.	0

No.	Question	Response and Comments	Score
21.	*How many pounds are there in a ton?*	Two thousand. [This correct response comes as a surprise, although Claire does well on both the Arithmetic and Digit Span subtests. Numbers appear to have a special meaning for her. Claire has failed the last eight questions, so that one would not expect her to know this answer. Although a psychologist may be fairly sure that a person is unable to answer further questions, it is often worthwhile to go beyond the five failures recommended by the manual. Even though the examiner may not be particularly interested in knowing whether a patient is able to achieve further credit, he may find it important to discover how the patient deals with questions as they become progressively more difficult to answer.]	1
22.	*What is the capital of Greece?*	I don't know.	0
23.	*What does turpentine come from?*	I don't know.	0
24.	*How far is it from New York to Chicago?*	I don't know. ("What would you guess?") (She shrugs her shoulders.) ("Make some kind of guess.") I just simply don't know. [With the exception of the "American man" question, Claire is reluctant to take a chance, to make a guess, because she is so afraid she may be wrong. The rest of the Information questions were not administered. Claire almost certainly would not know the answers, and it seemed important, at the beginning, to avoid a situation in which she would experience too much failure.]	0

RAW SCORE: ___12-13³___

WEIGHTED SCORE: ___6___

COMPREHENSION

No.	Question	Response and Comments	Score
1.	*What is the thing to do when you cut your finger?*	Put a Band-Aid on it.	2

³ A figure following a hyphen represents an alternate score. It is assumed that this score reflects what the subject could optimally achieve, in the absence of repressions, regressions, anxieties, temporary inefficiencies and other intelligence-inhibiting or intelligence-disrupting impairments.

No.	Question	Response and Comments	Score
2.	*What is the thing to do if you lose one of your friend's dolls?*	Replace it. [This response shows a surprisingly fluent use of words.]	2
3.	*What would you do if you were sent to buy a loaf of bread and the grocer said he did not have any more?*	I'd just go on and tell my mother what the grocer said. [Claire demonstrates helplessness in relying on her mother rather than using her own initiative. The solution of going to mother for direction is usually found in younger children.]	1
4.	*What is the thing to do if a girl much smaller than yourself starts to fight with you?*	Well, I'd just tell her mother on her.	1
5.	*What should you do if you see a train approaching a broken track?*	(She claps her hand over her mouth.) Oh! I gotta think! . . . . Well, you just . . ah . . ah . . try and fix it before the train comes. [Here she is more active, but unrealistically so.]	0
6.	*Why is it better to build a house of brick than of wood?*	I don't know. ("Could you think of some reason?") No, I don't know. ("Well, just give me any reasons you can think of.") Because . . ah . . ah (she hits the table) when the wind comes, it might blow the house down, and it wouldn't with the bricks. ("Any other reasons?") M'm. [Again, Claire is able to give a scoreable response when she is firmly encouraged. Were one to accept her "I don't know" at face value, one would accept her wish-fear to be considered more limited than she is.]	1
7.	*Why are criminals locked up?*	Cause they might steal something you have.	1
8.	*Why should women and children be saved first in a shipwreck?*	I don't know. ("Can you think of any reason?") M'm.	0
9.	*Why is it better to pay bills by check than by cash?*	Uh-uh.	0

No.	Question	Response and Comments	Score
10.	*Why is it generally better to give money to an organized charity than to a street beggar?*	You might not know the street beggar. . . . ("And why shouldn't you give him money then?") Well, he might start chasing after you. [Claire's fearfulness is triggered off by a question which ordinarily is handled without affect. She reacts emotionally to a situation which most persons can handle objectively.]	0

(The remaining comprehension items were not administered because they were too complicated and hence threatening.)

RAW SCORE: ___8___

WEIGHTED SCORE: ___4___

ARITHMETIC

(Claire does amazingly well and efficiently here. She can do twelve of the sixteen problems, most of them in less than three seconds. She is goal directed and does not attempt to lead me away from the test. Her helpless mannerisms have dropped away, and she takes obvious pride in her ability.) [This is the kind of surprise for which the examiner should be prepared. Arithmetic is so often the nemesis of retarded children. So often they do not have a concept of numbers; most frequently they have had discouraging experiences with them and try to avoid them. This subtest shows how wrong it would be to understand a "retarded" child as equally retarded in all abilities. It is not rare to see the degree of test scatter which Claire demonstrates. Her relatively intact arithmetical ability is of a kind that may offer a basis on which to build a program to educate or train her. One can hardly overestimate the importance of this kind of scatter. One should view these islands of higher ability as more than an accident. Although Claire had had special training in arithmetic, it is significant that she has been able to make use of it. Apart from its "ability" significance, Claire's capacity to work so effectively with numbers may well reflect such characteristics as a sensitivity to relationships and an alertness to her surroundings.]

RAW SCORE: ___12___

WEIGHTED SCORE: ___10___

DIGIT SPAN

(On Digits Forward, Claire repeats five digits on her second try. She becomes confused on six digits and says that she cannot do them.

(She repeats four Digits Backward on the second try. When she is given five digits, she can do only the first three both times; then she says, "I don't get the rest of it.")

RAW SCORE: ___9___

WEIGHTED SCORE: ___8___

SIMILARITIES

No.	Items	Response and Comments	Score
1.	*Lemons-sugar*	Sweet.	1
2.	*Walk-throw*	Hands.	1

THE INTELLECTUALLY LIMITED

No.	Items	Response and Comments	Score
3.	Boys-girls	Women.	1
4.	Knife-glass	Cut. [These first four questions require that verbal completion, rather than a true concept, be offered in answer.]	1
5.	Plum-peach	They're shaped the same way. ("How do you mean?") (She shakes her head.) (I give examples of concepts that would fit.)	1
6.	Cat-mouse	They . . . are animals.	2
7.	Beer-wine	They're liquor.	2
8.	Piano-violin	They're instruments. [Claire is able to conceptualize on this level.]	1
9.	Paper-coal	I don't know. ("Can you think of any way?") Uh-uh.	0
10.	Pound-yard	(She shakes her head right away, without permitting herself to think about the question at all.) [Claire combines a tendency to give up without giving herself a chance (probably because of fear that she *might* fail) with a true inability to solve a problem because of intellectual limitation. She illustrates the intermingling of ability and motivational factors. Could she do better if she were willing to take the risk of failure? So often retarded children are doubly penalized: first, by their retardation and, second, by the anxiety which inhibits them from learning what they could, even with their limitation.[4]]	0
11.	Scissors-copper pan	(She shakes her head; then she thinks about the question a moment; she shakes her head again.)	0
12.	Mountain-lake	(She shakes her head right away; then she thinks a little about it, and then she shakes her head again.)	0
13.	Salt-water	They're both minerals.	0
14.	Liberty-justice	I don't know.	0
15.	First-last	I don't know.	0
16.	The numbers 49 and 121	(Not administered.)	–

RAW SCORE: 10

WEIGHTED SCORE: 8

[4] The author once witnessed a retest increment of 30 I.Q. points in an eleven-year-old boy whose anxiety was so reduced by medication that he could permit himself to try intellectual problems which he had previously angrily rejected.

PICTURE COMPLETION

(Claire is able to get the first eight completions without significant difficulty. She gets two of the next four and fails the rest.)

No.	Item	Time	Missing	Response and Comments	Score
9.	Scissors	—	Screw	I can't find anything wrong here. (25") (She shakes her head.)	0
10.	Coat	3"	Buttonholes	Buttonholes.	1
11.	Fish	3"	Dorsal fin	His fins. ("Where should they be?") On the other side. ("Would you see them?") (She shakes her head.) [This is not an unusual failure for a young or retarded child. At first it seems that Claire has the correct answer, but she means that the side fin (which would be invisible to an observer) rather than the back one, is missing.]	0

(She solves the *screw* item, but on the others she says, "I can't find a thing wrong with them." On the last, *house,* item she says, after 11", "I think the sun is setting in the wrong direction." ("How do you mean?") "East, it should be over this way (to the side)." [Claire is aware that this is the last item of the subtest. She realizes that she has not been doing well and wants to "give" me some kind of answer to make up for her failures. Although she cannot do what is required, she does not want to leave me with a poor impression of her. She changes the sun's directions in order to give me at least a symbolic something, even though I had asked what was missing, rather than what was wrong with the picture.]

RAW SCORE: __10__

WEIGHTED SCORE: __7__

(The testing was interrupted at this point and resumed the following day.)

PICTURE ARRANGEMENT

No.	Item	Correct Order	Time	Arranged Order	Story[5] and Comments	Score
1.	Fire	FIRE	27"	FIRE	It was about a fire. ("Tell me all about it.") And . . ah . . and . . ah . . ah. . . . . This little boy was playing with matches, and he knew he wasn't supposed to. And then he . . . and then gets himself caught on fire, and he burns the house down, and his mother	4

[5] The patient is asked to tell the story she has sorted, after the cards have been removed.

No. Item	Correct Order	Arranged Time Order	Story and Comments	Score
			calls the fire department, and . . ah . . . and then they get the ah . . ah . . . . . fire hose out	
2. Burglar	THUG	26″ UTHG	The story is about a villion . . villain. . . . . . The . . . (she smiles, obviously embarrassed and unable to go on). . . He finds something to do . . and then . . he . . ah . . goes to the house. He opens up the window, goes in, and finds this . . ah . . man, and sees him get in . . . and then he arrests him. [Claire does not appear to understand this sequence at all. The story reflects her difficulty in grasping continuity. She is unable to bridge the gap between individual pictures in order to assume the "as if" of the cards representing a continuous story. Although the same character is represented several times, Claire sometimes feels that each representation is that of someone else. Is her own life equally fragmented?]	0
3. Farmer	QRST or SQRT	8″ QRST	About this man who . . ah . . its . . who plants these seeds for corn . . to . . . . he can't . . . . then he gets this corn all planted out . . . And then, after he gets it all planted out, he sees a scarecrow in there. And then . . then after a while he decides he'll pick some. And then after he gets done, he goes to his truck, a whole load, and the . . and drives away.	6

No.	Item	Correct Order	Time	Arranged Order	Story and Comments	Score
4.	Picnic	EFGH or EFHG	38″	EFGH	It was about a dog. And he smells the chicken. And then he finds out it *is* a chicken. He . . grabs the . . ah . . ah . . chicken away from this man and woman. And they walk along and walk along. And they find that their chicken is missing. And that's it. ["And they walk along and walk along" is an immature way of saying something like, "and they walk along for a while." Claire's manner of telling a sequence of events is highly immature. It consists of a chain organization whose elements are connected by "and." No element stands out; no portion is more significant than another; everything is of equal importance, as in the stories of very young children. In this way Claire demonstrates her difficulty in indicating a cause-effect relationship.]	4
5.	Sleeper	PERCY	21″	EPRCY	Well, it was about this man. And he was asleep. And . . ah . . this dern alarm clock rang off, it just gave him fits . . . . Soon he gets up, gets dressed, goes down to eat, and his wife tells him he's almost late for work . . So he gets down to his office and starts in sleeping again . . And his boss finds out he's sleeping and fires him. He was a dummy to do a thing like that. [Significant here is Claire's moralistic end-	0

No. ·Item	Correct Order	Arranged Time Order	Story and Comments	Score
			ing. According to her view, behavior is either right or wrong. It is "wrong" to fall asleep at work. Since "bad" behavior must be punished, Claire invents a punishment. She demonstrates her lack of sophistication, her inability to grasp humor, her (probably identificatory) need to assign moral values to behavior, as well as her tendency to modify reality to make it into what she needs it to be.]	
6. *Gardner*	FISHER or FSIHER	35″ FSIHER	It was about the man. Soon he . . no, soon his wife tells him to fix the fence, and to hoe the garden, or something. So he goes out and . . he hoes for a while, and then he decides he'll go fishing. So, after a while, when he gets down to the lake where he's sitting, he . . ah . . finds . . he soon finds out that he . . decides to go to sleep while he's fishing. He was a dummy, too. ("Why is that?") Because his wife told him to hoe that garden, and he didn't want to. [Again Claire fabulizes. Possibly because elements are not held firmly enough in her memory, she contaminates the present sorting with the preceding one and has "the man" go to sleep. This is the second time she uses the phrase "he's a dummy," and one begins to understand the extent to which being	4

No.	Item	Correct Order	Time	Arranged Order	Story and Comments	Score
					a dummy means being "bad," and to what extent she is very probably referred to as a "dummy" and as "bad" at home.]	
7.	Rain	MASTER MSTEAR ASTEMR	38″	MASRTE	Well, his wife. It's about the man. And his wife tells him . . . his wife goes out to find that it's raining. So after a while the man finds out he has to take his umbrella, so he fools around and fools around and fools around, until finally he decides he'll go out. So he goes out. . . And that's it. [This is the third time that Claire talks about "the man," and although the men of the last three sequences are obviously different, it seems that Claire considers them to be the same, possibly because they are all "dummies." She is unable to make a coherent story here, but once again one meets her judgmental, moralistic tone. One begins to see the extent to which Claire sees men as "dummies"—to what extent she may be repeating comments about the way her father is seen at home and to what extent her tendency may represent both a projection and a retaliation. Suggesting that others are "dumb" is undoubtedly somehow reassuring to Claire.]	0

RAW SCORE: 26

WEIGHTED SCORE: 8

BLOCK DESIGN

(Claire was given credit for Items A and B. On Item C she had a block rotated. She corrected her error when I asked if her blocks were just like those on the sample and therefore received full credit on the item.)

(She is eager to turn the Block Design cards before I am ready.) [Claire tries to deal with the anxiety of the unexpected by attempting to prevent its becoming unexpected. She must not let herself be surprised—i.e., unprepared—because then she is more likely to fail. She may well also experience difficulties with impulse control.]

No.	Time	Accur.	Description of Behavior and Comments	Score
1.	18″	Yes	(She has no difficulty, although she is somewhat slow and tentative. She begins to turn the card for the next item.)	5
2.	27″	Yes	(Again she experiences no difficulty.) Is that right? (She peeks at the following item.)	4
3.	80″	Yes	(Much trial and error at the beginning, with some confusion. Once she overcomes her initial difficulty, she completes the design fairly quickly.) That looks right.	0-4
4.	44″	Yes	It looks like a diamond in the center. There we go! (Triumphantly.) It ends up looking like a diamond, in the center of it. I followed right what it says here. You notice I use all four of the dots (blocks), ah, four dots . . red ones. [Claire's wish to have me think well of her is apparent. She uses a familiar shape—a diamond—in an effort to concretize and so facilitate the task.]	4
5.		No	(When she first sees the design:) Hmmmm! It's kind of complicated! (She gets the general idea fairly quickly. She changes two upper corners which she has reversed, but she leaves them still somewhat incorrect and then changes them to correct. At 2′ 35″ she has the design correct, except for the last corner block, which is reversed.)	0
6.	2′ 57″ (over-time)	Yes	(She does this one very slowly and with some errors, but she corrects her errors. She proceeds slowly but purposefully. She does the design correctly, but after the time limit. Then she peeks at the next design.)	0-4
7	3′ 24″ (over-time)	Yes	(At first it looks as if she could not possibly construct this design, but gradually, bit by bit, with many corrections, she manages to put it together.) [Although Claire achieves a weighted score of only 8-9 on this subtest, it is important to recognize that, sooner or later, she is able correctly to complete almost all designs. She is not able to work speedily. Sometimes she needs a good deal of time, but once given it she	0

No.	Time	Accur.	Description of Behavior and Comments	Score
			can do the tasks fairly well and quite accurately. Once she overcomes her initial planlessness and confusion, she is able to proceed in a fairly well-organized way. Again, this particular "eventually coming through" quality should be considered when Claire's future is planned.]	

RAW SCORE: 19-27

WEIGHTED SCORE: 8-9

OBJECT ASSEMBLY

Item	Time	Accur.	Description of Behavior and Comments	Score
Man	19″	Yes	(As with Block Design, she takes her time to get the parts to fit neatly.) [Frequently the somewhat retarded child attempts to make up for lacks in certain abilities by being particularly neat.]	5
Horse	60″	Yes	(She is slow but sure.)	6
Face	3′	Partial	Will this make a person? . . . . This is a complicated one. I'm afraid it's a little too complicated. (She does much contour fitting, not knowing what the pieces will make.) (At 3′ the two hair pieces are properly attached, as is the nose. She has the mouth in the chin area. She is able to do the entire face after I help her fit the eye piece.) It's kind of complicated, but I did it! It turns out to be a face. [Claire does not realize she is putting together a face until she is well along with it. Had she had an early appreciation of what she was to make, she could have avoided much contour fitting and other trial-and-error behavior. Claire finds this kind of visual-motor coordination task difficult, but her main problem appears to be the cognitive one of discovering what she is supposed to be doing. She organizes correctly, almost as an accidental afterthought.]	2

(We had to stop testing at this point and resumed later that afternoon, after Claire had completed her appointments at the laboratory.)

| Auto | 2′ 50″ | Partial | (As she enters the office:) You may think I look like a scarecrow when I take my scarf off. [Again, the wish to be pleasing to me and the tendency to be apologetic.] (She has the first three and the last two pieces together at 2′ 30″ but does not know where to place the two center pieces. At 2′ 50″ she has all pieces | 5 |

Item	Time	Accur.	Description of Behavior and Comments	Score
			fitted correctly, except for the door piece which is inverted.)	
			RAW SCORE:	18
			WEIGHTED SCORE:	6

VOCABULARY

No.	Word	Response and Comments	Score
1.	Bicycle	Something you ride on. [Claire demonstrates her concrete orientation. She does not describe a bicycle abstractly; she describes both it and what follows in terms of functions that can be performed.]	2
2.	Knife	Well, it cuts.	2
3.	Hat	You wear it.	2
4.	Letter	You mean, the kind that you write to? You write one.	2
5.	Umbrella	You . . ah . . . (There is a long pause during which she smiles at me.) . . . . . You ah . . hold it. ("How do you mean?") So you won't get water on your head.	2
6.	Cushion	It might mean the cushion of the finger. ("What is that?") The little soft part here. (Shows me.) [This is an idiosyncratic definition.]	2
7.	Nail	You pound on it. You pound it into something, in other words.	2
8.	Donkey	Something you ride on. Ride on. (She speaks in slow, measured tones, ostensibly so that I can keep up with her as I write.)	2
9.	Fur	As . . well, it's something you wear. ("Can you tell me more?") No. ("What is it?") It might be the coat of an animal.	2
10.	Diamond	Well, it's something real shiny. ("Can you tell me some more?") No. ("What's it for?") Some special occasion.	2
11.	Join	Well, it connects. [Claire makes an unexpected leap into the more abstract. Her ability to make such a leap suggests that both ability and preference are involved in her choosing more concrete ways of expressing herself.]	2
12.	Spade	I don't know . . I'm afraid I can't answer that. ("Have you ever heard of it?") Uh-uh.	0
13.	Sword	. . . I don't know. ("I bet you've heard of that word.") It's something you fight with. ("Can you tell me any more?") Oh, it's real sharp in the tip end of it. [Here again is an illustration of the error one could fall into if one accepted Claire's "I don't know" at face value.	2

No.	Word	Response and Comments	Score

With firm encouragement she gives an adequate response.]

14. *Nuisance* — That puzzles me. ("Any idea?") No. ("Have you ever heard of it?") (She shakes her head.) ("Do you sometimes say 'I don't know' when you really do know?") In a way. ("When?") Off and on. [Originally, the examiner speculated that *nuisance* was a loaded word for Claire, that she might be called "nuisance" at home and that therefore the word aroused so much negative affect that she could not or would not define it further. A little later (see *nonsense,* word 16) it becomes apparent that Claire has defined "nuisance" as "That puzzles me." The examiner first thought that Claire was responding with her reaction to a word she found too difficult to define; only later did it become clear that she was actually giving her definition of the word. In this way false examiner hypotheses are sometimes made and discarded. Perhaps Claire is conveying her confusion about what people might mean when they call her a "nuisance." Possibly she wonders why people call her that and what they mean by it when they do.] — **0**

15. *Brave* — Well, if you know you're brave, you're intelligent. [Here again, it seems as if all "good" things are lumped together under the heading "intelligent"; all "bad" things under the term "dummy."] — **0**

16. *Nonsense* — I just told you that. ("Where's that?") On the last page. ("What did you say then?") It puzzles you. [Claire has apparently confused *nonsense* and *nuisance* (word 14). It may be that when something puzzles her she behaves in such a way that her behavior is described as "nonsense" and she as "a nuisance."] — **1**

17. *Hero* — You're real brave, and you know lots of stuff, I guess. [Again, a "good" thing is associated with being intelligent.] — **1**

18. *Gamble* — It means you want to take something up. ("How do you mean?") . . . . Let's see . . . . . ("What do you have in mind?") I don't know. — **0**

(Claire did not know the meanings of the remaining words.)

RAW SCORE: 26

WEIGHTED SCORE: 5

CODING B

(Claire works slowly and intensely. Her figures are accurately drawn. She is able to complete only one line of symbols. Once she becomes lost; once she skips spaces in order to fill in those that she knows well.) [Time once again is the villain.]

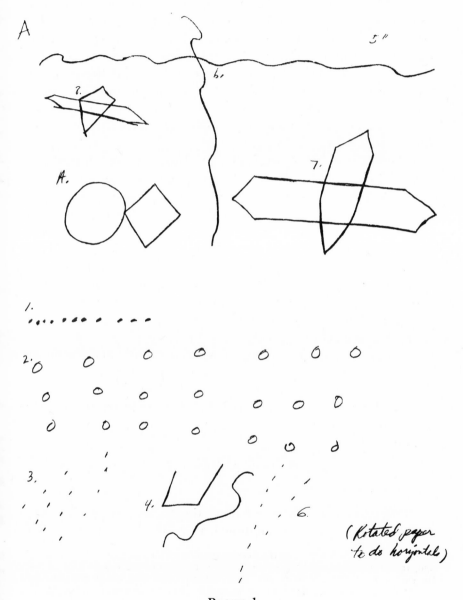

PLATE 1

THE BENDER GESTALT TEST[6]

[Part A (Plate 1, p. 37) demonstrates what happens to Claire's visual memory when it is not reinforced by a present stimulus: geometrical patterns become primitivized, reversed and simplified, and at times the gestalt becomes distorted. Claire's graphomotor movements demonstrate irregularities of speed, pressure and rhythm. She tends to be sloppy and has difficulty making her lines come to a point. Sometimes her drawings develop a shapelessness (see Nos. 3 and 5). Particularly notable is her poor organization: she begins in the middle of the page, drifts toward the bottom and then goes to the top and fills in empty spaces wherever they are available. At times she oversimplifies a drawing and creates one which is very different from its model (see Nos. 7 and 8).

[Claire is able to do better on Part B (Plate 2, p. 39) where she can study and copy the stimulus and thereby reinforce her visual-motor capacities. Even on this part, however, we see strong evidence of Claire's tendency to primitivize and simplify. Primitivizations appear markedly in Design 1; poor organization and poor motor control are evident in Design 2; simplifications of dots into dashes in Design 5; fragmentation of the gestalt in Design 4; impaired wrist-hand coordination in Design 6; distortions of the gestalt in Design 7, and gross inaccuracies of execution in Design 8.

[These drawings are consistent with the preceding findings that Claire functions intellectually at a lower level than one would expect of a girl whose chronological age is thirteen years, one month. Her performance on this test is consistent with her weighted score of 4 in Coding on the WISC.

[Clearly, the visual-motor coordination required for drawing and writing appears to be among the least developed of Claire's abilities.]

THE DRAW A PERSON TEST[7]

PART I (PLATE 3, p. 40)

("What is the girl like?") I don't think she's real good. I don't think she's the type of girl I'd draw if I was drawing a model. ("How

6 Bender (1946). On Part A of the Bender, the subject is encouraged to study each design; the card is removed after 5″, and he is asked to draw the design from memory. On Part B, he is given as much time as necessary to copy each design from the card.

7 Machover (1949). On Part I, the person is asked to draw a person. On Part II, he is asked to draw another person, of the opposite sex from the one he has just completed.

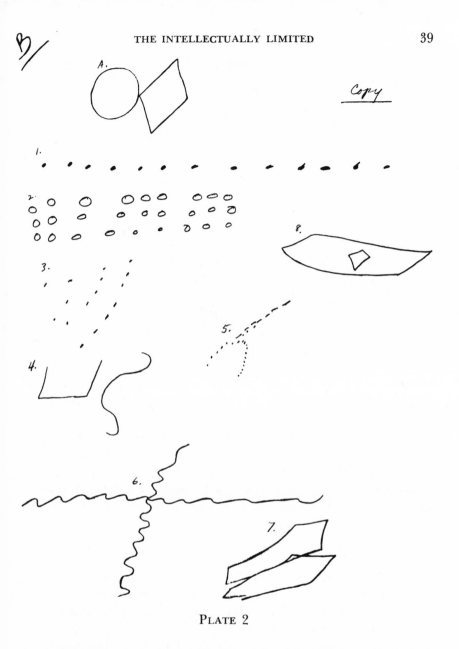

PLATE 2

would that be?") As far as drawing a model from a side view, I'd do it real artistic. ("What kind of girl is this?") I think she's a teenager. ("Anything else?") She looks like a woman. ("Can you tell me any more about her?") No.

[Claire's drawing is done primitively. The figure of the girl is poorly differentiated: there is no distinction between neck and

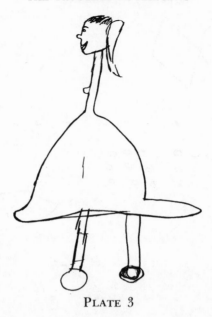

PLATE 3

shoulders; there are no arms; the feet are immature circles and the legs are of different thicknesses. The drawing could have been made by a young child.

[Claire seems somewhat aware of the inadequacy of her drawing when she says, "I don't think she's real good."[8] One is amazed, however, that she is not more taken aback by the inadequacy of what she has drawn, that she is not more self-critical. It is difficult to know whether she is consciously aware of how poor the drawing actually is.]

PART II (PLATE 4)

Well, about the boy . . if I were drawing him, it wouldn't be too artistic, but on the other hand, if I were drawing a model, it wouldn't be like this, I'll tell you. ("How would it be different?") Well, it's a different sex. It just isn't too good. ("What kind of a fellow is he?") A girl that goes with him. Oh! A boy that would go with the model I drew. ("What would he be like?") Hmmmm . . a teenager. ("Anything else?") No. ("What is that bump at the bottom of his shirt there?") His hands.

8 Unfortunately, I neglected to find out precisely what Claire meant—whether she had made a drawing which was "not good" or whether she had drawn a girl who was "not good" (i.e., herself).

[This drawing is even more primitive than the first. Once again, the facial features are differentiated, a characteristic which suggests Claire's attentiveness to the faces of others, her sensitivity to expressions which she uses as a gauge by means of which to adapt her actions.

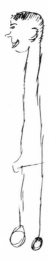

PLATE 4

[One should not leap to the conclusion that Claire experiences significant sexual confusion because of the slip in her description of the boy she has drawn. Confusion of pronouns is frequently encountered in retarded children. It is also often noted in adolescents, in whom it reflects a time-limited uncertainty about sexual and other identity. Before one becomes concerned by signs of identity confusion, the signs should be present in greater profusion than here. An examiner becomes concerned not only at meeting such signs in quantity, but by qualitative aspects, such as the degree to which the expression of identity confusion results in more severe and general disorganization. Most adolescents experience sexual confusion in their development toward adulthood; obviously, most are eventually able to make the appropriate choices.

[That Claire tries to deny sexual interests is suggested by her attempt verbally to undo the outline of the male genitals she has drawn. Claire's sexual interest is probably characterized by just such quick and inconspicuous expressions, followed by just as complete a denial.]

RORSCHACH TEST[9]

RORSCHACH SCORING SHEET

Number of Responses: 25 (1)

Manner of Approach (Location)

W	6
DrD	1
D	14
Dr	3 (1)
S	1
DC	0
Total	25 (1)

Groups of Contents

A	9
H	8
Hd	3
Obj.	1 (1)
Pl.	1
Shadow	1
Ground	1
Architect	1
Total	25 (1)

Location Percentages

W%	24(23)
D%	56(54)
Dr%	16(19)
De%	0

Determinant and Content Percentages

F%	76(77)/92(92)
F+%	32(30)/32(30)
A%	36(35)
Obj.%	4(8)
P%	4(8)-(4)((8))
A+%	0
H%	44(42)

Form, Movement, Color and Shading Determinants

F+	3		
F−	7		
F±	4		
F∓	5 (1)		
M+	1	M∓	1
FC−	1	FC∓	1
CF	1		
C′F	1		
Total	25 (1)		

Qualitative Material

Popular	III(VIII)
Combination	VIII IX X
Fabulized Combination	(1)
Fabulation	8
Confabulation	4
Peculiar	4
Perseverated	6
Symmetry	2
Castrative	1
Vague	4
Arbitrary	3 (1)
Projection	1
Aggression	4
Frightening	2
Self-reference	1

EXPERIENCE BALANCE: 2.0/3.0

[9] Rorschach (1921).

RORSCHACH PROTOCOL[10]

Card #	React. Time	Score	Protocol	Inquiry and Observations
I	6″	WF∓A	1. It looks like a bug. ("Anything else?") (She looks at me instead of the card.)	1. ("What did it look like?") I can't describe it. ("Tell me as you remember it.") . . . . . . ("Tell me whatever you remember.") (She shrugs.) I remember it's a bug. ("What makes it look like a bug?") The shape. ("What about the shape?") The head. ("How do you mean?") I don't know. (When she is shown the card again, she is able to describe such aspects as "little points," the wings and tail.) [Claire's response is consistent with her test protocol up to this point. Her "bug" is an easy, undifferentiated, nonreflective response, about which she can say almost nothing. She is apparently trying to get rid of the card as quickly as she can. Her looking at me instead of the card further reflects her wish to avoid, as well as her uncertainty about how I would like her to proceed.]
			It might be a . . . (She looks at me again and smiles.) . . . (She picks up the card and looks at it some more.) It's just a bug.	[It is difficult to tell at this point whether Claire is truly giving herself a chance to see something more or whether she is going through the ritual of looking, primarily to please me.]
II	4″	DF±Hd	1. It might be a head . . two heads. (Again she looks at me instead of the card.)	1. ("What do the heads look like?") They're persons' heads. ("And what else do they look like?") (She shrugs.) They don't look like much of anything. ("What kind of persons do they seem to be?") Live persons. ("What else?") Ah . . oh . . . . ("Do you know what I

---

[10] The Rapaport administration, briefly, is as follows: The subject tells the examiner all the percepts he sees on each card. When the subject has finished, the examiner removes the card and selectively, during inquiry, asks the subject to clarify some responses, from memory.

React. Card # Time Score	Protocol	Inquiry and Observations
		mean?") Uh-uh. (I give examples, e.g., old or young?) Old. ("Old what?") Persons. ("Are they men or women?") Men. ("What makes them look old?") The shape of them. ("Where?" I show her the card.) Near the front. ("What about the front?") The nose and lips. (She points vaguely.) (Black D's.) [Apparent again is Claire's passive resistance in the service of anxiety. She will not "give" unless she is pushed; even then she responds reluctantly. Her percept is vague, undifferentiated and immature.]
DF±A Vague	2. It might be a bug. (She looks at what I write and looks at me.)	2. ("What kind of bug?") Just a big bug. ("Can you tell me a little more about it?") No. ("Is it like the first bug you saw?") (She nods.) (Lower central red "butterfly.")
DF−H Vague Pec.	3. It might be a person. That's all.	3. ("Could you tell me about the person?") It was hidden in there. ("How do you mean?") The shape of it. (She indicates that the person can't be seen because it is hidden. She is getting more restless.) ("How is it hidden?") In the body of the bug. ("What is it doing there?") I don't know. (She is puzzled.) [Because inquiry with Claire is so confusing, one cannot tell whether she briefly saw the "ballerina" in the center space. Possibly because of the inconstancy of her perceptual memory and possibly because of her resistance, the percept seems to have disappeared.]
III 3″ WM+HP	1. It looks like two people are dancing. Well, they were holding hands . . dancing, I guess.	1. ("What kind of people?") Oh . . . . . just people, I guess.

React. Card # Time Score	Protocol	Inquiry and Observations

DF—A
Persev.
Pec.

2. The . . . in the center of it, there's . . there's the bug of it. (She turns the card to the side.)

2. ("What kind of bug?") A little one. ("What more can you tell me about it?") Nothing. I just saw the bug there. (Red center D.) [One notes first the easy "bug." This percept apparently represents a filler, an emergency response which is available until Claire finds something better. The "bug" response worked for Claire on the last card and apparently represents a way out of difficulty. "There's the bug of it" is a peculiar verbalization. It is as if Claire believed that the essence of each blot is its "bugness."]

DF+A
Symm.
Cast.
Persev.

3. On this side of it . . ah . . it's a bug . . . (Taps finger.) Rooster. Then on the other side (turning it again) it's the same thing.

3. ("And the rooster?") Part of his back end was cut off. ("As if?") As if a knife had just come down and slashed it. (Side red D.) [Claire's perceptual processes seem to have gone ahead of her associative ones; she outlines a percept but is unable to capture an association to it, so she falls back on her ubiquitous, easy "bug" before she is able to think of a rooster. The "as if" question is often valuable in bringing about worthwhile association.]

DrC'F
Shadow
Pec.
Arb.
Confab.

4. The center of the people . . their shadow . . . . that's it.

4. ("What made it look like the people's shadow?") I don't know . . it just did. ("Can you tell me any more about it?") (She shakes her head.) [Had a response of this type been obtained from an adult person of normal intelligence, one would immediately wonder about a schizophrenic disorganization. Where inquiry is so little responded to, scoring often constitutes educated guesswork.]

46   THE TROUBLED ADOLESCENT

[One rather frequently finds highly arbitrary responses among the intellectually retarded and among young children. One cannot interpret this arbitrariness to mean the same as if it were given by a nonretarded or older person. Often,
of course, retarded children and adolescents are seriously emotionally disturbed
as well as retarded. It may then be difficult to distinguish the lack of organization caused by immature thinking from disorganization caused by emotional
factors.

[Often children are called "psychotic" or "schizophrenic" because of peculiar,
confused, disorganized thinking. This diagnosis is frequently made on a phenotypical basis—the patient's thinking is superficially similar to that of the severely
emotionally disturbed person. Because of this superficial similarity, an erroneous
leap is made and a diagnostic label, neither parsimoniously conceived nor accurately thought through, is applied. The diagnostician must remember that persons of limited intelligence frequently give the superficial appearance of severe
emotional disturbance because of poorly organized thinking. The lack of organization can often more correctly be referred to disability rather than to other
causes. If a person with limited intellectual ability is given a task which requires
well-organized thinking, the results of his *un*ordered thinking may approximate
the *dis*ordered thinking of severely emotionally disorganized persons. The dy-
namics of the two conditions are not at all the same, however.]

Card #	React. Time	Score	Protocol	Inquiry and Observations
IV	3″	WF≠A Frightening Project. Persev. Vague Fab.	1. It just looks like a bug! (She looks to see what I write.) ("What do you think about my writing?") I don't think they're too good. ("How do you mean?") Because of your handwriting. (She turns the card over and hands it to me, looking as though frightened by it. She stands up.) Can we work on the Dictaphone today? ("Is this kind of scary?") Uh huh. . . . . Are they ink blots? ("Yes they are. What about them is scary?") Just the whole thing itself. ("In what way?") I can't very well describe it, but . . . . ("Just try.") I just can't describe it at all.	1. [The Rorschach cards are frequently frightening to children, and Claire reacts the way many younger children do. It is often not evident what about the blots is frightening. Probably the child makes preconscious associations which may never achieve full consciousness. He is aware only of something vaguely disturbing; he cannot define what is disturbing and therefore deal with it more clearly. Probably the poor structure of the task is an additional source of anxiety; perceptual-associative integration requires that much effort be put forth for the organization of what, particularly to the retarded child, often appears fragmented and chaotic.]

Card #	React. Time	Score	Protocol	Inquiry and Observations
V	3″	WF∓A Persev. Fab. Frightening	1. The same as the other one.	1. ("The same thing?") It's just a bug. And that bug has to be underlined. ("Why is that?") Well, it's just scary. I don't know . . it's just an odd-looking bug. Just an odd-looking bug. [Even the previously "safe" bug has become infected by frightening affect.]
VI	2″	WF−A Arb. Persev.	1. The same as the other one, a bug. ("Try to see something else.")	
		DrF∓H Fab. Symm.	2. (She turns the card sideways.) From a different view I can see a person standing near the water. (She turns the card over and returns it to me.) Right in the center of the picture.	2. ("What kind of a person?") A real ugly one. (" Like what?") I don't know. ("Man or woman, etc.?") I think it was a man. (The lower side projection.) [Another "negative" male.]
VII	6″	DrDF± Hd Fab. Self-ref. Agg.	1. It looks like two blabbermouths. Do you want me to light that cigarette for you? (She does so, and she blows out the light. She starts to reach for my stopwatch.)	1. ("Tell me about the blabbermouths.") (She opens and closes her fingers as though she were talking a great deal, and she keeps on doing this.) ("Tell me about it.") Their mouths stood open. ("Like who?") Like some of my friends. ("Do they do that?") Oh, do they ever talk about . . . . someone! I don't like it special, very good. They just talk too much. ("About you?") No, about other people. (When shown the card, she is able to point only to the mouth area of the popular head.)
		WF−A Persev.	2. And then, too, it looks like a bug.	

Card #	React. Time	Score	Protocol	Inquiry and Observations
VIII	6″	⎧ DF∓A(P)	1. It looks like two little squirrels climbing up a tree.	[Claire's two squirrels climbing the tree are almost popular, but not quite. This response demonstrates her tendency to distort even the usual a little bit. The fabulized tree that looks as though it were going to fall down any minute reflects Claire's insecurity. With a more verbally-cognitively precise person, one would ask why the tree looked as though it were "going to fall down." By now, though, it is apparent that Claire cannot deal with such a question productively. To ask the question, therefore, would be simply to go through an empty ritual.]
		DF+tree Fab.	2. The tree looks like it's going to fall down any minute. ("What kind of tree is it?") A pear tree. ("What makes it look like that?") It just looks like a pear tree. I don't know in what way though. Yes, it just looks like the pear tree of olden days.	
		W Comb.		
		⎩ DF-ground	3. This orange part here looks like .. like .. the ground. That's all.	
IX	13″	DFC−H Fab.	1. The pink part looks like a real pretty girl. She was .. oh, was a real pretty one.	1. ("What parts of the girl did you see?") I don't know. [Claire reacts in exclusively emotional terms. The area is a "pretty girl" because the coloring is pink.]
		DF+Hd Fab.	2. The green part looks like an ugly man.	2. [Are men ugly and girls pretty?]
		⎧ DrM∓H Fab. Agg. add:	3. The orange part looks like the man killing another man. That's all in that one.	
		Comb. ⎨ (DrF∓ obj.) Fab. comb. Arb.		

Card #	React. Time	Score	Protocol	Inquiry and Observations
X	2″	DF—Architect Fab. comb.	1. It looks like a king's palace.	(No inquiry was made on these responses, primarily because they were so fabulized, had such a fairy-tale quality and seemed so little related to the formal characteristics of the blot. In general, I felt I could obtain very little on inquiry which would clarify the responses.) [Claire seems to have lost intellectual self-discipline and to have given herself up to a fairy-tale mood. She is no longer attempting seriously to elaborate and create meaning out of the blot. She has let herself go and has entered a make-believe world, peopled by figures from songs and stories. Claire practically ignores reality, as sizes, positions, colors, textures and shapes are arbitrarily squeezed into her never-never land. She seems to have given up trying to make intellectual sense out of what apparently is chaotic to her. But she is *permitting* affect to take over as an organizer—she is not helplessly swept along by it.]
		DF∓H	2. These (two top gray D's) are the king's helpers.	
W Comb.		DF—H Fab. Agg.	3. These two are the men that come fighting. (The usual crabs.)	
		DCF Obj. Fab. Arb.	4. With green torches.	
		DF—H? Confab. Agg.	5. The yellow part . . I guess it's green. Anyhow, they come to kill those men that's come to fight the king.	
			6. The pink one here is the girl . . is the queen. This part here is the lady. The blue is what she's wearing . . and the pink also. That's it. That's all of that one	
			I forgot to mention this tall part here is the palace. (The uppermost D.)	

Children's Apperception Test[11]

Card 1 (Chicks seated around a table on which is a large bowl of food. Off to one side is a large chicken, dimly outlined.)

Ah . . it's about these little birds. The father and the mother and the child . . . . . are having their supper. And this rooster peeks over

[11] Bellak and Bellak (1949).

them. And they don't like it. After a while they get . . . too nervous, and then they find out that the rooster is invisible. That's all my story. ("Why does the rooster peek?") He wants something to eat. ("Why does it make them nervous?") They just get tense. ("How do you mean?") They have a fear of somebody's looking over them. (She looks out the window.) They fear he's going to take it away from them. ("How come he's invisible?") Ah . . they don't know. ("How do they feel about his being invisible?") That makes them want to feel . . . the . . . . has somebody looking over them. [Claire is reflecting the tension she feels about having her activities overseen. The "invisible rooster" suggests that Claire always carries with her the vague feeling of being watched, that "being watched" hangs in the air she breathes. This may be how she experiences her home atmosphere, the testing atmosphere, as well as moral injunctions from within and without. Again, she evidences an immaturity of form and content, a fragmentation of thinking and a tendency to fabulize. Sometimes the fabulization is in the direction of what is familiar, e.g., the story of *The Three Bears*.]

Card 2 (This is presented after Card 9.)

Card 3 (A lion with pipe and cane, sitting in a chair; in the lower right corner a little mouse appears in a hole.)
   That's a sad old little lion. He's setting in a chair with his cane alongside of him. He don't know it, but this little mouse comes out . . . . . and scares him half to death . . . . He goes on smoking his pipe and ignores the little mouse. That's all to that one. ("How did the mouse scare him?") He scares him by coming up towards him. ("How did that scare him?") He don't know who it is. ("What does the mouse do?") He looks around and looks around . . . until finally the lion . . . stops smoking his pipe, and . . gets away from the little mouse. He *scares* that little mouse to death. That's that. ("Does the mouse mean to scare the lion?") No. [What appears big and strong is easily frightened by the innocuous and by what does not even mean to frighten. Claire apparently tries to maintain composure in the face of fright. A further solution to avoid fright involves frightening the frightener. This and the last card raise questions about the

strength and significance with which the father is viewed within the family.]

Card 4 (A kangaroo with a bonnet on her head, carrying a basket with a milk bottle; in her pouch is a baby kangaroo with a balloon; on a bicycle, a larger kangaroo child.)

It's about this kangaroo with her two little ones. They are going to town . . and this little . . this other one . . is riding his tricycle. The other one is in its mother's pouch. And that's all of that one. ("What happens?") They get their groceries and start home. ("Which one of the little ones appears to be happier?") The one in the pouch. ("How come?") He has a balloon. ("How does the other one feel?") He don't have a balloon. ("How does he feel?") He don't feel too happy about it. ("Which one is the mother happier with?") I guess both. ("Does she like one better than the other?") No. [Claire is unable to deal with rivalry. The baby who is close to the mother is happier because "he has a balloon." Claire apparently needs to deny the younger child's satisfaction about being so close to his mother. Only the balloon counts.]

Card 5 (A darkened room with a large bed in the background; a crib in the foreground in which are two baby bears.)

It's about these two little bears and their mother and dad. And they're sound asleep. And something comes along that this one little bear wakes up and gets his other . . pal to wake up. So the two of them wake up and go out and get something to eat. While they are out, their mother and father wake up and come out after them. When they get out there, they find these two little pests and put them back to bed. And they say to them, "You get back in bed and stay there!" That's all. ("How do the kids feel?") They don't feel too good about that one. (How do you mean?") They don't like their mother to shout at them. ("Why did their mother shout?") Because they did *not* do as she said. ("Why are they pests?") I don't know why she call *them* little pests. ("What does the father think?") He was thinking to do something drastic about it. ("Like what?") Spanking them, but good. ("Does he feel the same as the mother?") Yes. [Once again Claire identifies herself with, and at the same time deeply resents, the negative label which the parents place on her.

One wonders to what extent Claire needs to provoke negative reactions from them.]

Card 6 (A darkened cave with two dimly outlined bear figures in the background; a baby bear lying in the foreground.)
Oh boy! This is a good one. It's about this little bear . . and his mother and father are in this cave. And they . . his mother and father are asleep. But he is awake, and he doesn't know what to think about it. He gets up and finds out that the mother and father . . . . are awake. As soon as he gets out of the cave, his mother and father come after him. He runs and runs and runs . . for his life. And that's all of that one. ("Why does he run for his life?") He wants to get free. ("From what?") His mother and father. ("Why is that?") Because his mother and father thinks he's been bad. ("What do they think he's done?") He's kept them awake. ("Are they mad?") Yes. Uh-huh! Boy! ("How come?") Their mother and father snored like the dickens . . . that's what kept them awake. He snored back at them. [Again Claire expresses the theme of revenge: her parents do something to her, so she does it back to them. She feels that her parents are extremely unfair, that they punish her for what they themselves do, and they never see themselves as being wrong. She openly expresses the wish to get away from them, quite possibly because of anxiety (panic?) regarding their intimacy.]

Card 7 (A tiger with bared fangs and claws, leaping at a monkey which is also leaping through the air.)
(As I show this card, Claire asks if she can go to the bathroom. When she returns, she says:) Have you looked over it? Does it tell a good story? ("Have some of these cards been kind of hard?") Yeah. ("Shall we wait until tomorrow for the rest of them?") Yeah.
(We discontinue the testing for the day. The next day, instead of looking at the card, she looks at me and smiles. She keeps looking at me. Finally she looks at the card.)
It's about a lion that chases this little monkey. . . He scared him until he ran up the tree . . . and that was all of that one. ("How does the monkey feel?") He didn't feel too good. ("What did the lion want to do?") He wanted to chase him. ("Why?") I don't know. ("Did he want to catch him?") Yes. ("What would he have done then?") I don't know. [Claire apparently finds the emotions which the highly aggressive theme of this card evoke so frightening that

she gets rid of the stimulus as quickly as she can. She is unable to say what the tiger's eventual motive could be. She sees herself and others as destructive, but she cannot let herself think about the potentially destructive outcome of this mutual ill will. She does not know and does not want to recognize the motivation for all this anger.

Claire finds it increasingly difficult to tell spontaneous stories; I have to ask many questions, and Claire answers most of them with uninstructive monosyllables.]

Card 8 (Two adult monkeys sitting on a sofa drinking from tea cups. One adult monkey in foreground sitting on a hassock talking to a baby monkey.)

It's about these monkeys. . . One of them is talking to his little son about something, while the others are talking to each other. The father . . . tells this little monkey to go upstairs and go to bed. And that's all to that one. ("What does the little monkey do?") Ah . . he . . does what his father says to. ("Does he want to go upstairs?") No. ("Why not?") He wants to stay up. ("Why?") He just *wants* to stay up. ("Who are the other monkeys?") They're company. ("Where's the mother monkey?") She's talking to the son. ("Where's the father?") I guess he's out of town. [The instability of Claire's perception is again illustrated by the ease with which the monkey she has called the father becomes the mother. She does not need to justify this switch and may not even be aware of it. What is becoming increasingly clear is that Claire sees her parents as not giving help, support, softness or warmth. Any encounter between child and parents involves one making a demand on the other. A parental request is usually an unfair and stern order. The child irritates the parents by not easily obeying their wishes.]

Card 9 (A darkened room seen through an open door from a lighted room. In the darkened one there is a child's bed in which a rabbit sits up looking through the door.)

It's about this little rabbit. His mother and father are in bed . . . and he decides he'll stay up for a little while . . So he stays up until he *finally* goes to bed. (She nods with emphasis.) ("Do the parents know he stays up?") No. ("How would they feel?") They wouldn't feel too good. ("What would they do?") Scold him. ("Why does he want to stay up?") He wanted to see what was going on. ("Is he afraid to go to bed?") No. ("Does he dream?") No. [Again, the child is doing something "forbidden." Again the "naughty" child identifies with his parents—"he finally goes to bed." Again the parents are dissatisfied with the child and don't feel "too good." As before, the child wishes to see "what's going on." Claire probably feels left out whenever she correctly or incorrectly thinks that her parents are intimate with each other.]

Card 2 (One bear pulling a rope on one side while another bear and a baby bear pull on the other side.)

It's about these bears, and they're having a rope fight. (She sighs.) These two bears on the right-hand side are pulling . . . the other one, on the left-hand side . . is pulling. And I believe that's all on that one. ("Who wins?") It was just those three bears. ("And which side wins?") The two on the right-hand side. ("Who are they to one another?") Friends, I guess. ("They're not related?") (She shakes her head.) ("How come they're pulling rope?") I don't know. [The usually described intrafamiliar conflict is threatening to Claire so she has the tug-of-war participants be "just friends."]

Card 10 (A baby dog lying across the knees of an adult dog; both figures with a minimum of expressive features. The figures are set in the foreground of a bathroom.)

It's about these two dogs. . . The mother dog is trying to get the little dog to go to the bathroom, and he won't do it. He . . she forces him to do it, but he refuses . . . . . . (She smiles.) . . . . She is *real* angry . . and *makes* him do it . . but he still refuses. Obviously he just won't do it . . . . (She looks at me.) That's all to that one. (She smiles again.) Do you have any more? ("How does this story end?") It ends up fine. ("How?") He *finally* does it. [This story represents the classical prototype—the child who stubbornly withholds and refuses his mother's efforts to "make him do something" on the toilet. Claire's smile reflects her pleasure about being able to triumph over her mother—and the examiner—through passive resistance. This resistant way of dealing with people will, of course, play a major, encumbering role in any treatment program to be set up for Claire. The major potential treatment obstacle will involve the angry, impotent reactions of the persons trying to establish helpful relationships with Claire.]

SENTENCE COMPLETION TEST II[12]

(The stems of this test were dictated to Claire, and she completed the sentences verbally.)

She hoped that when she grew up she wishes she could do it. ("What?")[13]. . . . ("She could do what?") What she wanted to do. [Claire's anxiety results in a lack of openness; she reveals as little about herself as she can. The completion also expresses her generalized sense of impotence and inadequacy.]

When she saw what the other kids were doing she decided to do what they were doing. [She uses others as models to find out how to act.]

When she compared herself to her friends they noticed her. [Probably negatively.]

She was sad whenever she thought of misbehaving. ("How do you mean?") I don't know. ("How would she act when she misbehaved?") I don't know. [When she "misbehaves" her parents become particularly angry.]

When she was asked about her aches and pains she didn't tell 'em. ("Why not?") I don't know. ("Why might she not have told them?") Cause they make fun of her. ("Who does?") Her friends. They go off to their other friends and laugh . . like the dickens. [Claire's loneliness, her isolation and feeling of being lost among other children are clear.]

The person she admired most was her aunt. ("How come?") She was well dressed. [Claire does not say she admires either of her parents. She admires her aunt, but for an external characteristic.]

Her sister did the same thing.

When her mother came into the room she noticed what the girl was doing. ("What did the mother do or say?") She scolded her. [!]

When she was with her brother they went into a store.

At school they worked hard.

When she looked at the work the others were doing the teacher scolded her. ("Why?") Because she was supposed to do her own work.

---

12 The content of this test was developed at the Menninger Foundation.

13 Although one must face the probability of adversely affecting future responses, the author thinks that too much is lost (particularly the affective atmosphere of the moment) when one waits until all stems are completed before inquiry is begun. In order to avoid a response's growing "cold," inquiry was always instituted after a puzzling completion was offered.

[Here is another scolding adult in authority. Claire so far has not once described an adult as understanding or even pleasant. She perceives and uses her disability as a great and heavy albatross.]

She was very happy when her mother came home. [This response represents the other side of Claire's anger toward her mother. For the first time Claire expresses positive feelings for her mother.]

The thing she found hardest to do was her work. [An open admission.]

Whenever certain things really bothered her she got so nervous she flew into pieces. [This completion describes the degree of Claire's disorganization when she feels under stress.]

Her dreams made her unhappy. ("How was that?") Did you hear that pop? ("What was it?") Electricity. [Claire started to expose her anxiety, seemed to become frightened because of this revelation, and attempted to divert me. The examiner did not pursue the "unhappy dreams" because the area seemed to arouse emotions with which Claire could not adequately deal.]

She liked what she was given. ("What was that?") A present. ("Who gave it to her?") Her aunt. [Again the aunt, not the parents.]

When she saw that the man had left the money behind she ran and picked it up. ("What did she do then?") Gave it to him.

She thought that her father was mad as could be. [Once more, the angry father.]

Whenever she and her family disagreed they . . . . flipped.

When she was very little she cried like the dickens. ("Why did she cry?") She had . . I guess she had a rash. [It is highly doubtful that "she" cried because she had a rash, but Claire finds the conflict-related reasons for crying impossible to tell about.]

Her best friend was . . I guess Eileen.

She was unhappy with her mother when she . . f-f-flew on the airplane. ("Why was that?") I don't know. ("Was she afraid?") No. [A probable reaction formation to the wish to have mother hurt.]

She never thought she would be able to do the work she was told. (She yawns.)

She always hoped that she could live on a farm. [Because life on a farm is less complicated?]

Her parents disagreed with her.

What she liked best about herself was the way she acted. [Claire makes frequent use of the mechanism of reversal.]

Her mother was more likely than her father to play with her. [Again Claire lets us glimpse her good feelings toward her mother.] (The test was stopped here and continued the following day.)

Her brother said he did not want to do it. ("What was that?") I don't know. [?]

When she had nothing else to do she . . ah . . went to visit her friends.

She thought that her intelligence was not so good. [Although Claire uses denial, she is nevertheless occasionally able to face her disabilities somewhat.]

What she liked best about school was the way she got to go out for recess.

When she couldn't see a way out she *pried* the door open.

She saw the cockroach on the wall and . . . . took it down.

Her teacher says she *must* do the work, or *else!* [Claire is having a very bad time at school. She feels forced to learn, although she is obviously unable to do the work her schoolmates can.]

Whenever she got angry she f-f-f-f-flew up into pieces.

She remembered that when she was little she got to do the things she didn't want to do. ("How do you mean?") Hm . . make beds. ("What did she think of that?") She hated it. [She picks what is probably a prototypical early memory which suggests that she views herself as having been treated badly all her life.]

When the kids invited her to go to the hiding place she accepted.

After school she usually went home.

She admired her mother when she did the things she wanted. ("Who did the things?") Her mother. ("Like what?") I don't know.

She and her sister went uptown.

She thought that her body was dirty . . so she washed it off. [Claire describes a self which she considers repugnant but which can be fixed.]

When she had a lot of homework to do she . . got busy and *did* it. [Frequently when Claire emphasizes words, as she does here, they seem direct echoes of what she has been told by adults.]

What she disliked about school was her work.

Whenever she spoke about her problems to someone . . . She didn't do it. [Claire expresses her inability to accept help from others.]

When she entered the haunted house she . . was frightened.

She didn't like her mother to scold her.

When the baby arrived it cried.

Whenever she didn't do what she was told she got scolded.

What would make her angriest was she didn't want to do the things she was supposed to do. [A vicious circle seems to exist in the relations between Claire and her parents: Claire is angry and does not do things she is supposed to do; her not doing these things results in an angry parental reaction; this reaction makes Claire angrier and more resistant; the increased resistance results in more parental irritation. And so it goes, on and on.]

In her spare time she went to the grocery for her mother.

What troubled her most was the problems she had. ("What was the worst one?") Hmmm . . like washing the dishes. [Again, as several times before, Claire begins to express herself openly, only to cloak what is really on her mind with an innocuous substitute.]

When she was alone in her room she cried for help. [!]

What scared her most was the *way* . . she did *not* do the way she was supposed to do. [Claire is perhaps frightened by her parents' anger when she does not do what they want. She may be frightened because she has so little control over her negativism, which creates such anger in others.]

She disliked her mother when she got mad at her . . that is, her mother.

She thought that her looks were horrible.

The thing she could do best was the work. [This and the previous sentence form a significant sequence: a frightening admission, followed by a denial. Claire would feel too vulnerable if she admitted to looking "horrible" without undoing the admission by protesting her good work.]

When she saw the boy she knew . . he . . she knew she was in love with him.

She had no respect at all for her mother.

She always enjoyed the movies . . that is, the films. [A pathetic effort to sound "proper," to use the "right" word.]

She had a very uncomfortable feeling when she . . went to bed. [This discomfort could result from any of a number of factors.]

She found it easiest to do the work.

THE PSYCHOLOGIST'S REPORT[14]

Claire is a deeply dependent thirteen-year-old who needs passively to cling to whatever adult is nearby. Side by side an incorporative mode of relating herself to others is an extremely strong, passive-resistant tendency. One can see how Claire is engaged in a constant power struggle: she feels under obligation to obey, to produce, to bow under to the will of others; and she tries constantly to resist these pressures (which she also partly desires). This resistance to pressure is dramatized in her Children's Apperception Test story to two dogs pictured in a bathroom:

> The mother dog is trying to get the baby dog to go to the bathroom, and he won't do it. She forces him to do it, but he refused. (She smiles.) She is *real* angry . . and *makes* him do it . . but he *still* refuses. Obviously he just *won't* do it. ("How does the story end?") He finally does it. ("Why doesn't he want to do it?") Because he just doesn't feel like doing it.

Claire's view that adults pressure her is also reflected in such Sentence Completions as: *Her teacher* "says she *must* do the work, or *else*." A theme of "misbehavior" runs through the test material. Claire is convinced that her mother, in particular, reacts angrily to what she interprets as Claire's unwillingness to do what she is supposed to. One can almost feel the battle of wills which has developed between mother and daughter, raging around such matters as doing the daily chores.

Claire not only expresses her anger about being pressured to "behave," but she tries to sabotage others' efforts to make her do so. So, for example, in spite of my repeated requests that she stop, she continues to look ahead to see what test problems will be coming next. In this way she gives herself extra time, which cannot be taken into account in scoring her test performance. The openness with which she bends rules suggests that she expects and apparently wishes some sort of negative reaction from others.

14 The psychologist's report was presented at each adolescent's final conference, and for that reason it usually does not contain all the author's points, made throughout the course of each chapter, since the author's comments are often intended to serve a didactic function. Sometimes reference is made to test material which was either abbreviated or omitted altogether. Material was condensed or omitted whenever it did not seem to offer much that was new or revealing.

Claire functions at a Borderline level of intelligence. On the Wechsler Intelligence Scale for Children, she achieves a Total Intelligence Quotient of 75-76; a Verbal Quotient of 79, and a Performance Quotient of 76-78. With the exception of Arithmetic, on which she performs adequately for her age, none of her subtest scores reaches a level appropriate to her age. Her range of weighted scores extends from 4 to 10, but these scores may not be an accurate gauge of her day-to-day ability. For example, although her word usage is surprisingly good in everyday situations, she achieves a weighted Vocabulary score of only 5. She finds it difficult to assume the necessary abstract attitude on this test and resorts to the most concrete definitions. Thus, she defines *umbrella* as "You . . uh . . you hold it," and *nail* as "You pound on it." *Fur* is "Something you wear" and and *diamond,* "Something real shiny." In other words, when Claire is in a position to organize things in her own way, she can handle herself a good deal more effectively than when she has to comply with conditions laid down by someone else. In this connection, one should mention Claire's need to appear more limited than she actually is. She may well fear the increased independence which usually follows in the wake of greater ability. Although she resents being helplessly ordered about, she apparently finds this resentment easier to deal with than the anxiety which would accompany greater autonomy.

Claire's intellectual limitations are particularly apparent on tasks involving perceptual and motor skills. Her drawings are distorted, fragmented and primitively constructed. Her perceptual helplessness is seen on the Rorschach, where she perseveratively interprets many differently constituted blots as a "bug."

Her intellectual and affective immaturity emerge not only when, for example, she describes the Fourth of July as "firecracker day" but, more significantly, on the Comprehension subtest, when she sees the solution to relatively simple problems as requiring the advice of her mother. Emotional and intellectual immaturity are strikingly apparent in her tendency to create a sort of fairy-tale reality. This tendency reaches major proportions on the less-structured Rorschach, where she attributes elaborate meanings to infinitesimal perceptual specks. Perceptual and integrative organization occasionally become highly arbitrary; she may, for example, interpret some area as a "person" who, on inquiry, cannot be seen because he is "hiding." Apparently much of Claire's tendency to confabulate is related to her awareness of her cognitive deficiencies. On the Rorschach she seems unable perceptually and intellectually to differentiate anything much more complex than a bug, but she feels an implicit coercion to come up with a more intricate percept. Since she is unable to create the more differentiated one, she makes up the sort of thing she thinks I want her to see. Such a tendency is undoubtedly apparent in her everyday behavior, too; i.e., when she feels unable to deal realistically with a situation, she may well *invent* something—behavior which could easily account, in part, for the history of her "lying."

Claire's fearfulness and aggressiveness is another prominent feature. She finds the projective tests vaguely "scary" and many frightening and destructive themes occur to her as she deals with them. On the Rorschach, for example, she sees a rooster, part of whose back end is cut off, as though a knife had come down and "just slashed it." She sees two squirrels climbing a tree which is about to fall down any minute. She confabulates a man killing another. Asked why a person should give money to an organized charity rather than to a street beggar, she partly answers, "Well, he might start chasing after you." On Sentence Completion, she says, *Whenever certain things really bothered her* "she got so nervous she flew into pieces"; and, *Whenever she was alone in her room at night* "she cried for help." That much of Claire's fearfulness and anger involve feelings toward her parents is suggested by a number of projective themes which deal with the anger, punitiveness and destructiveness which she experiences as coming from her mother and father. In one Children's Apperception Test story, for example, a little bear wakes and leaves his cave. "His parents follow him. He runs and runs and runs . . for his life. ('Why does he run?') He wants to get free. ('From what?') His mother and father. ('Why?') Because his mother and father think he's been bad." The "badness," in this particular case, seems to be the child's desire for revenge: he tries to act toward the parents in the way he feels they have acted toward him. Prominent, too, is the little bear's apparent panic. But while Claire complains about the constant, angry struggle that goes on between her mother and herself, she makes very clear how much she needs her mother and how much she fears being left by her.

Being called "bad" and being a "dummy" emerge as pretty much one and the same. Being a "dummy" is also equivalent to various other kinds of moral deficiency, particularly to disobedience. Being "intelligent," on the other hand, is the same as being virtuous, brave and as having other "good" attributes.

Claire's self-image emerges clearly. Reluctantly, but relatively unequivocally, she has incorporated what she senses to be her parents' and other adults' evaluations of her. She thinks of herself as a "little pest" whose intelligence is "not so good," whose body is "dirty" and whose looks are "horrible." She is a lonely, unhappy, isolated girl who feels ridiculed by others her age and who is reluctant to let on to them about her sad feelings because "they make fun of her . . her friends do. They go off to their other friends and laugh . . like the dickens." But while Claire is unhappy about the angry skirmishes that take place between herself and others, she apparently tries to keep them going; an angry relationship appears to be better than none.

In summary, Claire is an adolescent of Borderline intelligence, whose strange clinical behavior seems, in part at least, to represent her effort to compensate for the intellectual limitations which she tries to deny but of which she is nevertheless aware. One of the major trouble spots in her life involves a perennial power struggle, primarily between herself and her parents, but between herself and others as well. She feels she can maintain her individuality only by passively, but obdurately, resisting the demands she feels from others. She *reacts*, rather than acting independently for herself. She will find it difficult to achieve the kind of autonomy which growth into adulthood requires, because she deals with adults in this reactive fashion. Rather than establishing new, more horizontal relations with peers, she maintains the older, predominantly vertical ones with her parents and parentlike persons.

DISCUSSION

Although Claire is not severely retarded, at least by intelligence test standards, she needs to represent herself as rather seriously intellectually disabled. She avoids growing into adulthood and shirks what should be a task of adolescence—the beginning resolution of early dependency. Claire needs to remain a very young, very passive and very resistant child who feels that nearly all people are throwing difficulties in her path. Although she toys with the thought of leaving what she feels to be angry, demanding, unreasonable, ridiculing parents, she can not take this important psychological step as other children her age begin to do. She considers herself too disabled to deal with independence, to face the world without the presence of those who have nurtured her through her life (no matter how badly she may feel they have done their job). She denies her budding sexual wishes and assumes, instead, a mask of what she considers to be adolescent seductiveness.

Although her ability is in fact limited, she exploits this inability and exaggerates it. Others with her degree of impairment are able to lead a more independent life. While she would undoubtedly experience considerable difficulty if she were on her own, the thought of even a small degree of independence seems out of the question. Claire's internal and external emotional environments make it impossible for her to approach, let alone resolve, any significant aspect of adolescence. Her needs to cling to childhood, reinforced by limited intelligence, make it emotionally impossible for her to take further steps toward psychological growth. The question is, in other words, whether Claire's Borderline intelligence is as much a true limitation as she needs to convey, or whether she uses this limitation to meet her needs to be taken care of and to avoid a situation where she will no longer be taken care of as a little girl. Claire's Borderline intelligence and emotional needs are so intertwined that one cannot assign either factor as "the" cause of her immovability from the position of young childhood.

Claire's emotional difficulties are severe, but not nearly so severe as Stan's, part of whose test battery follows. Stan is significantly more disorganized than Claire. He has to deal both with a Borderline intelligence and with an uncertainty, disorganization and confusion that are a great deal more severe than Claire's. Claire is in almost unbroken contact with her surroundings (except when they become unbearably difficult to handle). She is convinced people treat her unfairly, but she is constantly aware of them, and she always tends to adapt her behavior to theirs, either fulfilling their expectations or (more frequently) frustrating them.

Stan's test material, which follows, differs significantly from Claire's. It reflects how Stan, on occasion, psychologically takes leave of areas which create relatively minor difficulties between himself and persons and things. Instead of trying to deal with a reality which he considers to be unfair, he simply repeals it; he nullifies aspects of the world which are too complex. Unlike Claire, who laments her life, Stan simply does not allow himself to be aware of what is too painful. When he does remain in contact with the world, however, he functions more effectively than Claire.

CLINICAL SUMMARY: Stan

Stan is fourteen years old. A speech defect, increasing learning difficulty and poor school adjustment have been problems for several years, but Stan's persistent and frequent sex play with his five-and-a-half-year-old sister have recently led to psychiatric evaluation elsewhere. Stan has another sister, aged eleven.

For the last seven years Stan's parents have been concerned with his speech difficulty, his learning problems, and his poor adjustment in school. Intelligence Quotients on Stanford-Binet tests given eight, seven and four years ago were 73, 76, and 70, respectively. Because of "undesirable conduct and undesirable play with other children" the patient was referred for a psychiatric examination five years ago. This examination indicated that he was "emotionally insecure and rather disturbed," although it was thought that he could continue in school in an ungraded class. Stan was given a psychiatric work-up on an inpatient basis last year. Since then he has been seen by a private psychiatrist who believes that Stan shows marked "inability to handle his anxiety and has a severe ego disturbance."

Shortly after her marriage, the mother became pregnant with Stan. During the nine months of pregnancy she experienced nausea, vomiting, and severe coughing which increased existing family tensions and conflicts. The delivery was difficult, and labor was medically induced. Nothing of significance was reported about Stan's birth condition other than "weakness." His sleeping a great deal in infancy was believed to be the result, in part, of the fact that he was breast-fed while his mother was taking opium pills for a cough.

Stan was born abroad, and when he was five years old he and his parents were caught in bombing raids. At one time, part of the room they occupied was destroyed by bombing.

Toilet training was started at the age of seven months. Day control was established by eighteen months, but Stan was enuretic until at least the age of six years. English was not spoken in the home during Stan's childhood, and the parents frequently do not speak English at home at the present. Even abroad, Stan was slow in learning to speak; he was three years old before he began to use isolated words. His parents say that, after he came to America, he "quickly learned English and forgot all the foreign words he knew." When he was in the fourth grade, at about the age of ten, he suddenly began to stammer. While the parents feel that Stan has always been a very heavy sleeper, Stan himself claims to have had severe nightmares and bad dreams since at least the age of nine.

The mother, with Stan and his older sister, came to America in 1948. They were followed two years later by the father, who had remained behind to finish his required army service. When Stan was eight years old and his mother was pregnant with the younger sister, the school authorities noted that he showed sexual interest in girls; he would try to kiss them, pulled at their dresses and attempted to lift their skirts. In the past year he has been observed engaging in mutual sex play with his younger sister.

Learning has been a problem since Stan entered public school. Special help by the mother and by hired tutors has resulted in some improvement in selected subjects. Stan has found it difficult to make friends and has been withdrawn and shy. He has complained of headaches, which have not been relieved by glasses, for a number of years.

Physical and Laboratory Findings: Physical, hematological, neurological examinations, skull and chest x-rays, were all within normal limits.

THE PSYCHOLOGIST'S DESCRIPTION

Stan quickly established a friendly but anxious relationship. He wanted very much to please, smiled frequently in a somewhat embarrassed manner and was eager to demonstrate his good intentions. Always, after our first meeting, he smiled and waved from afar when he saw me.

Stan's stammer increased as his anxiety mounted. On the Children's Apperception Test, for example, his blocking became so pronounced that the rhythm of his speech broke down almost completely. He experienced speech as painful at such times, but he continued to talk, even though he found the going very difficult. Sometimes Stan had difficulty finding words, and at these times he made do with inadequate substitutes. When I asked whether he was sometimes unable to think of an easy word which might be at the tip of his tongue, he smiled and agreed.

Stan was afraid of this examination because he thought we would take him from his family and put him in the hospital without giving him a chance properly to say good-by to them all.

WECHSLER INTELLIGENCE SCALE FOR CHILDREN

Name : Stan   Age: 14-1

	RS	WTS	0	1	2	3	4	5	6	7	8	9	10	11	12	13	14	15	16	17	18	19	20
COMPR.	9-11	4-6					•		×														
INFOR.	11-12	5						•															
DIG.	8	6							•														
ARITH.	11	8									•												
SIMIL.	5	4					•																
VOCAB.	28-29	5						•															
P. A.	27	8									•												
P. C.	11	8									•												
B. D.	10-14	5-6						•	×														
O. A.	8	1		•																			
CODE	44	8									•												

TOT. VERB.	26-28
TOT. PERF.	30-31
TOT. SCALE	56-59

VERBAL I.Q.: 70-72 LEVEL: Borderline

PERFORMANCE I.Q.: 72-74 LEVEL: Borderline

TOTAL I.Q.: 68-70 LEVEL: Defective—Borderline

INFORMATION

No. Question	Response and Comments	Score

(Stan gets the first ten questions correct, without difficulty.)

11. *What are the four seasons of the year?* — You mean you want January, February, March? (I repeat the question.) Twelve. ("What comes after winter?") Winter, summer, fall, spring. [Once Stan is put concretely on the track, he can continue correctly; without such help, he is uncertain about what is expected.] — 0

12. *What is the color of rubies?* — It could be any color. ("Any color more than another one?") It could be red. — 0-1

13. *Where does the sun set?* — I think it sets in the south. — 0

No.	Question	Response and Comments	Score
14.	What does the stomach do?	(He smiles.) . . . . (There is a long pause.) Well, the stomach . . could do most everything. It could sometimes . . hurt you . . you could have pains . . I guess that's it. [Stan has apparently reached the limits of his ability. He has become unsure of himself and fills in his intellectual gaps with whatever information he can think of (whether relevant or not). Not unexpectedly, his first reaction tends to be an affectively colored (frightened) one.]	0
15.	Why does oil float on water?	Don't know.	0
16.	Who wrote Romeo and Juliet?	Uh . . (He frowns as he apparently tries to remember. There is a considerable pause during which he is thinking.) I know his name, but I can't think. Maybe you can give me the initials. ("Can you think of other books he might have written?") He wrote a story about a king and he wrote poems and stories. ("Does the initial S help?") No. ("Does W.S. help?") Oh . . William Shakespeare. (He smiles.) [Again, once he is concretely put on the right track, he can remember.]	0
17.	What is celebrated on the Fourth of July?	Well, like the Fourth of July . . . . . . Well . . uh . . we can celebrate . . like . . uh . . for instance, that we can go to a party or dance, that you can enjoy yourself. Go to a parade? ("Can you tell me anything else about the Fourth of July?") No. [With help, he correctly offers the author of Romeo and Juliet, but he is unable to say even very generally what is celebrated on the Fourth of July!]	0
18.	What does C.O.D. mean?	Cash on delivery. [As with Claire, a surprise out of the blue. A success occurs after six failures.]	1
19.	How tall is the average American man?	Very tall. ("How tall?") He could be about six feet one inch or five feet nine inches or six feet . . or six feet five inches. ("How tall are you?") I don't know. I guess I'm about five feet or something. [Since he does not know the answer, Stan gives various alternatives. "About five feet or something" tells much about his poorly differentiated conception of himself, particularly since he is about five feet six inches tall.]	0
20.	Where is Chile?	Don't know.	0
21.	How many pounds are there in a ton?	Sixteen.	0

No.	Question	Response and Comments	Score
22.	What is the capital of Greece?	(Omitted.)	
23.	What does turpentine come from?	(Omitted.)	
24.	How far is it from New York to Chicago?	I'd say about seven or eight miles. ("How far is it from New York to Topeka?") Well, it could be .. it could be about five miles. [Stan arrived from New York only the preceding day; it is evident that he has no conception of distances.]	0

(The remaining questions were omitted.)

RAW SCORE: 11-12

WEIGHTED SCORE: 4-6

COMPREHENSION

No.	Question	Response and Comments	Score
1.	What is the thing to do when you cut your finger?	Well .. you .. you can .. put medicine, or see a doctor right away .. or get a bandage or some kind of treatment to stop the blood.	2
2.	What is the thing to do if you lose one of your friend's balls?	It .. um .. te-te-tell him .. that .. you were sorry .. or .. get him another ball .. or .. or .. just give him the money. Or treat him to whatever he wants to have. ("Which would you choose?") I'd say, pay him. [As Stan's tension mounts, his stammering becomes more evident.]	2
3.	What would you do if you were sent to buy a loaf of bread and the grocer said he did not have any more?	I would go home and tell my mom he didn't have any.	1
4.	What is the thing to do if a fellow much smaller than yourself starts to fight with you?	Well .... (He shrugs.) ... Uh .. well, the .. only thing you must do is fight back, defend yourself. [Stan's answer is expressed in an adult fashion; he is probably repeating what his parents have instructed him to do. He may well have done a poor job of defending himself in the past, and his parents may have encouraged him to "fight back."]	0

No.	Question	Response and Comments	Score
5.	What should you do if you see a train approaching a broken track?	Well . . I would either . . . wa-wa-wave a flag or holler for it to stop . . or change a switch. ("Which would you do?") Ch-change the switch. [Although Stan has previously given the response which would give him full credit, he picks an unrealistic answer after he reflects on the possibilities. The poor choice demonstrates inability to choose the most appropriate of various alternatives. While he may have the best answer at his disposal, he does not recognize it as best.]	0-2
6.	Why is it better to build a house of brick than of wood?	Well, because . . uh . . brick would b-burn. I mean . . wood would burn easily and start a fire . . and . . and . . and . . brick would last longer and brick wouldn't start any fire or damage. [Stan is able to recover after the two preceding responses which he could not handle well. It is possible that the "fight" question created so much anxious turmoil that Stan became immobilized then and on the next two questions, not recovering until now.]	2
7.	Why are criminals locked up?	So they shouldn't do any more da- any . . any harm to anybody. [Stan reconsiders the word "damage" and uses "harm" instead. Apparently he fears that he will have too much difficulty trying to say "damage."]	1
8.	Why should women and children be saved first in a shipwreck?	(He smiles.) . . . . I don't know. ("Can you think of any reason?") . . . . . . Because . . uh . . uh . . . . (He smiles again.) Because . . maybe the women and children . . are ascared of the water . . or maybe they don't want to drown or be drowned or dead or anything. So that's why . . uh . . uh . . they should . . uh . . uh go first.	0
9.	Why is it better to pay bills by check than by cash?	Because . . uh . . uh because a man could . . could read . . what he has to pay in cash and by . . uh . . uh by a check. ("So why is it better to pay by check?") Like for instance, he doesn't remember how much it cost . . he could either find out by the check, and so then he could remember how much it cost. [Stan actually does fairly well here. Through the confusion there eventually emerge rather sound ideas.]	1
10.	Why is it generally better to give money to an organized charity than to a street beggar?	Well . . be-because so that . . so that he can have food, clothing and medicine for the sick and . . and nice homes and apartments, and things like that.	0

No.	Question	*Response and Comments*	*Score*
11.	*Why should most government positions be filled through examinations?*	(Omitted because it seemed so doubtful that Stan could understand the question. To ask it would only unnecessarily face him with his intellectual shortcomings.) [Particularly with younger children, as well as with older intellectually retarded persons, the examining psychologist frequently walks a fine line as he decides how far to go in testing limits and creating the accompanying anxiety. As important as it may be diagnostically to find out how a person deals with a problem he finds very difficult to solve, the psychologist must decide whether the utility of this added diagnostic information is outweighed by the distress he arouses in the person who is unable to deal with his anxiety effectively.]	
12.	*Why is cotton fiber used in making cloth?*	So that you can be warm . . that's all I can think of.	0
13.	*Why do we elect (or need to have) senators and congressmen?*	(Omitted.)	
14.	*Why should a promise be kept?*	Because . . uh . . if it isn't kept . . in other words, it is punishing the child . . in other words, not telling the truth. [As in Claire's case, the thinking has become quite irrelevant from the point of view of logic, even though it is not at all irrelevant from an affective standpoint.]	0

RAW SCORE: 9-11

WEIGHTED SCORE: 4-6

DIGIT SPAN

(Stan correctly repeats five Digits Forward and three Backward.)

RAW SCORE: 8

WEIGHTED SCORE: 6

ARITHMETIC

(He receives credit for the first eleven problems, but he is unable to do the last five. His failures are not peculiar in any way. The solutions to the first eight problems never take longer than 2″.)

RAW SCORE: 11

WEIGHTED SCORE: 8

SIMILARITIES

No.	Items	Response and Comments	Score
1.	*Lemons-sugar*	Sweet.	1
2.	*Walk-throw*	Hand.	1
3.	*Boys-girls*	Women.	1
4.	*Knife-glass*	Is dangerous. [This unexpected "likeness" gives us a further indication of how disruptive Stan's phobic reactions can be. The degree to which Stan feels surrounded by danger causes him to distort reality and therefore to lose credit on an item which, judging by preceding and succeeding successes, he might be able to pass. The psychological impact of this aggressive and frightening idea is great enough to cause Stan to offer a grammatically peculiar response.]	0
5.	*Plum-peach*	Well . . they are both round, but they have different colors. (I explain what is meant by "similarities.") [Very young children, when they are asked to describe similarities of two items, frequently produce differences. Stan shows not only the quantitative impairment of abilities reflected in his Scattergram, but also a qualitative characteristic which alerts us to the degree of his inability.]	1
6.	*Cat-mouse*	They are alike by their growth . . one is big and the other one is small. ("How are they alike?") You mean, in other words, they have tails and they have feet. [Once again Stan is torn between giving differences when he is asked for similarities.]	1
7.	*Beer-wine*	Well, beer is sort of . . sweet and wine is sort of sweet and sour or strong. In other words, there could be many different kinds of wine . . could be brown, or any sort of color. ("How are they alike?") They are alike . . by . . well, they don't have the same cans. [A vivid example of an inability to conceptualize a similarity.]	0
8.	*Piano-violin*	Well . . a piano does not have strings and also a piano does not have what . . you . . uh . . uh . . sort of like an arm, and . . uh . . a violin doesn't have any keys or a stand. (He yawns.) ("Can you tell me how they might be the same?") Hmmm . . No. [The yawn gives evidence of rising tension.]	0

No.	Items	Response and Comments	Score
9.	Paper-coal	Well, paper and coal are .. uh .. are used for .. like for writing and for .. and for heating, like .. uh .. like when you start a fire you crumble up the paper and throw it away in the fire or whatever it is. ("How would you say they are alike?") They're alike in different homes, you know.	0

(Subsequent items of this subtest were not administered.)

RAW SCORE: 5

WEIGHTED SCORE: 4

PICTURE COMPLETION

(Here, more than anywhere else, Stan shows how much difficulty he may experience in finding words. For example, he refers to the missing comb tooth as a "handle." At other times it is also obvious that he is reduced to a poor substitute whenever he cannot find the right word. On Item 10, for example, he can not think of "buttonhole." Instead, he says, "A .. like a hole. I forget what they call it." On the screw item, after 7″ he is able to say only, "A .. like a line. ('You mean a groove?') Yeah."

RAW SCORE: 11

WEIGHTED SCORE: 8

PICTURE ARRANGEMENT

(Stan's performance here is not remarkable except for the FIRE sequence, where he tells the story of a mother who gives her boy a match and tells him not to play with it. He receives no credit on the last three items.) [Stan's FIRE story reflects his feeling that his mother, under the guise of discipline, actually seduces him into committing self-destructive behavior (e.g., in the present case, setting the room afire).]

BLOCK DESIGN

(Stan performs with sporadic successes and failures. His solutions are not usually bizarre; they are occasionally rather peculiar and desperate efforts arising from impotence to find a workable solution.)

RAW SCORE: 10-14

WEIGHTED SCORE: 5-6

OBJECT ASSEMBLY

(Stan's very low score here is the result of inability, uncomplicated by bizarre or even unusual solutions. He simply cannot put the objects together correctly.)

RAW SCORE: 8

WEIGHTED SCORE: 1

VOCABULARY

No. Word	Response and Comments	Score
1. *Bicycle*	It's . . what you ride. [The relatively immature functional definition is noteworthy.]	2
2. *Knife*	A weapon. [This is an unusual aspect of *knife* on which to focus. As with the Similarities item, "a knife and a piece of glass both," the word triggers off a fearful, defensive reaction. Interestingly, the functional mode has given way to a more abstract one.]	2
3. *Hat*	What you wear. [Again, the functional definition.]	2
4. *Letter*	What you write. ("Could you tell me a little more?") What you write . . uh . . w-with your pen. ("What do you do that for?") For good news; you haven't heard from them all day. [As with the very young child, we see a time diffusion. A passage of days, of weeks, of years is characterized by the child as happening "yesterday"; something that takes a very long time may be described by the child as taking "all day."]	2
5. *Umbrella*	It is a . . protection . . for getting wet. If it's a rainy day you just open up your umbrella. [Stan's conversation is filled with words related to attack and defense.]	2
6. *Cushion*	What you sleep. ("How do you mean?") Well, a cushion is when you go to sleep, you just rest . . on top. It's sort of a pillow.	2
7. *Nail*	A nail is used for homes and things. ("How is it used?") Like when you hang something like a picture or a . . or a . . or you want to hang curtains or something like that.	2
8. *Donkey*	An animal . . stubborn.	2
9. *Fur*	To keep warm on a cold day. ("What is it exactly?") All I know is, it comes from an animal.	2
10. *Diamond*	Pardon? It is a . . uh . . hm . . sort of like a . . gift you know, what you wear on your finger. Or it's something . . precious. ("What does it look like?") It could look . . it could be shiny, or it could be very d-dear to anybody wearing it.	1
11. *Join*	Like together . . a group.	1
12. *Spade*	A spade is . . uh . . is used to . . uh . . to . . in the field. ("How is that?") For wheat or corn. ("What does it do?") Like you want to spread it out more	0

No. Word	Response and Comments	Score
	and give it some room. [Stan may have a correct idea, but he can not express it precisely enough to earn a score.]	
13. Sword	A weapon.	2
14. Nuisance	Somebody who's b-b-bothering you. In other words, won't leave you alone.	2
15. Brave	Somebody who is . . uh . . who won't be scared, who's willing to do it.	2
16. Nonsense	I don't know.	0
17. Hero	Uh . . one who can . . do . . things without getting killed . . or . . uh . . just being not afraid of anything. [Fear plays a prominent role in Stan's thoughts.]	0-1
18. Gamble	Like . . uh . . gamble for money. ("What does that mean?") You want to win a good deal or a plan. ("How do you mean?") Like buy a ranch or a store.	0
19. Nitro-glycerine	I don't know.	0
20. Microscope	What you look through. ("How do you mean?") Like at the moon.	0
21.-27.	I don't know.	0

RAW SCORE: <u>28-29</u>

WEIGHTED SCORE: <u>5</u>

CODING B

(Stan's performance is neat and accurate. He makes no errors. He achieves a weighted score of 8 because he is unable to complete more symbols.)

RAW SCORE: <u>44</u>

WEIGHTED SCORE: <u>8</u>

[So far Stan's performance does not impress us as peculiar. He is limited and fearful, but his thinking is not particularly strange. There are suggestions of Stan's preoccupation with being attacked and with defending himself, but it is a preoccupation to be expected in someone who is so limited in his attempts to handle the expectations placed on a growing youth.]

THE TACTUAL FORM TEST

(This is a test of touch recognition. In Part I [Plate 5], the subject is asked to feel the outlines of the Seguin form-board shapes without being able to see them. When he indicates that he knows the outline of the form he is tactually examining, he is asked to draw it. In Part II, the subject is permitted to study each form visually and is then asked to copy the sample while looking at it.)

[Stan's performance reflects the inadequacy of his tactual-kinesthetic perception. Most children of Stan's age rather quickly recognize the Seguin forms and are able to draw them quite accurately. Although Stan is able to grasp some of the simpler shapes, such as

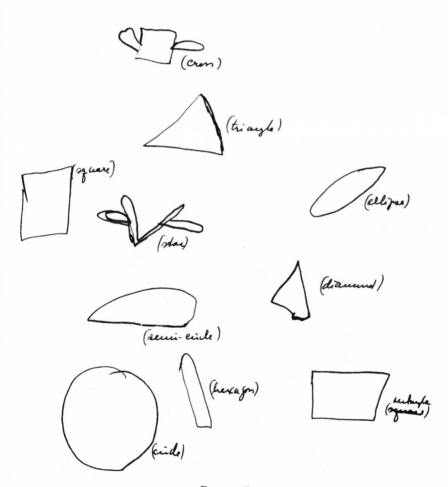

PLATE 5

the circle, square, rectangle, ellipse and triangle, his difficulties mount as the forms become more complex. His drawing of a star is probably the most poorly made. He misses the essential gestalt and reacts only to a "pointedness." Similarly, his cross is a rectangle with "ears." His diamond is a damaged triangle, and his hexagon has lost the characteristics of this form. Stan's problem, in part at least, involves an inability to grasp the form in its entirety; it is hard to know whether he loses part of what he has already recognized because of poor memory or whether he explores inadequately.]

THE BENDER GESTALT TEST

[Stan's performance on the 5″ Exposure (Part A, Plates 6 and 7) is immature. His drawings are irregularly spaced and occasionally moderately misproportioned; dots become dashes or circles; circles vary in size; distortions occur where lines should touch; overlapping figures become fragmented; angles are poorly differentiated; wavy lines are jagged. There is an improvement when Stan copies the figures (Part B, Plate 8), except for Designs 1 and 6, which become worse on the copy. Improvement is usually expected on Part B because, although performance tends to be lowered as a result of psychological and physiological fatigue, the help of the model's visual availability usually outweighs the hindrance of fatigue.

[Although Stan's Bender is not well drawn, it is done much more effectively than Claire's. Stan rarely fragments his gestalten, except for Design 7 of the 5″ Exposure and, to a minor degree, Design 4 of the copy. In the perceptual-motor realm, therefore, Stan seems better organized and integrated than Claire.]

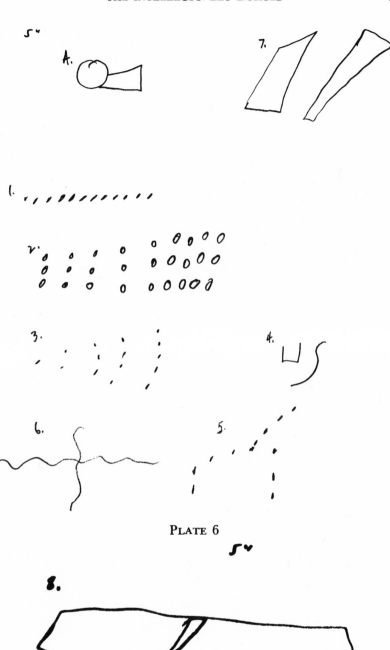

PLATE 6

PLATE 7

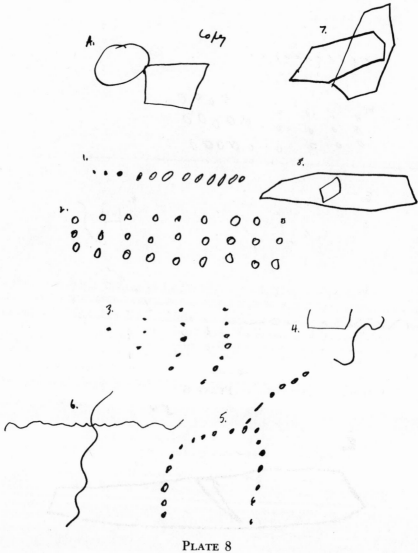

PLATE 8

RORSCHACH TEST

Number of Responses: 21

Manner of Approach (Location)

W	7
D	12
DrS	1
S	1
Total	21

Location Percentages

W%	33
D%	57
Dr%	5

Form, Movement, Color and Shading Determinants

F+	4
F−	4
F±	2
FMC′+	1
FM−	1
FM+	1
FC±	1
FC−	3
CF	2
C	2
Total	21

Groups of Contents

A	13
H	(1)
Obj.	1
Pl.	1
Cloud	1
Geol.	2
Fire	2

Determinant and Content Percentages

F%	48/81
F+%	60/50
A%	62
Obj.%	5
P%	14(19)
H%	5

Qualitative Material

Popular	I(V)VIII X
Combination	II III VII VIII
Arbitrary	2
Fabulation	3
Fabulized Combination	2
Confabulation	3
Peculiar	3
Contamination	1(?)
Confused	1
Vague	1
Autistic	2

EXPERIENCE BALANCE: 1.5/6.5

Card #	React. Time	Score	Protocol	Inquiry and Observations
I	3″	WF+AP	1. It could be a butterfly. ("Anything else?")	
		WF−A	2. It could be some kind of ant. That's all.	2. ("What did the ant look like?") It has sort of bug antennas and its arms, you know, and the tail. (W.) [Although not infrequently seen as a bug, the card is rarely seen as an "ant." Objectively, the blot has no characteristics which

Card #	React. Time	Score	Protocol	Inquiry and Observations
				could make one see an ant. The very things which characterize an ant—the delicacy and length—are missing in this blot. It is also odd to speak of an ant's legs as its "arms"— nor, of course, do ants have "tails." This is a poor response but not a really peculiar one.]
II	3″	DFMC′ +A	1. This could be like two cubs kissing.	1. ("What kind of cubs?") Bear cubs. ("Could you describe them?") They're black.
	W. Comb.	DC Fire	2. And it could also be fire on top of their heads.	2. ("How about the fire?") It was sort of like orange with red mixed together. ("Could you tell me more?")
		DC Fire Fab. comb.	3. And . . uh . . also fire under them.	3. It was sort of burning. [Stan's responses are beginning to be strange and farfetched. While the red D's are often seen as fire, it is rare to place them on top of the bears' heads. This is a "position" response: the fire is on the bears' heads and under them because that is the location of the red, on top of, and below, the black. Stan makes no effort to justify the logic of this percept.]
III	23″		Do you have it the wrong way?	
	Comb.	DFM−A	1. This could be an ant that is cooking their meal	1. ("Tell me about the ant.") Well, the sort of bodies . . their bodies. ("What about their bodies?") They had sort of little . . uh antennas on top of their heads and uh . . in their figure. (Tiny Dr areas that are sticking out of the "bodies.")
		DFC−A DFC−A Arb. Pec. Fab. comb.	2. and birds are flying around them.	2. ("And the birds?") There were sort of like pigeons. ("Could you tell me about them?") They were sort of orange. (He is referring to all the red D's.) [Now Stan is be-

React.			
Card #	Time Score	Protocol	*Inquiry and Observations*

coming thoroughly arbitrary. Not until Card X did Claire begin this kind of loose, confabulized storytelling. Stan makes up a story which has little to do with the construction of the blots. He does not permit himself much hesitation or confusion; instead, he blindly goes ahead, weaving a tale in which animals behave like people. Stan's percepts are not bizarre or horrible, but their very arbitrariness indicates that they are not born of reality testing so much as of an imagination which is internally fed and which barely makes use of external actuality to confirm or deny its accuracy.]

IV   25″

(He starts to turn the card and looks at me as though to gain my permission. I encourage him to do whatever he wishes, and he turns the card upside down.) ∨

WF—A
Fab.
Confab.
Vague
Aut.

1. This is sort of like a different kind of animal. And it's sort of like a butterfly . . that has arms and legs. That's all.

1. ("Why did it seem to be different?") Because it was crawling on the ground. ("How do you mean?") Like a mole. ("What kind of animal was it?") It was like a butterfly. ("Was it a butterfly or a mole?") A mole. ("Why is that?") Because it was crawling on the ground, and it had legs. ("And what about it made it look like a butterfly?") Because . . do you want to give me the picture? ("Try it without.") Because her arms were spread out. [Stan shows severe obsessive confusion. He is unable to make a choice. He can not decide whether his percept is that of a mole or of a butter-

Card #	React. Time	Score	Protocol	Inquiry and Observations
				fly, so he tries having both. It is impossible to tell to what extent the confusion one experiences as one tries to participate with Stan is the expression of his retardation and to what extent it is the result of the disorganization which apparently accompanies it.]
V	3″	WF± A(P)	1. This is sort of a butterfly . . that has ears and . . and wings.	[Stan seems to have lost his critical faculty. He accepts things at their face value, regardless of whether they make sense. He did not demonstrate such impaired judgment on the WISC, and one therefore recognizes that his present poor judgment must emerge because of the lack of structuring of the Rorschach cards. It is Stan's uncritical acceptance of strange and arbitrary percepts which makes one aware of being in the presence of more than just lack of ability.]
VI	7″	WF− Geol.	1. Well, this is sort of a mountain . . and the rocks are . . are spread out and sharp. That's all.	1. It was sort of round, and . . uh . . and it had a little . . rocks sticking up.
VII	5″	W. Comb. { SF− Clouds DFM+ (H) Fab.	1. These are sort of clouds and in the middle	1. ("What about the clouds?") It was sort of white and it was sort of like a circle.
		DrSF+ Obj. Confab. Contam.?	2. is a house. And the clouds are . . are talking to each other . . that's all.	2. ("How about the house?") It was white. ("How does the house happen to be in the middle of clouds?") It was a very bad storm, and the wind was just blowing so hard that it lifted it to the clouds. ("Could you tell me about the clouds talking to each other?") They were sort of looking at

Inquiry and Observations

each other, sort of like whispering. ("Did the clouds look like something?") Yes, like people. ("What kind of people?") Sort of like Indians. (When I ask Stan whether clouds usually talk to each other, he smiles and says, "No.") [If this response were given by an adult of normal intelligence, one would feel immediately, and probably rightly, that one was dealing with a severely disturbed person whose thinking was vague, confused and contaminated enough to be labeled "psychotic." What does such peculiarity mean when one finds it in the protocol of a person of borderline intelligence? Probably it is not so severe an indication of pathology; still, it is more severe than Claire's efforts to make the environment hang together through relatively innocuous, more reality-relevant fabulizing. One can ask what difference it makes whether "contamination" is the result of "schizophrenia" or of borderline retardation. The impairment is the same; it may be that the psychic and cerebral damage it reflects is also the same. Chances are, however, that the similarities are phenotypical only and that genotypically the two processes stand on altogether different ground. What someday will be the treatment of choice in one case may be of little or no help in the other. One's best guess now is that Stan lies on the border between the child who is simply retarded and the one who is "psychotically" disorganized.]

		React.		
Card #	*Time*	*Score*	*Protocol*	*Inquiry and Observations*
VIII	3″	⌈DF+AP Comb.⟨ Confab. ⌊DCF rocks	1. Well, this is a certain kind of an animal that likes to eat honey, and he's trying to find some honey, and he climbs up a rock, and .. and later he finds some honey. That's all.	1. ("What kind of animal?") Bear. ("How do you know about the honey?") That's a good question. (He smiles.) Well, because his friends told him that if he could find some honey, he would get something. ("What do the rocks look like?") They were white and orange. [Again Stan's answer reflects a good deal more than the reality of the blot. He creates a rather complex story out of very little. He perceives two areas which are rather commonly seen as climbing animals, and he elaborates this simple percept so that it becomes only distantly related to what is directly given by the blot. He is not in the least fazed by my questions (e.g., how the bear knows about the honey), which I ask to see if he is aware of his confabulatory tendencies. Instead of being taken aback, he pauses momentarily, makes a small joke ("good question") and goes on to give an "answer" which does not seriously deal with the question at all. Stan shows great unconcern about adhering to reality; he is not disturbed by his logical inconsistencies being pointed up; he simply side-steps them, ignores them and continues undisturbed.]
IX	14″	WCF pl Aut. Arb.	1. This is about .. all trees. And there are many different kinds of trees . . . . That's all.	1. ("Tell me about the trees.") They were green and white. ("Anything else?") And pink. ("What makes you think of trees?") Well, because it was standing on a log .. I mean on a .. sort of like a .. on a stand. And they were on top of that stem, and they looked like trees. ("How did they look?")

Card #	React. Time	Score	Protocol	Inquiry and Observations
				They were sitting on it. [The feeling of handling quicksilver remains as one tries to pin down Stan's response.]
X	9″	WF±A Confab. DF+AP Fab. DFC±A DFC−A	1. Ah, the last one. (He smiles.) This is an all group of animals . . mixed together. And they are hunting for food. And also they are looking for homes to live, and that's all.	1. ("What kind of animals did you see?") Fishes, crabs and butterflies and beetles. ("Would you show them to me?" I give him the card.) These (side blue D's) were crabs. And also mark down snakes. (Lower central green D's.) ("What did the snake look like?") It was green. ("What did the fish look like?") Yellow. ("What made you think of a fish?") Because they had like fins . . . fins. ("And why did they look like crabs?") Cause . . uh . . they had snappers and also . . uh . . the way they look. ("How do you mean?") Well, the body were flat and sort of scary like. (He was unable to point out the butterflies or beetles he had first mentioned.)

A comparison of Stan's test performance so far with Claire's illustrates a number of similarities. Both, for instance, obtain an Intelligence Quotient which places them in the Borderline range of intellectual ability. Yet there are major differences between the two. Although their obtained quotients are only a few points apart, the examiner feels that he is dealing with altogether different persons. While Claire throws herself helplessly on others' mercy, constantly making it clear that she feels badly treated, Stan apparently finds others considerably less important to his welfare. He needs them less. He proceeds at his own pace and does not seem to care very much what impression he makes on adults or what they demand of him. He seems to evade solving the adolescent problem of growing up by bypassing it. He does not want to stay young, like Claire. Instead, he proceeds at his private pace and constructs his own reality. Claire looked at any problem long enough to want to avoid it and stay away from it; Stan, however, seems not even to recognize that there is a problem to solve. He does not admit that a problem even exists. He does not deal with reality by modifying it somewhat, as Claire does; instead, he occasionally refuses to admit its existence. He does not respond to a reality which is there—he prefers to construct one which fits his momentary needs.

THEMATIC APPERCEPTION TEST[15]

[One begins to see the seriousness of Stan's pathology as he tells TAT stories. A few of these are picked at random to illustrate how Stan becomes progressively more disorganized as efforts are made to find out what he means. Stan's first story, to Card 1, is brief, realistic and relatively well organized. His stories to Cards 18 BM and 16 (the blank card) are rambling, almost impossible to follow, and characterized by the sudden unexplained appearance of disjointed and rather pointless elements. It becomes increasingly difficult to pin Stan down to what he means. His stories become quicksilver, fleeting and intangible, uncertain and elusive.]

Card 1 (A young boy is contemplating a violin which rests on a table in front of him.)

Well, this boy's thinking how to play a violin, and he hopes then that maybe he'll grow up to be a good musician. ("How did he happen to take up the violin?") Well, his uh . . uh . . cousins . . brought it to him. [This story is well organized, probably at the expense of creative elaboration. For organization, Stan has to pay the price of constriction.]

Card 18 (A man is clutched from behind by three hands. The figures of his antagonists are invisible.)

The man . . is . . dreaming that-that-that he was taken away and . . and he thought uh . . that . . by . . uh . . by being unscared . . uh . . he would fight, so he started fighting, and his mind was on something else, so . . uh . . he killed a man who was . . who took him away, and . . and . . and . . when he got home uh . . hm . . uh . . he saw that everything was dark, and so he looked around and . . and . . all of a sudden uh . . uh he was scared so . . uh so he ran and as he fell . . and . . and . . then he awoke and it was all gone, you know sort of a nightmare. ("Stan, you say that he was taken away. Where

15 Murray (1943).

was he taken to?") Well, uh . . in a hideout. ("Why?") Because uh . . uh he uh killed somebody. ("I wonder about something else, too. He was fighting, but his mind wasn't on it, so he killed the person?") Yes. ("How do you mean, his mind wasn't on it?") Well, his mind was on . . on something else . . . to go home, you know. So he was scared, you know, that . . that this man who took him away would kill him, so he was starting to stop fighting and . . and uh . . and he killed him. [Stan tells this story as though it were not *about* a nightmare, but as though he were *in* one while telling the story. The story seems to be told almost in primary-process terms with all parts so vague that it is impossible to take firm hold of any of its elements. In trying to make things more clear, interrogation succeeds only in making them more confused, more uncertain and more open-ended. Stan may well use having his "mind on something else" to try to absolve himself of responsibility, perhaps when he is discovered in sex play with his younger sister. Are the two situations, of sexual excitement with consequent parental blame, and the nightmare attack involving murder, phenomena that are effectively similar for Stan?]

Card 16 (Blank card.)
    ("Now Stan, here's a card that has nothing on it. I'd like you to make up a picture and then tell me a story about it.") Of a man who . . who . . who is, who went to the store and . . and all of a sudden hm . . uh . . he felt in his pocket that there was . . that he forgot to take his . . uh his wallet and so . . uh . . he told the cashier as he went back, he would be back in about fifteen minutes, so when . . uh . . when he got out it started to rain and . . and he couldn't go home because he . . because his umbrella, so . . . so all of a sudden he saw . . uh . . uh . . a man who . . who was walking by and . . and . . uh . . and he told him if he can have two dollars because that's how much he got from the things that he bought, so the man gave it to him and . . and the man said that he would pay him back so . . uh . . so he gave it to the cashier and . . and . . uh . . he walked home, and all of a sudden there was the same man who gave him the money, so he told him and . . that . . he . . that he couldn't have . . the . . give him the money because his wife wasn't home, so he waited a little while. There was about an hour or two hours in all. All of a sudden he saw he . . he saw some money that was lying on the ground and . . uh when he got there there were two dollars. So

he picked it up and gave it to the man and . . uh . . they were happy then. [This story represents an even more striking example of primary-process thinking than the previous one. Things happen chaotically, illogically, with little beginning or end. Events are jumbled; they have no readily understandable reason for being. It is evident that, as Stan has less external support and consequently must depend more on inner controls to give order and structure, he becomes increasingly disorganized. The disorganization, although present to a severe degree, nevertheless appears to arise out of inability, as in Claire's case. The disorganization is not so much the result of over-valent ideas which distort and warp; rather, it appears to result from Stan's inability to create order. He simply appears to lack the power to build his psychological organizations on sound foundations, well-differentiated substructures and solid boundaries.

[As we saw him perform on the Rorschach, however, another aspect of his thinking became apparent: he does not fabulize simply to make external elements more coherent, as Claire did; rather, Stan's fabulizations are direct wish contributions from within, contributions which color the world in a highly unusual, frequently bizarre and altogether private fashion. Stan's Rorschach performance, in other words, reflects not only a lack of ability; rather, it reflects this lack *plus* a strange private way of viewing the world.]

THE PSYCHOLOGIST'S REPORT

Stan's severe stammer is intimately affected by his anxiety level. Occasionally he has difficulty finding words, and he tries to make do with substitutes which he knows to be inadequate. Trying to think of the word "buttonhole," for example, he says, "Coat . . like a hole . . I forget what they call it." His use of such sophisticated words as "famine," "protection," "astonish" and "adore" emphasizes how the unavailable words are frequently not beyond his intellectual grasp. The possibility of mild aphasia must certainly be considered.

In line with test results obtained at other centers, Stan at this time functions in the Borderline to Defective range on the Wechsler Intelligence Scale for Children. His Verbal Quotient is 70-72, his Performance Quotient 72-74 and his Total Quotient 68-70. The considerable scatter of his subtest scores suggests that, even at this limited level, his abilities are inconsistently developed. Subscores range from 1 on Object Assembly to 8 on four other subtests. Although he claims arithmetic to be his worst school subject, he achieves his highest verbal score here, an achievement probably resulting from the special tutoring he has received.

Stan has a tendency to become so enmeshed in the concrete that he finds it extremely difficult to deal with such abstractions as size, weight and distance. When I ask how far it is from New York to Chicago, he says, "I'd say about seven or eight miles." He estimates the distance from Chicago to Topeka to be "about five miles."

His concreteness is frequently self-centered. Thus, when I ask, "What does the stomach do?" he answers, "It could sometimes . . hurt you. You could have pains." Stan's Similarities performance further illustrates his tendency to become entangled in, and unable to transcend, concrete aspects. When I ask how wine and beer are alike, he explains, "Well, beer is sort of sweet, and wine is sort of sweet and sour . . or strong. In other words, there could be different kinds of wine. They could be brown, or any sort of color. ('How are they alike?') They are alike by . . well, they don't have the same cans." Stan's relative inability to be objective results in ineffective judgment. When I ask, for example, why women and children should be saved first in a shipwreck, he replies, "Because . . uh . . because . . uh . . maybe the women and children are ascared of the water."

Stan's ability to analyze and integrate perceptually is also severely impaired. On Object Assembly, for example, he is reduced to impotent trial-and-error placements; he fits items vaguely, randomly, without goal or purpose. The same type of ineptitude is apparent in his Block Design performance. Stan tends to give up quickly on most performance tasks, sometimes at the first sign of difficulty. When he is encouraged to keep on trying, however, he is usually able to do more, sometimes reaching a successful solution.

Areas of greater competence include rote memory, which is less impaired than other functions. Further, he is alert to happenings which go on around him, and he is able to stay with activities which require only repetitive, noncreative effort.

But the more Stan is forced to rely on his creative and interpretive resources, the more he tends to become arbitrary, unrealistic and, at times, autistic. On the Rorschach, his thinking frequently becomes peculiar and vague. His confusion only becomes greater when attempts are made to clarify meaning and to sharpen perceptual organization. Stan's reaction to Card IV illustrates the point:

he sees "sort of like a different kind of animal. And sort of like a butterfly . . that has arms and legs. ('What makes it different?') Because it was crawling on the ground . . . like a mole. ('How about the butterfly?') It was *like* a butterfly. ('Is it a butterfly or a mole?') A mole. ('What makes it look like a mole?') Because it was crawling on the ground, and it had legs. ('What made it look like a butterfly?') Because his arms were spread out." It is difficult to determine how much of the confusion characterizing this response is the result of Stan's disorganization, how much is the result of easy suggestibility, and how much the result of his extremely limited ability to integrate. Stan's private fantasy often arbitrarily distorts reality. Thus, he sees Rorschach Card VIII as, "A certain kind of animal that likes to eat honey, and he is trying to find some honey, and he climbs up on a rock, and later he finds some honey. ('How do you know he's looking for honey?') That's a good question. Well, because his friends told him that if he could find some honey, he would get something." It is apparent here how Stan's craving to be orally gratified intrudes on slight provocation.

His thinking occasionally becomes so fluid that perception and cognition fuse. For example, he describes Rorschach Card VII as, "Sort of clouds, and in the middle is a house. And the clouds are talking to each other. ('How do you mean?') They were sort of looking at each other. ('As if?') Sort of like whispering." In other words, two percepts which are ordinarily seen separately—(a) Clouds, and (b) Indians talking to each other—have fused and become contaminated, so that Stan interprets the area as two clouds talking to each other. Stan's TAT stories tend to be similarly confused, so that the listener is frequently at a loss to understand which person is doing what to whom and why. While Stan's jumbled presentations reflect the severity of his disorganized, "retarded" thinking, one cannot help wondering to what extent the confusion may at times be motivated, so that it serves evasive, denying and repressive purposes.

Stan's intense fearfulness and timidity are almost everywhere in evidence. His projective test material is filled with statements which reflect his pervasive apprehensiveness. He gives, for example, the following Sentence Completions:

He saw the cockroach on the wall "and he was afraid."

When invited to go to the hiding place, he thought "it would be dangerous. ('Why?') He thought it would be like wild animals."

When he entered the haunted house "he was scared."

When he was alone in his room at night "he was scared. ('Scared of what?') His nightmares scared him."

A possible clue to the partial etiology of Stan's fearfulness can be found in the following Sentence Completion: *What scared him most* "was his father. ('Why was he scared?') He thought that his father would beat him up. ('Why was that?') Because . . uh . . because he told a lie."

Stan wonders to what extent his fears are realistic. He tells a Thematic Apperception Test story in which a woman is frightened of something. She calls the police, but when they arrive they find nothing. She discovers the frightening object to have been an illusion, created by a play of light. The listener is not sure, however, whether the woman really believes that what frightened her does not in truth exist—i.e., whether she can accept the policeman's explanation. Other TAT themes further underscore the flimsiness of the boundary which separates Stan's nightmares from his reality. To the "Hypnosis" card, he tells the story of a boy who is attacked by a friend. While Stan explains that the assault was really only part of a nightmare, he never makes clear whether the entire story is no more than a dream from beginning to end.

Stan thinks of his mother as someone constantly trying to bargain in order to get her way; the bargains often break down because one or the other does not keep his end of them. Stan complains that his mother accuses him falsely of doing "bad" things with girls when, he insists, he is only talking to them. It is apparent that he sees his mother as actually tempting him to express destructive impulses under the guise of wishing to control him. On Picture Arrangement, for example, Stan's story to the FIRE sequence includes the following: "His mother gave him a match and told him not to play with it." Anger toward his mother emerges in disguised fashion in his TAT stories, which feature mothers who are sick and in need of surgery and hospitalization. With the exception of the Sentence Completion item already mentioned, Stan rarely speaks of his father, an omission the meaning of which is difficult to pin down. Stan is not seriously aware of other people, except as they enhance or interfere with his needs and pleasures. Much of his life is spent in a world peopled with fantasy figures and things—some of them gratifying and many of them fear and frustration provoking.

In summary, Stan functions in the Borderline to Defective range of intelligence. His capacity to conceptualize his experiences is severely limited. He is markedly fearful and apprehensive, and this may be one major reason for his limited capacity to form adequate relations. When forced to depend on his own intellectual resources, the resulting arbitrariness, confusion and fluidity reach profound proportions.

The third battery of tests in this chapter is George's. Although his Total WISC I.Q. (50-51) is considerably lower than that of Claire and Stan, his Verbal Quotient of 70-71 approximates their Total WISC I.Q. While George's total performance is significantly more impaired than Claire's or Stan's, it nevertheless appears that he will have an easier time growing into adulthood than they will.

CLINICAL SUMMARY: George

George is fifteen years old. He has been recognized as being different, and probably retarded, all his life. At present he is presenting no new problems; rather, he shows the ones he has always shown, such as slowness in learning, difficulty in motor coordination and an excessive dependency on his parents.

George was born when his mother was thirty-nine and his father forty. During pregnancy, George's mother had nausea and a threatened miscarriage at four months, and also some spotting and pain, which necessitated a week in the hospital and a considerable restriction of her activities. After this, the pregnancy progressed to full term without incident, and George was born after normal labor. Soon after his birth, the family became concerned because he was cross-eyed. He had severe eczema and markedly bowed legs. When he was one and a half years old, the family began to question his mental state. He drooled considerably, constantly held his mouth open, and said nothing but "mama." Speech began at three and a half years, but he could not speak in simple sentences until he was seven and a half years old. Bowel training was begun at fifteen months and established by two years, with night wetting ceasing at four years. His main difficulty during early childhood involved his lack of coordination.

George's parents have made tremendous efforts within their own family and the community to influence, direct, support, encourage, train and, in general, to meet his special needs. In school, George has been passed from grade to grade; although he has not come up to the standard level, it was felt better for him to be promoted than to be kept behind. George is not part of any social group at school, yet his peers seem to accept him with the idea that he is different.

George's mother is a rather pleasant-looking woman who appears to be about her stated age of fifty-four. She gives the impression that she is a stable, comfortable person who has found security with her family. The father looks somewhat younger than his age of fifty-five. He appears to be in robust health and gives the impression of intelligence and directness. George's siblings are all college graduates, and both of his brothers are lawyers. He is the youngest of four children, with a sister aged twenty-eight and twin brothers aged twenty-five.

Physical and Laboratory Findings: Physical examination reveals a marked amblyopia and generalized discoordination. The neurological examination suggests no focal neurological signs. The EEG is an abnormal one, compatible with diffuse brain disturbance, with major abnormality over the anterior right hemisphere.

The Psychologist's Description

George does his utmost to be pleasing during the test sessions. He attempts all testing tasks, even those that are extremely difficult for him. Although tense during our first meeting, he becomes much more at ease during later sessions. As is true of many retarded children, he asks innumerable questions—about me, the clinic, his schedule, the laboratory procedures, the other doctors he is seeing and so forth. But he displays a maturity, facility and social comfort which are much more developed than one would expect in a boy with his degree of retardation.

Frequently it is difficult to understand George. He is unable to pronounce many sounds: he substitutes s for sh, ts for ch, r for l, and distorts many vowels. Because of this speech immaturity, sheep becomes "seep," chimney becomes "tsimney," blossom becomes "brossom," and burn becomes "booan."

Although George never drops his friendly willingness to comply with a request, he frequently seems unable to understand what is expected. Sometimes when I give him directions, he merely sits and looks at me, at a loss to understand what I intend. I often find it necessary at these times to draw his attention away from my face and toward the task I would like him to do. Even when problems are too difficult for him, he attempts to deal with them somehow, although his limitations usually cause him to handle them inadequately. For example, after I demonstrate the bead stringing on the VI-year level of the Stanford-Binet, I ask him to copy my design. Instead, he looks at me with a puzzled half-smile. When I encourage him, he tries to comply, but he simply places the beads in front of him and, obviously puzzled, asks whether this is what I want him to do.

WECHSLER INTELLIGENCE SCALE FOR CHILDREN

Name:　George　　　Age　15-9

	RS	WTS	0	1	2	3	4	5	6	7	8	9	10	11	12	13	14	15	16	17	18	19	20
COMPR.	13-15	7-8									•	x											
INFOR.	7-8	2			•																		
DIG.	9	7								•													
ARITH.	10	7								•													
SIMIL.	9	6							•														
VOCAB.	26-27	4					•																
P. A.	8	1		•																			
P. C.	1-2	0		•																			
B. D.	2	0	•																				
O. A.	0	0	•																				
CODE	29	4					•																

TOT. VERB.	26-27
TOT. PERF.	5
TOT. SCALE	31-32

VERBAL I.Q.:　70-71　　LEVEL:　Borderline

PERFORMANCE I.Q.:　Not in Table　　LEVEL:　Retarded

TOTAL I.Q.:　50-51　　LEVEL:　Retarded

George's WISC Scattergram reflects how much more poorly he solves Performance than Verbal tasks. He performs so poorly on the Picture Completion, Block Design and Object Assembly subtests that his scores cannot be included in the test's Table of Equivalence Scales. In fact, he does less well on these subtests than a child aged five years, two months. George's Total I.Q. of 50 can be misleading unless one keeps in mind the highly discrepant subtotals which make up his final score. It will become apparent that George, even with his inadequate Performance scores, reads and writes at a level consistent with his Verbal, rather than his Performance, abilities.

The extreme Verbal-Performance discrepancy in George's WISC performance immediately raises questions whether his functioning is neurologically impaired. It is usually easier to think about what is meant by "organic" when one is dealing with the performance of a patient whose usually competent functioning is interrupted by unaccountable gaps in ability, gaps which reflect lacks rather than distortions. What about the person whose abilities are *generally* impaired? Is it legitimate to distinguish between "retarded," on the one hand, and "organically damaged" or "neurologically impaired," on the other? Is it even a question of "either/or" or is it always a question of how much of the one and how much of the other? Do we mean by "retarded" only the three percent who constitute the lowest point of the normal distribution? If we think of retardation as involving all performances below a certain I.Q., then the definition would have to include many "organics." If we define retardation as a "disease," then we cannot very well include the lowest three percent of the *normal* distribution. George's neurological examination shows that he suffers from certain developmental, neurologically significant stigmata and that he has an abnormal EEG tracing. Do these findings mean that George is "organic" *rather than* retarded? Does the distinction between "organic" and "retarded" always make sense? Perhaps it will, once we develop different methods of help based on validly conceived differential diagnoses. At present we seem able to do about the same amount of good, in about the same ways, for retarded (whatever that is) as for generally impaired "organic" (whatever that is) persons.

George has developed capacities which do not depend primarily on visual-motor coordination. His less severely impaired verbal abilities permit him to make a fairly adequate social adjustment. He is able to hide or disguise some disabilities, so that they do not stand in his way too seriously. He has been able to develop skills, such as reading, writing and arithmetic, which will be useful and necessary to his future functioning. Unlike Stan, to whom reality at times seems irrelevant, George tries to adapt himself to the external environment. He does not value it negatively, as does Claire. By accepting it, he comes to terms with it, within the considerable limits which his inabilities set.

INFORMATION

No.	Question	Response and Comments	Score
1.	How many ears have you?	Two. (He laughs.) We're getting into the body now. Probably it's the only one I know about the body. [He is "setting the scene," outlining the conceptual area, to help himself function more effectively.]	1
2.	What do you call this finger? (Show thumb)	Thumb?	1
3.	How many legs does a dog have?	(He smiles.) I've had dogs, but . . . . . (he smiles again.) . . . . . ("Could you try and tell me?") (He is thinking hard.) They have more than people. ("How many do people have?") Two. ("And how many do dogs have?") Do they and cats have the same? They don't, do they? Four? ["I've had dogs" represents George's efforts to use a memory image to help himself come up with information which should be immediately and automatically available.]	0-1
4.	From what animal do we get milk?	Uh . . . . cow	1
5.	What must you do to make water boil?	. . . . . . Uh . . . . uh . . I don't know. ("Can you think of any way?") You mean . . put something in it? ("How do you mean?") You put it in a cup. ("And how do you make it boil?") Oh . . you find a . . you find out . . to put it in . . uh . . water? (He is very tense.) [George's answer illustrates how a person may achieve a score on, say, an eight-year level, and yet not function as an eight-year-old ordinarily would. After all, a fifteen-year-old with a mental age of eight has been around almost twice as long as a "genuine" eight-year-old. For that reason, the intellectual organizations of a fifteen-year-old with a mental age of eight and of an eight-year old with a mental age of eight cannot be identical. The eight-year-old with normal intelligence is developing as a growing boy should; the fifteen-year-old with a mental age of eight is developing at about half that rate. Learning at the proper speed, at the proper time, with the proper equipment, is accompanied by an intellectual organization which has only the thinnest similarity to that of someone who achieves the same scores at a significantly later or earlier time of life. When we say someone has the mental age of a person chronologically older or younger, we do not mean the two have the same mentality;	0

No.	Question	Response and Comments	Score

we mean only that both can do tasks which persons of that age can ordinarily do. A score usually reflects a final product. It may say little or nothing about how the product has been achieved. Yet the *quality* of a performance often tells more than the score, which attests only to the correctness of the end product. Most seven- or eight-year-olds know how to boil water. According to his total Information score, George's available information is at the seven- to seven-and-a-half-year level; yet he can not answer a question which five-year-olds can often handle. Once again it is apparent that "mental age" is an abstraction that has very little to do with "real" age. The M.A. was never intended as more than an abstraction, but even psychologists tend to forget this fact.]

6. *In what kind of a store do we buy sugar?*

Oh . . just a minute . . uh . . Any store that most towns have? ("Tell me one.") Is it a special store? I mean . . uh . . ("Where do you go?") . . . . . (I give him alternatives; a laundry, filling station, hardware store, etc. To each wrong one he says, "No.") ("So where would you go?") The Johnson store? Do you have a Johnson store in Topeka? Is it pretty big? Have you lived in Topeka long? [George does not think of a class of stores, but of a specific, concretely conceptualized store. Facts which should be well established are turned into questions. He rarely permits himself an unequivocal declaration. It is apparent that he experiences safety through the asking of questions. He does not ask questions merely to avoid having to answer them; rather, he assumes the identity of "the question asker." As the naïve interrogator, he walks through life with less fear of being attacked.]

Score: 0

7. *How many pennies make a nickel?*

Five?

Score: 1

8. *How many days in a week?*

Days in a week? Seven.

Score: 1

9. *Who discovered America?*

(He smiles.) Uh . . Conumbus (*sic*). Christopher, was it? What year was that? ("What year was it?") Was it eighteen-something? When did he die, do you know? Was he pretty young then?

Score: 1

10. *How many things make a dozen?*

Twelve things.

Score: 1

No.	Question	Response and Comments	Score
11.	What are the four seasons of the year?	Uh . . summer, winter, is it? Uh . . fall? . . . . . . ("And what's the other one?") What is it? Is it anything that school goes on? ("Is it?") I don't know. (He smiles.)	0
12.	What is the color of rubies?	I don't think I've ever seen it. Aren't they what cats have? ("How do you mean?") Some cats have them in their ear, don't they? ("What for?") Scratching too much?	0
13.	Where does the sun set?	In what place . . or in what time? (I repeat the question.) Night time? ("What place? What direction?") That's one thing I don't know.	0
14.	What does the stomach do?	(He whispers "Stomach.") You mean what do you do with it? ("What does the stomach do?") I don't know. ("Do you have any idea?") Uh-uh.	0
15.	What must you do to make water boil?	(Repeat.) Put it in a cup? Is that an accident do you think? (He is referring to a passing ambulance with its siren going.) Could it be taking someone to the hospital? Can you tell? They could be arresting somebody, too. [When an examiner feels tension may have interfered with optimal performance, it often pays to repeat an item or even an entire test. In this case, Question 5 was repeated because it appeared that George's tension interfered with his ability to answer this easy question. By the time he finished the Information subtest, it seemed he had relaxed sufficiently for tension no longer to be such a disorganizing agent. On readministration, he did no better with Question 5 than he had done the first time, however.]	

RAW SCORE: 7-8

WEIGHTED SCORE: 2

COMPREHENSION

No.	Question	Response and Comments	Score
1.	What is the thing to do when you cut your finger?	Cut any part? Go get some tape and tape it on . . if you have some.	2
2.	What is the thing to do if you lose one of your friend's balls?	We've had that happen . . (He smiles.) You mean a good way? A friendly way? Tell them you'll probably buy one? We always have a lot of balls and they always get thrown in the busses (bushes). We have kind of a big lawn.	2
3.	What would you do if you were sent to buy a loaf of bread and the grocer said he did	(He laughs.) . . Oh . . uh . . . . if who sent you? (He laughs.) ("What would you do?") You mean, go to another store and see if they have one or not. Ellands (errands) is that what we're doing now? [George does not have the intellectual flexi-	2

No.	Question	Response and Comments	Score

not have any more?

bility to adapt easily to things as they come, regardless of the conceptual category into which they might fit. He tries to achieve security by categorizing every activity.]

4. *What is the thing to do if a fellow much smaller than yourself starts to fight with you?*

(He laughs.) . . . . . . Much smaller? What about their age? Who started? You mean he started? ("If a boy much smaller than you started it.") What should you do? Say you don't want to fight because you might hit him . . hit him, and something might happen . . they're smaller and younger. I don't think they'd do too much . . I mean, they're little. Is that what you mean? [George constantly needs to pin down, to make sure, to have the precise conditions stated. Only when he knows the meticulously defined nature of the terrain does he feel free to enter and explore it.]

Score: 2

5. *What should you do if you see a train approaching a broken track?*

Train. There'd be two things I *could* do. If it's coming right at it? Or far away? ("All we know is that it's approaching a broken track.") Go in front of it and motion, or go where the man sells tickets and tell him.

Score: 2

6. *Why is it better to build a house of brick than of wood?*

I think I ought to know that. I live in a brick house. Why is it better? I don't think it'd have anything to do with tornadoes, like Redmont had. It could be if a tornado hit it, it might do more damage. We went past there when we came here, and it did lots of damage. ("Where's that?") Redmont. That's not a big town. There's just 466 population. (He gives the statistics on the dead and injured.) You can even have that happen to a big town. ("Which is better off?") A brick house. They said it might rain in Kansas City. I'm going to see the ball game. I'll see the A's play. Do you like sports pretty well? (He tells me about the ones he likes and doesn't like.) [The length and colorfulness of George's response indicates that "bricks," by way of bricks→safety→tornadoes→ danger, have triggered off easily aroused anxieties. Anxiety causes George to become less focused and to bring into his discussion topics that are only distantly related.]

Score: 1

7. *Why are criminals locked up?*

(He smiles.) Younger people, too? ("Criminals.") It doesn't matter what they are? They're locked up because they have done something wrong . . stolen or something. They have a place here in Topeka for boys. Do they have a place for girls? They caught those boys from Hutchinson. (He is referring to some boys who had run away from the Boys Industrial School.) [Again the effort to

Score: 0-1

No.	Question	Response and Comments	Score

pin down precisely: younger, older, bigger, smaller, all have significance for George. He compares himself to those who are bigger and older, very much as a little child compares himself to adults. George is well informed about things which have the smell of danger. Thus, he knows precisely how many people were killed and injured in the tornado. He knows that some boys have escaped from the Industrial School, but they have been caught and can no longer harm him.]

8. *Why should women and children be saved first in a shipwreck?*

Shibreg? (*sic*) (I explain.) Because they can't do as much as men. I mean, they're not as strong. [It is apparent that many of the examiner's efforts to clarify a patient's thinking do not coincide with recommended (i.e., standardized) forms of inquiry. The psychologist collides with an old testing conflict: does he want a truly "accurate" I.Q., but at the expense of not discovering *what* and *how* his patient is thinking? While final scores which the patient achieves when the examiner uses freer forms of inquiry are not derived from standardized methods, they may give considerably more complete information. A more exhaustive inquiry permits an examiner to find out information which might be of much more help than an "undistorted" intelligence figure. With well-phrased questions and clarifying help, the examiner can attempt to test the limits of his patient's abilities, disabilities, blockages, disorganization and so on. The patient's entire psychological structure, rather than only his intelligence, is being tested. In order to carry on this type of examination effectively, the examiner must occasionally ask pointed questions and give explanations when, according to the instructions in the test manual, he should remain quiet. The examiner must forever choose the times he considers it wise, or even necessary, to transgress the bounds of standardized inquiry.]

1

9. *Why is it better to pay bills by check than by cash?*

(He smiles and repeats the question.) . . . . I don't know.

0

10. *Why is it generally better to give money to an organized charity than to a street beggar?*

Oh . . my mom has told me something. Because a brind (blind) beggar might not be brind at all. He could make like brind and get all the money. Does that ever happen? Does it happen a lot? What do they do? [George's mother spends much time with him, explaining rather complicated

1

No.	Question	Response and Comments	Score
		ideas. She is patient and tries to tell about the world so that he will comprehend it better. Although he appears to have trust in what she tells him, he nevertheless needs to check up on her, to verify whether other people believe as she does. He wants to make certain she has told him what is "really" so and that it coincides with the experience of others.]	
11.	*Why should most government positions be filled through examinations?*	(He doesn't understand this question at all.)	0
12.	*Why is cotton fiber used in making cloth?*	Fiber? What fiber? ("Why is cotton cloth used?") Why is that now? (I repeat the question.) You mean like women, mostly? ("Why do they use it?") Is it to make it more neater?	0
13.	*Why do we elect (or need to have) senators and congressmen?*	(Omitted.)	0
14.	*Why should a promise be kept?*	Any kind? ("Any promise.") Oh, because . . some . . because if you don't keep a promise, something bad might happen. Like I promise you that I might go out and eat and . . . . . Oh, no, you might promise a man to go out and eat, and a woman, and if you don't keep your promise, they don't know what to do. You might just cook food for them and all, the way they usually do. [This garbled explanation, with its concrete examples, apparently describes a real incident.]	0-1

RAW SCORE: 13-15

WEIGHTED SCORE: 7-8

ARITHMETIC

(George achieves credit on the first ten problems. He solves several of the simpler ones in one or two seconds.)

No.	Problem	Time	Response and Comments	Score
11.	*A workman earned $36; he was paid $4 a day. How many days did he work?*	28"	A workman did what? (I repeat the question.) Oh, about . . it wouldn't be a week. About two days. ("How do you do that problem?") Subtract? To find out how many days he worked. You couldn't add, because you get four days.	0
12.	*If you buy 3 dozen oranges at*		What was that now? If you buy thirty dozens . . . . (I repeat the problem.) Oh . .	0

No. Problem	Time	Response and Comments	Score

30¢ a dozen, how much change should you get back from $1.00?

seventy? [George no longer has a conception of how to tackle these more complex problems. So long as arithmetic problems involve only a simple, one-step procedure, George responds automatically and correctly. As soon as a problem involves two procedures, however (e.g., *multiplication and then subtraction* in Problem 12), George's thinking becomes hazy. The complexity of the problem is so great that George contaminates its elements. Thus, "three dozen oranges at thirty cents a dozen" becomes "thirty dozen."]

RAW SCORE: 10

WEIGHTED SCORE: 7

DIGIT SPAN

(George repeats five Digits Forward on the second try. When he tries to repeat six, he either omits a number or confuses the sequence. He is able to repeat four Digits Backward, but when he attempts a series of five, he either reverses adjoining numbers or omits a number.)

RAW SCORE: 9

WEIGHTED SCORE: 7

SIMILARITIES

No.	Items	Response and Comments	Score
1.	*Lemons-sugar*	Sweet.	1
2.	*Walk-throw*	Arm.	1
3.	*Boys-girls*	Women.	1
4.	*Knife-glass*	. . . . Uh . . what now? (I repeat the question.) Broken? [George, in a sense, is "broken."]	0
5.	*Plum-peach*	They're not the same coror (color). And they don't taste alike. A plum is popperl (*sic*), isn't it? And a peach is yellow. ("Can you think of any way in which they are alike?") (He shakes his head.) (I give him some examples.)	0
6.	*Cat-mouse*	They're both animals. [When given help (from completion to conceptualization), George is able to abstract. On the *Plum-peach* problem, he makes the typical error of the immature or retarded person: he is unable to ignore differences between the two items and cannot overlook superficialities so as to abstract essences. When he is shown how to do it, however, and helped to "shift," he is able to assume the abstract attitude at least for a short while.]	2

No.	Items	Response and Comments	Score

7. *Beer-wine* — (He smiles.) Uh . . they're both something that you drink. Beer is stronger than wine, isn't it? [He is still somewhat caught up by the difference, so that he can not quite leave it be.] — 1

8. *Piano-violin* — You can play at them. That's what my sister does. She plays the piano, but not the violin. The boys play sports. (He talks about this type of boy-girl *difference* at some length.) [Again, after giving a similarity, George is compelled to say how the items are *not* alike—i.e., his sister plays one instrument but not the other. Notable is his effort to differentiate between what boys and girls do. This need to clarify the distinction between what his sister does and what "boys do" represents George's effort to clarify his identity. He is probably not certain about the essence of maleness and femaleness; he uses relatively peripheral criteria to distinguish between men and women, very much as young children use long and short hair to differentiate between boys and girls.] — 1

9. *Paper-coal* — Newspaper? (I repeat.) No, I don't know that one. — 0

10. *Pound-yard* — You measure with both of them. [This unexpected, high-level response comes as a great surprise. How could George suddenly organize himself to come up with this very fine response?] — 2

11. *Scissors-copper pan* — (He misunderstands "pad" for "pan." I explain the word.) You mean like you put food in? I don't know that. — 0

12. *Mountain-lake* — A mountain you climb up, and you swim in a lake. And you can't swim in a mountain. You don't have to swim in a lake; you can go fishing. We go fishing in Minnesota. Do you like fishing? What do you fish? ("Can you think how a mountain and lake are alike?") Uh-uh. — 0

13. *Salt-Water* — You can taste both of them. [Although he has the wrong concept, he understands that he is to find a similarity and is not diverted from this task by the concrete differences. George's performance on this subtest suggests a waxing and waning of ability, possibly related to a waxing and waning of available energy; he can do things one moment which he is incapable of doing the next. This waxing and waning is frequently found among retarded, brain-damaged children and among adolescents.] — 0

RAW SCORE: 9

WEIGHTED SCORE: 6

PICTURE COMPLETION

No.	Item	Time	Missing	Response and Comments	Score
1.	Comb	15″	Tooth	I probably won't know . . . . ("What is that?") That's a comb. Oh, it's the thing right here. (He points correctly to the missing tooth.) ("What do you call that?") Lettuh? (sic) Or a point?	1
2.	Table	25″	Leg	There's a lot of things, isn't there? The thing right here (points correctly to where the leg should be). ("What do you call that?") That's a figure, but I don't know what kind it is. ("What is it used for?") For a table. That's a table. ("What do you call this?" I point to the leg of his chair.) A leg? ("So what is missing on the table?") A leg? [Words which should easily be available are not; they become available only with help. Here is another example of the value of modifying the test administration for the purpose of finding out important information—in this case, information about how easily words can become available to George when he is helped.]	0-1
3.	Fox		Ear	(He laughs.) That's . . a cat, I think. It doesn't have a cleah (clear) tayul (tail) I think. Is that a cat? A dog? I know it's an animal. (He laughs.) What time do you close here? ("Do you see anything else missing?") No, but . . oh! The legs would be down here, farther right here. Are you busy at night? Do you have TV at home? [While it is not surprising that George is unable to recognize a fox, one is nevertheless taken aback when he toys with the idea the fox might be a cat. The juxtaposition of the severe perceptual inability and George's many personal questions furnishes a major clue to a preferred way of handling the recognition of his disability: he becomes intensely person-oriented. Objects often have little meaning to George—frequently he does not recognize them, and often he cannot manipulate them or do	0

No.	Item	Time	Missing	Response and Comments	Score
				anything else productive with them. Ordinarily, people, unlike objects, change as their environment requires. When one deals with a person of such limited ability as George, one modifies himself to meet unusual needs. For this reason, George finds it desirable to orient himself, at times almost exclusively, toward persons.]	
4.	Girl		Mouth	(He laughs.) Uh . there's supposed to be something right here. (He points to the neck region.) The nose isn't right. ("How is that?") It should be . . up . . further up. ("Anything else?") No.	0
5.	Cat		Whiskers	(He always looks at me before looking at the card.) [This is a further example of George's person-directedness. He looks to people for guidance, direction, approval, encouragement and orientation about how to proceed.] This (the back leg) isn't down far enough.	0
6.	Door		Hinge	That's a house. [His mistaking a door for a house reflects the degree of his perceptual impairment.] It's kind of mawked (marked) on there . . scratched. ("Anything else?") No. (He keeps looking at me whenever I ask him a question.)	0
7.	Hand		Fingernail (polish)	(He counts the fingers on the hand.) There's supposed to be another finger. ("How many are there?") Five. There's supposed to be six. ("Do you have six?") Oh! Ten!! There's supposed to be four more. [It is truly amazing to find this degree of confusion and disability in someone who is able to say that a pound and a yard are alike because "you measure with both of them."]	0

(The remaining Picture Completion items were not administered.)

RAW SCORE: __1-2__

WEIGHTED SCORE: __0__

PICTURE ARRANGEMENT

No.	Item	Correct Order	Time	Arranged Order	Story and Comments	Score
A.	Dog	ABC	12″	ABC	(He begins but is not sure of himself.) This is just putting things together. [Again, the orientation.] Did you get these from some place? Do you like boxing? [A probable contamination: the objects are taken from a box—"boxing."]	2
B.	Mother	TOY		YOT	What am I supposed to do? Make what? (I present the cards again, and he arranges TOY correctly.) Like this?	0
C.	Train	IRON		INRO	They're getting kind of hard. What is this? [George's inability to recognize what should be familiar again indicates the degree of his perceptual impairment.] (After his incorrect arrangement, he keeps looking at me to see whether I approve of what he has done.) What is it? A train? (I give him the sorting again.) Is this right so far? (He has the first half of the engine and another car put together; he finally sorts IORN.)	0
D.	Scale	ABC		ABC	(He laughs.) He is trying to look at that and that. It's a man trying to weigh himself, or not?	2
1.	Fire	FIRE	23″	FIER	("What was the story there?") The scale was it? ("No.") [George demonstrates how difficult he finds it to shift from one conceptual area to the next.] A fiah! (fire) ("And what was the story?") He was trying to put out a fiah . . in the house, I think. Do they evah (ever) have any fiahs out here?	0

No.	Item	Correct Order	Time	Arranged Order	Story and Comments	Score
2.	*Burglar*	THUG	43″	THUG	A man was looking at a policeman . . a cop. (He laughs.) C-o-p-y, is that how you spell cop? [Later he spells much more difficult words correctly.] And trying to talk to him. ("Anything else?") No. Am I supposed to remember all them things or not? I'm not supposed to get all these things right. You graduated in '52? [With youngsters such as George, who need to ask many questions in order to create an inner and outer equilibrium which permits them to feel more at ease, the examiner should feel free to answer some questions directly. Since testing is not therapy, and since direct answers to his questions will serve to reduce anxiety, it is better that the examiner adapt himself to some of the other person's needs. In a testing relationship, the examiner should not always expect the other person to meet only strict test demands. It is not wise to treat testing as though it were invariably a matter of unflagging earnestness, of life-and-death competition. Usually whatever helps to lower the anxiety level of the person who is being tested also helps him to produce qualitatively and quantitatively more competently. This is what is meant by "rapport." But rapport, once established, is not automatically maintained. Throughout the testing, rapport is frequently lost and must be re-established, sometimes over and over again. The	4

No. Item	Correct Order	Time	Arranged Order	Story and Comments	Score
				examiner must, of course, avoid losing control of the testing situation. He must find an optimal path between making testing go only his way and finding himself helpless in the hands of a person who so manipulates the testing situation that little of worth gets accomplished.]	
3. *Farmer*	QRST or SQRT	33″	QRTS	(While he is sorting, he looks at me every once in a while, apparently to see whether I consider his arrangement to be appropriate.) The man was trying to plant crops. He was a farmuh. ("What happened?") he went in a cah. He had a scayuh-crow theah, I think. [George's speech disability is growing worse as his failures mount. To what extent is the disability motivated, in the sense that George, probably unconsciously, is attempting to engage the examiner's sympathies?]	0
4. *Picnic*	EFGH or EFHG	32″	FEGH	A story? (He looks at me questioningly.) I *think* I know what it means. But I don't know what this is . a dog? Yeah, a dog.	0

RAW SCORE: __8__

WEIGHTED SCORE: __1__

BLOCK DESIGN

No.	Time	Accur.	Description of Behavior and Comments	Score
A-1		No	(He looks at me questioningly.) They're not the same colors, I think. (He makes a design altogether unlike the model and includes colors that are different from the model's.)	0
A-2		No	(He appears unable to distinguish the colors and doesn't grasp the idea of copying the design. I ask him	0

No.	Time	Accur.	Description of Behavior and Comments	Score
			to name the colors, and he identifies them correctly. He seems unable to grasp the idea of building his own design and instead keeps adding blocks to the one I built as a demonstration. He finally completes a design which looks nothing like the model. When I ask whether the two designs look alike, he appears confused. After we do the design together, block by block, he is able to do it by himself.)	
B-1	37″	Yes	(He seems puzzled about how to start, but then slowly and correctly places the blocks, checking each one carefully.)	2
C-1	28″	No	Yeah, but this is red and that's red, and that's red, and this is half red. (He is finished, but the design is completely wrong.)	0
C-2		No	(He puts down a full yellow block.) Is that right? . . . . . No. (He makes a design, using three full reds and one full yellow in the upper right-hand corner. Then, looking at me to test my reaction, he changes things around, so the full yellow is in the lower right-hand corner. He seems helpless about knowing how to go about all this.)	0

(The remaining items were not administered.) [George's helplessness and sense of confusion with a task which requires even a minimum of perceptual acuity and capacity for integration is evident.]

RAW SCORE: 2

WEIGHTED SCORE: 0

OBJECT ASSEMBLY

Item	Time	Accur.	Description of Behavior and Comments	Score
Manikin	1′45″	No	(He smiles. Before he begins to put the pieces together he says:) This is a gool (girl). (He strings all the pieces together, so that each is underneath the other. He makes no effort to fit them into a unity of any sort.) Have you been pretty busy today? (He indicates he has finished. I encourage him to continue and to make something. He does continue but again arranges one piece underneath the other, as before.) This won't be too easy, I don't think. (1′ 45″) (I demonstrate for him.) Oh! (He tries again but is only very slightly more successful than before. I demonstrate a second time, and he is able to make the correct assembly but has the legs reversed.)	0
Horse	—	No	Are you going to the KU graduation? Do the folks pay you or do you get other money? Does	0

Item	Time	Accur.	Description of Behavior and Comments	Score
			the lady downstairs (the receptionist) own this place and pay you? [This peppering with questions reflects the degree to which George's anxiety is mounting, probably because of the increasing difficulties he experiences.] I don't even know what this is. (He laughs.) I know this is a horse (referring to the head) and I have to put it up here. (Again, he strings the pieces together vertically, in haphazard fashion. Again I demonstrate for him. He asks what the different parts are: "The head? The hovess [hoofs], what he kicks with?")	
Face	—	No	What is it? (He smiles.) ("What does it look like?") It's not an animal. It's a human pooson (person), I think. Yeah, a human pooson. (Again, he strings the items vertically, without rhyme or reason, and he keeps looking to me for reassurance.) ("What does it look like it might make?") I can't .. it uh .. it's not a man though, and it's not what you'd ask in twenty questions. Oh, yeah, you can ask anything in twenty questions. Could you tell me at any time what it is? ("Could you make a face out of it?") Face? That's a body, isn't it? ("Could you put it together?") I don't think so, no.	0
Auto	—	—	(Not administered.)	

RAW SCORE: 0

WEIGHTED SCORE: 0

CODING B

(He fills in less than half the symbols. He tries to be neat, but his symbols are poorly drawn and occasionally go outside their allocated space. He makes seven errors: he omits two symbols, puts two in the wrong square, distorts the gestalt of two and reverses one.)

[Even though he does poorly here, he achieves his best performance subscore, with an age equivalent of eight years, ten months to nine years, two months. This achievement is consistent with George's writing ability, examples of which will be shown later.]

RAW SCORE: 29

WEIGHTED SCORE: 4

VOCABULARY

No.	Word	Response and Comments	Score
1.	Bicycle	You ride on it.	2
2.	Knife	Cut? [The concrete-functional orientation is apparent.]	2

No.	Word	Response and Comments	Score
3.	Hat	You weah (wear) . . you put on your head.	2
4.	Letter	You write a lettah (*sic*) to a sister or a brother or a girl friend in town . . or your folks. [It is as though George had a concrete image of each person to whom at some time in the past he has written a letter.]	2
5.	Umbrella	You have . . you put an umbrella on if it's raining hard. Some people take it when it isn't raining . . that stupid weather of ours. Do you have stupid weather, too?	2
6.	Cushion	You take a cushion to a ball game to sit on because it's comfortable, or you can buy it.	2
7.	Nail	Oh . . uh . . nail. A boy could . . a boy might go barefooted and get a nail caught. Something that hurts you pretty hard. ("What is it?") It's an object, isn't it? ("And how is it used?") You hit something against it, like, if you fix something. [Apparent again is George's alertness to situations of potential hurt.]	1
8.	Donkey	An animal. Something that you ride on.	2
9.	Fur	They make seep (sheep) out of fur. They shoot 'em . . or maybe they get old. Seep's an animal that they can make it out of. [George's understanding of cause and effect is inconsistent.]	1
10.	Diamond	A boy might get a girl if they're engaged. I think that's a diamond. ("Can you tell me some more about it?") Is it a gold thing?	0-1
11.	Join	You join together with something.	1
12.	Spade	Uh . . oh . . in the garden you use a spade to dig up things.	1
13.	Sword	People use swords in movies or acting. I don't go to the movies much. I have a TV. ("Tell me more about a sword.") It's a object . . a dangerous object . . you kill people pretty easy with it.	1
14.	Nuisance	(He laughs.) Uh . . people get in the nuisance. They like to tease. I kind of like to do that. Do you do that ever? Who to? Anybody? [Undoubtedly, George gets teased a great deal. He changes the unpleasant, passively experienced transaction into one where he is active. In this way, he makes it less noxious.]	1
15.	Brave	There's not two meanings, is there? There's a story . . if they don't have that, they're cowards. It doesn't mean fight, does it? Maybe stand up for your country. Who's that man who didn't like his country? We had him last year. Was the country as good then? (He asks whether and where I went to college, though I've told	2

No. Word	Response and Comments	Score

him before. He wants to know what I minored in and whether I found gym and health education easy courses.) [It is obvious that George does not care about my answers; he cares only about the *act of questioning*, about creating activity between us. Instead of answering my questions, a task he finds odious, he gives *me* some to answer. In this way he equalizes our positions somewhat. Asking questions and receiving answers is his major way of establishing a relationship with someone; it makes him feel less helpless when he tries to deal with tasks that are difficult.]

16.	Nonsense	It means . . not true.	2

17. *Hero* In sports it means to be a hero . . to win the game. It doesn't have to be in sports . . like you tell the police about the bad accident, or like the question you asked before about the railroad. [The test questions obviously have considerable significance for George, so that he remembers them over a long period of time. The questions have much more impact than first appears.] 1

18. *Gamble* That's what my brother . . it means taking bribes or taking money. Who do you think should be punished . . the one that takes or the one who gives? [This is the type of question discussed and argued in certain families. It is evident again how much George identifies himself with the sorts of preoccupations which are of concern in his home, even though he can not understand their full implications.] 0

19. *Nitro-glycerine* I don't know. 0

20. *Microscope* I think . . I think it's something that you can see how the pitcher is throwing the ball . . or someone in the bullpen, warming up. [Apparently George is exposed to a wide range of activities, and many of them he appears to enjoy.] 0

(He did not know the subsequent words.)

RAW SCORE: ___26-27___

WEIGHTED SCORE: ___4___

STANFORD-BINET SCALE, FORM L[16]

(George achieves a Stanford-Binet I.Q. of 52, M.A. 7-9, C.A. 15-9. His Basal Age is IV-6, and he passes no tests at the XI-year

16 Terman and Merrill (1937 and 1916-1937).

level.) [The Stanford-Binet is primarily intended as a check on George's WISC Intelligence Quotient. The scores from the two tests are almost identical, a phenomenon one rarely meets. The following is a very old story, but one which nevertheless bears repeating: there is no such thing as "the" I.Q. There are only different "intelligence" scores that are obtained with different tests. Since many intelligence tests correlate quite highly with each other, a score obtained on one test tends to be similar to that obtained on another. When, however, one test stresses verbal abilities, for example, while another stresses motoric, manipulative ones, the scores obtained from the two tests may have only a gross similarity. This situation is particularly the case when either verbal or performance areas are unusually depressed, as is true in George's case. Not infrequently I.Q.'s obtained on Wechsler-type tests and on the Stanford-Binet are ten, fifteen and sometimes twenty points apart. Hence, whenever one questions a patient's mental ability, it is important to evaluate his "intelligence" with several measures. Only in this way can one achieve a reasonably well-differentiated picture of "intellectual" functioning. Such a step insures against oversimplified thinking, with consequent oversimplified decisions.]

EXAMINING FOR APHASIA[17]

AGNOSIAS

Visual Agnosia

George easily recognizes actual common objects (such as a spoon, knife, key and comb); he recognizes pictures of common objects (although he calls the fork, "spoon"); he recognizes colors and reduced-size pictures of common objects. He correctly identifies some geometric forms, although he calls a triangle a "rectangle," and a square a "box." He is correctly able to read fairly complicated numbers; he accurately reads printed letters and printed words. He does less well when he tries to read whole sentences: although he correctly reads "I have a hat," he modifies, "The girl has a cat" into "The dog has a cat." He modifies "Persistence is essential to success" into "Prestiersance (*sic*) is external to success."

17 By Jon Eisenson. "The Record Form for Use with Chapter VI" in the revised Manual, *Examining for Aphasia*, The Psychological Corporation, Copyright 1954, is used.

Auditory Agnosia

With his eyes closed, George is able to recognize my coughing, whistling and handclapping as such. He calls my humming "singing" and is unable to recognize the sound of my scraping my foot. He calls finger snapping, "snapping your hands." He says he cannot whistle the way I can.

George shows significantly unusual behavior when tested for *Nonverbal Apraxia*. He is able to stick out his tongue according to my instructions, but when I then ask that he tap with his finger, he touches his finger to his tongue. When I ask him to slap the table top, he slaps his mouth. He is able to follow the command to close his eyes, but when I then ask him to show his teeth, he does so while keeping his eyes closed. [This last sequence graphically illustrates George's difficulty in shifting from and separating two areas which should be discrete. Areas which he should be able to keep isolated become fused. Such a "shifting" difficulty is seen frequently in the retarded and in persons suffering from organic insults of various sorts.]

APHASIAS

George is able to count correctly from one to twenty. Significantly, however, he does not stop at twenty, as he had been asked. He continues to count until he reaches twenty-three. [Evident is the perseveration which characterizes the behavior of the retarded and the organically damaged person.] He does a fairly good job of repeating the alphabet and omits only three letters. When he reaches Z, he says, "I can't say it. G . . like in gebra. I never have been able to say it." He is able to recite the days of the week in correct order. He omits only October when reciting the months of the year.

He is able to write numbers, letters, words and sentences from dictation (Plate 9). [It would be making a wild prediction to estimate that George could do even one quarter as well in spelling and writing as he turns out to do. While one can see his awkwardness of motor execution, he makes very few spelling errors and writes much more effectively than one would think possible. He misspells "occur" by adding an extra "r," and "June," so that it becomes "Jume." This last error, however, seems to be the result of a motor clumsiness, rather than of a spelling misconception. There is little one can offer to explain these writing phenomena; one can only watch with astonishment.]

He is able to do simple additions, subtractions, multiplications and divisions without error. [While this test further underscores the probability that George's problems are complicated by central neurological impairments (i.e., the rigidity, perseveration, word-finding difficulty, perceptual disability, memory impairment, and lack of motor control), one is equally, if not more, impressed by the positive abilities George has been able to develop in the midst of the major insults he has suffered.]

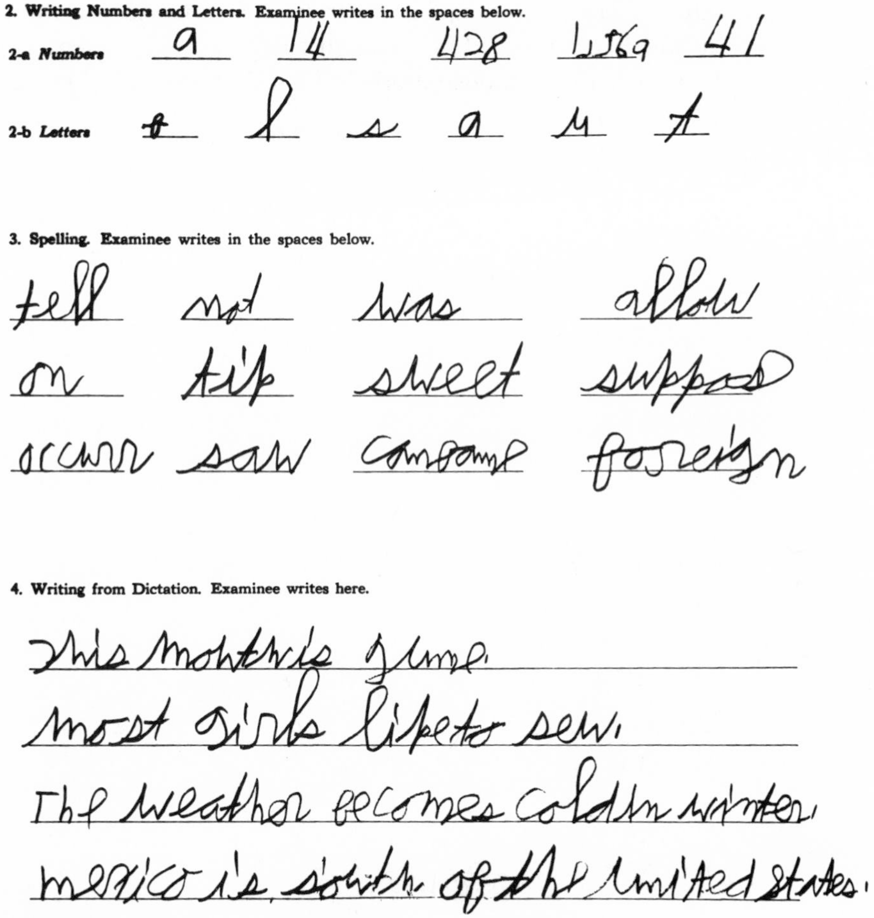

2. Writing Numbers and Letters. Examinee writes in the spaces below.

2-a *Numbers*

2-b *Letters*

3. Spelling. Examinee writes in the spaces below.

4. Writing from Dictation. Examinee writes here.

PLATE 9

The Bender Gestalt Test

PART A (PLATE 10)

Design A. (He draws this wordlessly.)

Design 1. I don't remember how many they were (dots). Was I supposed to count them? ("However you want to do it.") [George finds safety in counting. Visually perceived objects are extremely vague for him, but if he can count them, he can make them more definite. He asks for constant guidance and wants me to prescribe a precise way of behavior.]

Design 2. (He counts silently to himself. Again he keeps looking at me to check whether he is doing okay.)

Design 3. (He counts again. After he has finished:) I thought that you said that we could go through them and draw them again. ("We'll go through them once more.") That'll make it kind of easier.

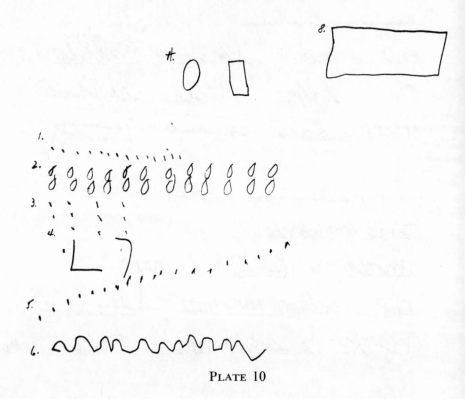

PLATE 10

Design 4. (He counts. He smiles.) I can't count that far. I'll probably be able to the next time, but not that time. [Implied is a promise of "better" performance in the future. To what extent does he need to appease me by promising me more in some indefinite future?]

Design 5. (Nothing remarkable.)

Design 6. How many more are there? Do you know? [It is interesting to speculate about the meaning of George's apparent naïveté. Does he think that I may not know much about what I'm doing, or does he want to make me into someone like himself, someone not well informed, so that he can feel more relaxed with me?]

Design 7. (He cannot draw this. He smiles:) I don't even remember that one. It's too hard.

Design 8. (He has no more room below his other drawings.) I'll put it up here. (The upper right-hand corner.) Is that okay? [Does George truly *not know* the answers to his simple questions? Does he wish to establish safety by renouncing independence and putting himself at the obedient disposal of a caring, knowing, more powerful adult?]

PART B (PLATE 11, p. 118)

Design A. Can I look at that? (He means his previous drawings on Part A.) ("Try to do it without looking.") I don't get to keep any of these? You write a lot down. Is that all you do. [Once again he demonstrates apparent naïveté. Might this also be a pseudo naïveté in the service of a wish to degrade me because I frustrate him?]

Design 1. I'll count how many there are first. (Counts.) I'll count them again. (He counts again.)

Design 2. (He starts to draw.) I got to count to see how many I have. (He smiles and looks at me. Then he counts a third time. Then he counts the ones he has drawn.) [Although the counting has the goal of making the world more precise, judging by his smile, it seems to have the further goal of trying my patience.]

Design 3. (He keeps looking at me to check whether I think he is doing all right.) Do you time me? [His questioning, in addition to the meanings already suggested, partially seems also to represent an attempt to flatter me by installing me as "the Wise One." He must know I am timing him, since I obviously glance at the stopwatch I am holding in my hand. Once again, he seems much less

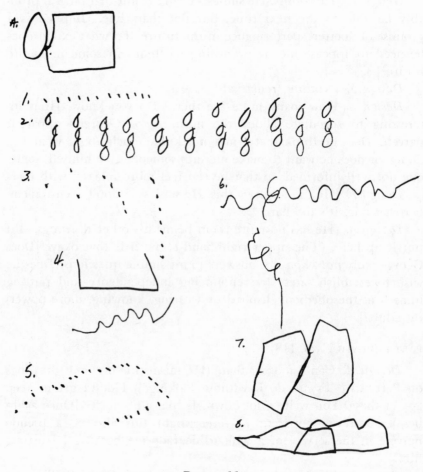

PLATE 11

concerned about the answers I give to many of his questions than about the establishment of a relationship in which he is the passive recipient of my sagacity. Perhaps he hopes that, once I realize how unknowledgeable (i.e., helpless) he is, I will not wish to harm him.]

Design 4. Most of this is timed. I couldn't draw this line (the curved one). What is that? [George has difficulty with abstract designs. He needs to make them into concrete, recognizable objects, just as on the Aphasia Test he needed to make the rectangle into a "box."]

Design 5. That's a lot, isn't it? (He smiles.) This chair is too comfortable. Maybe I'm too far away. (He moves closer to the desk.)

I'm afraid that . . . . . . this is going to take a while. (He counts the dots again and brings the card nearer to himself in order to copy it.)

Design 6. What is the next one? . . . . . A snake. I hate to draw snakes. Are you a real good drawer? Did you ever take arts and crafts in school? [His need to escape into the asking of personal questions may have been set in motion by his perception of "snakes."]

Design 7. This is seven and that was nine (looking upside down at No. 6). That doesn't make sense. Is this copyright by the same one? ("It's all the same test.") You mean, it doesn't have to be puhfec (perfect), does it? [Although this may be logically a *non sequitur,* his comments make a good deal of emotional sense.]

Design 8. I don't even remember that one from before. Do I have to put my name on this paper, too? And the date? Today is the thuhd (third), isn't it? April? I asked Bahton (Dr. Barton, the psychiatrist) if it's the thuhd, and he said, "Yes." [Why, if George has already found out that it is the third, does he ask again? As suggested before, his questioning is largely not real information seeking at all. The questions represent a way of relating himself and do not require an answer. In part, like Claire and Stan, George wants to check whether the adults who care for him are consistent and therefore dependable.] What's his fuhst name (Dr. Barton's)? What's yours? Do you have a middle name?

[George's drawings reflect his difficulties in perceiving, conceptualizing and executing abstract geometric figures. Problems with conceptualization emerge primarily in the form of an inability to draw a design until it is first translated into a concrete "thing." Without such a translation, George's drawings have little shape or coherence. He finds the abstract without a reliable frame of reference in which to place it, and he therefore finds it difficult to reproduce.

[Conceptual and perceptual functions are, of course, closely interlinked, and George perceives his environment in a thoroughly fragmented fashion. He does not see coherent forms, but only fragments of lines, circles, jagged ends and things which touch each other in some fashion. For these reasons, his drawings are chaotically and distortedly executed. He tries to insert some order by arranging neatly, but the end effect is nevertheless unharmonious. George has difficulty graphomotorically going in a certain direction. Lines which should be smooth and regular are jagged and out of proportion. What should be dots, ordered in a straight line, are hooked dashes, staggering up an incline.

[The extreme fragmentation of George's drawings adds to a suspicion that he suffers not only from uncomplicated retardation but also from a central neurological impairment of some sort. Strauss and Lehtinen (1947) suggest that organically damaged and mentally retarded patients differ in their gestalt perceptions: the perception of the mentally retarded person tends toward oversimplification and primitivization, while their figures maintain essential gestalt qualities; sensory-motor products of the brain damaged, however, lose their gestalt cohesiveness and become fragmented and chaotic, the way George's drawings do. Both the WISC and the quality of his Bender performance lead to the relatively certain conviction that his disabled condition is complex and probably involves some sort of "brain damage."]

The Draw a Person Test

PART I (PLATE 12)

(He looks at me for some time without saying anything. He seems either puzzled by the directions or reluctant to start something he feels he cannot do well. Then he says:) What did you say? A boy or a girl? ("Whatever you want.") I can't do it. ("Just try.") [Often a subject says he "cannot" draw a person. It is usually most strategic to avoid becoming enmeshed in a discussion whether he "truly" can. It works best for the examiner apparently to pay minimal attention to the other at this particular time, while making it clear that the drawings are expected to be done. If the examiner does permit himself to become involved in a long discussion, he will probably lose, or he will "win" over a resentful "opponent," or an impasse between the two principals is all that is achieved.]

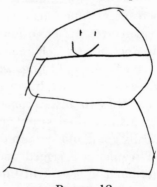

PLATE 12

(After George is finished, he says:) This is it. This isn't very good. I can't draw. I don't like to. It's the first time I drew since the first grade, and I'm a sophomore in high school now. Were you in the service? You must have been if you got your degree in 1952. [George is aware that more drawing is probably ahead. He knows he has not done well so far, so he asks far-removed personal questions to delay the inevitable.]

PART II (PLATE 13)

(After my instructions:) I can't ("Just do the best you can.") Do I have to draw a man, woman, boy, girl, dog, cat, house? [He indicates with this question that he considers my asking him to do all this as a major imposition.] (As he draws:) It's going to be about the same thing. Will there be others who see this? [Shame about what he probably considers to be an inadequate performance is evident here.] I'm going to make her fatter. (He laughs.)

[George's drawings are starkly primitive. They are consistent with what one might expect after seeing his Bender Gestalt productions and after noting his difficulties on the Performance section of the WISC. Judging by these drawings, one wonders how George conceives of and perceives people around him. Does he see them primarily as eyes and smiling mouths? About the only differentiation

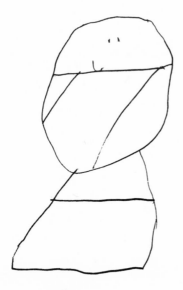

PLATE 13

apparent in his drawings of persons is in the head area; George portrays the mouth, the eyes and some lines whose meanings are obscure. An additional line occurs in the "woman's" midriff area, but George's entire drawing is so primitive that to place the usual interpretation here would probably be inaccurate. If we assume that what appears in the drawing is of first importance to the person drawing, then we must infer that, as is true of the very young child, George is primarily concerned with what others say to him and with how they look at him.]

RORSCHACH TEST

The formal summary of George's Rorschach performance reveals no surprises. His form level (F+%) is 33/40, reflecting his exceedingly limited capacity to perceive sharply or adequately what structure he does see. His Experience Balance of 0/7.0 underscores his inability to pause, to reflect, to wait, actively to organize and, instead, to be impulsive and rash. Affect, cognition and action do not cogwheel smoothly; each flashes in and out, on and off, the one with little regard for the other. George has only one adequate form-color response (FC+). The other color responses are: 1 C, 4 CF, 1 F/C— and 1 FC— response.

George's response to Card X, given in its entirety below, indicates the degree of his intellectual and emotional impoverishment.

Card #	React. Time	Score	Protocol	Inquiry and Observations
X	1' 50"		What's the X for? ("It's the Roman number ten.") Oh, a ten! How many X's make a hundred? (He asks a number of other questions. After a few more, I point to the card, indicating he should continue.) Oh, brother! This is going to take all year to do this! I don't think I know. (He is staring at me. At 75" I say "Does it look like anything?")	

Card #	React. Time	Score	Protocol	Inquiry and Observations
		Color-description	1. I know all the colors, but . . it's brue (blue) on each side, and two pink things.	
		DCP1	2. And he has brossoms (blossoms) right here. And the awtist (sic) designed these didn't he? Can you draw this good or not?	2. ("What made it look like blossoms?") The kind of different colors. ("Are they any special kinds of blossoms?") No.

CHILDREN'S APPERCEPTION TEST

Card 1 (Chicks seated around a table on which is a large bowl of food. Off to one side is a large chicken dimly outlined.)

Uh, just tell what they do? [Again, George needs orientation.] Uh . . these are animals, looking at a f-fish pond, and they have . . uh . . they have . . they have . . they have a spoon and they're looking at it, and had bowls down there. ("And what are they doing there?") They're just looking at it. And they've got something in the bowl. [The animals are passively "just looking," as George does. They can do little more.] ("What do they have in the bowl?") Uh, fish. [The unnamed animals are looking at a fish pond and at fish in their bowls. George's story setting makes no sense. His lack of logic and inconsistencies nowhere emerge more clearly than in these stories.] ("Who's that in the back?") Right here? (He laughs.) Uh . . uh . . a monkey? No, I don't know. [George is unfamiliar with even the most common animals. Although it is doubtful that he cannot recognize any animal at all, he so far has been unable to designate a single one by its correct name. It is difficult to know what this "ignorance" might mean. Could he have had some unfortunate experience with his children's stories?] ("What kind of animals seem to be sitting around there?") Uh, they're . . Could you have pets for them? . . . . . . Pets? ("What kind of pets?") Could they be pets you keep in your yard? (George wants to know whether one could have these pets in one's house. With considerable further questioning, he remains apparently unable to identify the baby chicks.)

Card 2 (One bear pulling a rope on one side while another bear and a baby bear pull on the other side.)

Bears tugging a rope, and another bear is doing it also, and the other bear was behind him doing the rope, trying to see how much they could get the rope. This one over here is smaller (the "mother" bear) and this one is bigger, and this is fust (*sic*), second and third. ("What are they trying to do with the rope?") Pull it. Just pull it away from this one. ("I see, and who are these bears?") Just animals. ("Are they related to each other at all?") Yes, this is papa bear, mother bear and little bear. ("I see. The papa bear and the little bear are trying to pull the rope away from the mother bear. And who wins?") Well them two. ("And how does mama feel when she loses?") She loses her temper. ("What does she do when she loses her temper?") She . . uh . . uh . . wants to eat him up. (He laughs.) ("What happens then?") (He laughs.) Uh, uh, she says she doesn't . . . she loses her temper, she doesn't like to lose. And she wants to try again. ("And who wins the next time?") The same thing happens. ("What does the mother bear do then?") She really gets, she loses her temper, and she says she's going to . . uh . . go get some food and eat a lot. ("How do papa and baby bear feel when they win?") They're happy and enjoy it. (When I have the dictaphone play back our voices, George wonders whether a person is inside the machine, speaking to both of us.) [George is not afraid to present intrafamilial discord. He teams up with his father against his mother, but he is not made anxious by describing his mother's anger. It is significant that mother takes her anger out, not against the father and baby, but against herself, i.e., by eating too much. While the intrapunitive is not a "healthy" way to express anger, it is a way which perhaps saves George from becoming too frightened. He is able to laugh at his mother's anger, a laughter which underscores the apparent lack of severe discomfort he feels in the face of maternal irritation. The fact that he chooses his father as a teammate suggests that George's masculine identificatory process is progressing.]

Card 3 (A lion with pipe and cane, sitting in a chair; in the lower right corner a little mouse appears in a hole.)

Hm . . a lion is sittin' there and it's got . . its cane and it's got a smoking . . and it's got a pipe, with its tail . . with its tail down, and it's kind of all messy around and everything. Sittin' in a chair, and it's mad. I don't know . . uh . . uh I don't know what it's mad about. ("Could you make up something it's mad about?") Uh . . it looks like it's real hungry, about starving to death. [George expresses conflict through oral modes. In the last story, the mother was so angry she ate a great deal. In this story, psychological deprivation is expressed through a "starving" metaphor.] ("So what is he going to do?") Go out and maybe find some bugs or something to eat . . or people or something . . either little deer, maybe a little deer or something. ("And how does he feel then?") Happy! He tries to get some seep (sheep) and then they kill him. ("Who kills him?") One of the ones that's trying to eat the little lamb . . uh . . uh . . they have a mother lamb and a papa lamb and a little lamb alike a bear, and they . . uh start. They have a . . uh . . Joe . . Joe . . that's a made-up name is . . is the keeper so he . . has . . uh . . go . . gets . . uh . . he goes . . gets a . . runs fast and gets a gun and kills this lion. [One would probably be correct to interpret George's story so far to mean that he identifies himself with the helpless, innocent "little deer" and with the "member of the lamb family" which finds itself helpless in the face of external threat. Not only George, but apparently his entire family, needs a protector, a keeper, who kills the lion—i.e., who protects the innocent family from a malevolent environment.] ("What's that in the corner?") Where? Right there? ("That's right.") (He laughs.) Uh . . I don't know. ("Could you make up what that is?") It's a little mice. ("What's the little mouse doing there?") Just looking at the lion. ("And what's the mouse thinking?") He's thinking that if the lion ever looks. ("He's thinking what?") That the lion might look. ("And what would happen then?") He would . . the mice would go back down, so the lion wouldn't eat him. [Even to be looked at by the external danger is dangerous.]

Card 4 (A kangaroo with a bonnet on her head, carrying a basket with a milk bottle; in her pouch is a baby kangaroo with a balloon; on a bicycle, a larger kangaroo child.)

How many are we having? ("We're having ten.") Good, I like these. [A probable denial.] Uh . . this . . this is a reindeer, along with a dog down here, and there's a dog trying to ride a bicycle. Here's some trees down here. And the reindeer's carrying a package with milk and food to eat, and they're going. ("What are they all doing there together?") Having a good time. ("How do they like each other?") They like each other. They're pretty fr-friendly. ("What do they do to have a good time?") They . . uh . . uh . . skip along and everything. [George again shows inability to identify animals. He calls kangaroos, reindeer and dogs. He avoids dealing with aspects of the pictures which might touch on proximity to his mother and potential rivalry with siblings for her affection. While he may prefer his father (cf. Card 2) to his mother, she must prefer no one to him.]

Card 5 (A darkened room with a large bed in the background; a crib in the foreground in which are two baby bears.)

These are getting kind of harder. [It is becoming difficult for George to maintain his denial.] Uh . . here's . . someone is in bed, and they have a rat in the house, and someone started to sleep, with the lamp over here, and got the covers over them. (He laughs.) And everything, and that's about all. ("Could you make up a story about all that?") Little . . the little two monkeys want to sleep in their bed. ("And who is that with the covers tucked over them?") Mother and father, keepin' care of them. They're lost. Cold weather. ("They're lost in the cold weather, and what happens to them?") They are going to sleep now. The folks are going to sleep. It's startin' to storm, but not much. Then it quit. ("And what happened to the two little monkeys then?") They went to sleep, and the mother thought they woke up, and she fed them. ("Do the mother and father keep them?") Yes, they like 'em. [This story attests to George's feeling of security. Although he may feel cold and lost "outside," he feels secure with his parents. They take him in from the cold, and while he sleeps, outside the storm abates. The mother feeds the strange little rat-monkeys, and both parents keep the monkeys there because "they like 'em." This exercise of George's imagination suggests that he feels himself to be a drifting, homeless monkey. His parents "take him in," however—they accept him and love him, even though he is different.]

Card 6 (A darkened cave with two dimly outlined bear figures in the background; a baby bear lying in the foreground.)

This little bear over here is sleeping, and another bear over there's asleep, and the rock, and . . uh . . a hill. It looks like kind of stormy weather, that's about that. ("What's the little bear thinking about?") He's not quite asleep. He's thinking he might wake up cause something might come there. The man might come and shoot him or something. [Although there is a fair amount of security at home while the "storm" is outside, the security is not complete. A stranger might break into the safety and harm George.] ("He's afraid a man might come in and shoot him. What does actually happen?") They wake up. The little bear wakes the big bear up and then goes and eats some bugs and insects and things. ("Are the big bears frightened, too, that a man might come and shoot them?") Yes. They never do. No one comes and hunts them. ("What would they do if a man came with a gun and shot them?") Run away. [It is becoming apparent that, while George feels safe, warm and protected with his parents, he nevertheless considers them to be fairly helpless. George does not feel impotent because of parental attack, as many retarded children do; rather, he feels part of a "seep" family which cannot protect itself against outside marauders—the world outside the family.]

Card 7 (A tiger with bared fangs and claws, leaping at a monkey which is also leaping through the air.)
    There's a lion right here, and he's . . uh . . trying to get out of the . . . . The lion is jumping and there's a monkey, and the monkey just gets in the air quick enough, and there's trees right here and (he heaves a big sigh), but the monkey finally gets away and gets out of the way and gets it. And he finally catches the lion and puts it in the zoo, and the monkey is in the zoo, too. ["He" is able to contain the lion's aggression. To assure total safety, however, the object of "the lion's" aggression, the monkey, also needs the safety of bars. Both the aggressor and the aggressed-against are isolated thus. In this way, force and anger are contained.]

Card 8 (Two adult monkeys sitting on a sofa drinking from tea cups. One adult monkey in foreground sitting on a hassock talking to a baby monkey.)
    Uh . . there's a monkey all friendly and all kind of laughing, and one of them looks like a Mutt and Jeff in the funny papers. ("And what's happening there?") They're talking and laughing. ("What are they talking about?") Talking how g-good of a time they're having. (There was momentary external interruption here.) ("Now what is it you said they were talking about?") What did you say then? (I repeat.) They were talking about they had a good . . real

good time. They're dr-drinking orange juice and things. ("Who are all these monkeys to each other?") They're friends. ("Who's that little one there?") Real good friends. ("This one?") He's a monkey. He's laughing, no, not laughing, but the other one is pointing. ("What's he pointing at?") At its head, the way its eyes . . . ("What are the two back there on the couch talking about?") (He laughs.) You asked me that. They're talking and having a good time laughing and drinking, and that's all. [With little exception, George presents a happy, uncomplicated scene, in which the family members are happy and enjoying each other.]

Card 9 (A darkened room seen through an open door from a lighted room. In the darkened one there is a child's bed in which a rabbit sits up looking through the door.)

Are we going to take all of these (other CAT cards)? We going to take all of them? ("Yes.") It's a little rabbit in his bed, and there's a door there, and a window there, and a big house, and the rabbits are awake. ("What's he thinking about?") The rabbit is thinking about what it, when he's going to get out. [It is not difficult to infer what the rabbit—i.e., George—wishes to get out of.] (What's he thinking about?") The rabbit is thinking about what it, when he is going to get out. ("How does he feel right now?") Pretty good. There's a bad storm outdoors and it's a bitter cold weather. ("Does he feel frightened of the storm?") Yes. ("What does he do when he is frightened?") He goes back to sleep. ("Does he have any dreams?") Yes. ("What kind of dreams are they?") (He laughs.) He dreams the storms might break out and they might hurt people, but he might try to get, he might still go to sleep. ("Where are his mother and dad?") They went out. They went some place. They went to the Far East. [Once more, the storm is raging outside while George is safe at home, in bed. Withdrawal into sleep often offers safety— except there may be dreams of danger.]

Card 10 (A baby dog lying across the knees of an adult dog; both figures with a minimum of expressive features. The figures are set in the foreground of a bathroom.)

There's a little dog and its friend down there. There's a toilet in the house, and its open, and there's towels on here, and that's about all I can say. ("What is the one dog doing with the other?") Rubbing. ("Why is the dog rubbing?") Down there rubbing and laughing, and he likes to open his mouth. He's yawning. ("What are they doing in the bathroom?") Sitting on a chair scratching each other. [George wishes to finish with this card quickly, possibly because he knows it is the last and he wishes to get through this difficult task, possibly because of the specific content of the picture. George interprets the spanking mother dog to be "a friend," and he interprets the interaction of the two dogs as their "rubbing" each other. Without more information, it is difficult to say whether George uses avoidance with this picture because of its arousal of disciplinary, anal or phallic anxieties, or whether he is actually telling about sexual activity he has had with some other child or adolescent.]

THE PSYCHOLOGIST'S REPORT

On the Revised Stanford-Binet, Form L, George achieves an Intelligence Quotient of 52. His abilities range from the IV-year, 6-month level, where he passes all tests, to the X-year level, where he passes none. On the Wechsler Intelligence Scale for Children, his Intelligence Quotient is 50-51. While his Verbal Quotient on this test is 70-71, his Performance ability is so limited that it cannot be scored. He achieves a total weighted Performance score of only 5, while a minimum total of 10 is required to enter the table. This minimum (which he does not reach) would be equivalent to a Performance Quotient of 44.

These figures reflect the degree to which George's verbal abilities are superior to those involving primarily perceptual, motor and sensory-motor functions. In the verbal area, he does best on questions that require commonsense judgment; he does least well on those which need the easy availability of factual information. He has difficulty, for example, explaining how many legs a dog has, saying, "I've had dogs, but . . . . . (he thinks hard). They have more than people. ('How many legs do people have?') Two. ('How many do dogs have?') Do they and cats have the same? They don't, do they? Is it four?"

George finds it hard to shift from one type of task to another. On the Eisenson Aphasia Test, for example, I first ask him to stick out his tongue and, later, to tap with his finger. He taps his tongue. When, subsequently, I ask him to hit the table with his hand, he hits his tongue. Similarly, when I read a Memory item on the Stanford-Binet, following the administration of some Verbal Absurdities items, he asks if I want him to tell "what is foolish" about the sentence I have asked him to repeat from memory. Each time a new type of test is administered, George needs explicitly to orient himself. He will say, "This is sums now, isn't it?" or "Is this putting things together?" or "This is about the body now." George's need for orientation requires he be given many additional specifications before he can deal with a problem. When he is asked, for example, what he should do if a child much smaller than he were to start a fight, he needs to know whether the child is not only smaller but also younger. When I ask him to give two reasons why children should not talk in class, he wonders whether I mean to include high school and college students, whether I mean "up to seniors in high school."

His difficulty in assuming an "as if" attitude emerges strikingly in his approach to certain hypothetical questions. He is asked why the following statement is foolish: "I read in the paper that the police fired two shots at a man. The first shot killed him, but the second did not hurt him much." After correctly explaining why this is foolish, George asks, "Why did the policeman try to shoot the man? . . Why?" When I explain that the item is only a made-up one, George says, "You mean none of them are true?" Such difficulty in assuming an abstract attitude may in part account for George's problem in comprehending the idea of a Dictaphone. Even after I very generally and nontechnically explain several times how one works, he continues to wonder whether a man or woman is speaking through it from downstairs. In line with his concrete orientation, George frequently wonders what something "really" is. When, for example, I ask him to do the Binet task of folding a piece of paper into a triangle, he asks, "Is it a kite?" Of one of the designs of the Bender Gestalt Test, he says, "Oh, that's a snake."

George demonstrates his major deficiencies in all tasks requiring motoric and perceptual functioning. His drawings of persons are exceedingly primitive and consist of a circle joined to a rectangle, without appendages of any sort. His fragmented Bender drawings are oversimplified, distorted, irregular and reflect George's strong tendency to perseverate. He has difficulty drawing an angle, and he finds it impossible to make one figure overlap another. In three attempts, he is able to copy a square only once correctly on a barely scorable (V-year) level. He makes a rectangle when I ask him to copy a pictured diamond shape. On three WISC Performance subtests—Picture Completion, Block Design and Object Assembly—his weighted score is zero. On Picture Completion, he can recognize no more than the first missing item (the tooth of a comb), and even that he cannot designate by name. On Block Design, he becomes confused when the *sides* of his real blocks show colors that are different from those pictured in the model. He can deal with Object Assembly items only by stringing the component pieces together in a haphazardly arranged, vertical line, disregarding all their meaningful connections. He is able to solve the simple *Manikin* item only after I twice show him how; even then, he reverses the legs.

Frequently he is unable to recognize the picture of an object. So, for example, he is not sure whether a drawn animal is a cat or dog, although he is fairly sure it is an animal. On the Children's Apperception Test, he does not recognize a table around which baby chicks are eating. He says it is a "fish pond," and he calls an adult chicken standing behind the table, a "monkey."

Considering his severe limitations, it is remarkable to see what George can do. He reads and writes simple material, and he computes easy arithmetic problems in a remarkable, altogether unexpected, fashion. So, for instance, he is able to spell correctly such words as "allow," "suppose," "weather" and "foreign," and he can correctly write simple dictated sentences. While the writing is large and irregular, it is quite legible. He is able to read a fairly difficult paragraph from the Stanford-Binet X-year level quite rapidly and without error, and he can retain some of the material he has read. He does simple addition, subtraction, division and multiplication with little effort—only when a problem requires him to figure out what arithmetical method to employ does he experience difficulty. George has apparently obtained excellent tutoring, and he seems quite comfortable functioning at this level.

George's Rorschach performance, too, while it manifests all the characteristics of retardation, is nevertheless a good deal more differentiated than one might expect. The content of his percepts is fairly varied and reflects his interest and pleasure in things he finds esthetically pleasing. While little is seen on the Rorschach to suggest that George is a fearful boy, there are occasional signs that suggest mild depression.

George's CAT stories demonstrate the extent to which he appears to experience security and protection at home. A number of stories deal with children who are cozily at home, while cold, stormy weather rages outside. In one story, a mother and father take two lost children into their home, and when the children wake from their secure sleep, the mother feeds them. While George's stories reflect the comfort he experiences at home, they emphasize at the same time "his perception of the outside" as cold and insecure.

Things at home are, of course, not invariably ideal. Sometimes, for example, mother loses her temper. Whenever she does not "win," she may become angry enough to feel she wants to destroy her husband and son. When she loses a second time (e.g., on the CAT "Tug of War"), she really becomes angry: "She says she's going to get some food and eat a lot."

Eating as a way of appeasing anger and other distress emerges as George's solution in several situations. The lion, who is extremely angry because he is almost starving to death, hunts some bugs, or people, or little deer, and then he feels happy. Eating associated with anger is sometimes followed by the severest punishment. The lion, for example, who goes to capture and devour some sheep, is killed by the man guarding them.

As secure as George may feel with his parents, he is not at all certain they can protect him. In the CAT story just mentioned, the parents are as frightened as their child; if the lion-killing hunter ever comes around the home, the entire family will need to run away. Significantly, however, the man with the gun never shows up. Another of George's solutions to external aggression involves both the aggressor and his intended victim. In a CAT story in which a monkey is chased by a tiger, the monkey first escapes but is then locked up in a cage, as is the tiger.

In summary, George is a friendly, pleasant, fairly comfortable fifteen-year-old boy whose performance on the intelligence tests places him on a Borderline to Retarded level. He shows many of the classical characteristics of the organically brain damaged: perseveration, rigidity, concreteness and extreme difficulty in solving tasks requiring perceptual and motor skills. While his fund of general information is exceedingly small, he is able to apply commonsense judgment to certain types of everyday situations. His relative social maturity, and his ability in the areas of reading, writing and arithmetic, reflect his capacity to benefit from the type of individual instruction which he has been given. He feels safety and security at home, but he considers conditions "outside" to be dangerous and destructive, both to him and to his well-intentioned parents. In general, one may consider George a "well-adjusted," mild to moderately retarded adolescent.

DISCUSSION

George is extremely dependent upon the good will and guidance of others who he feels know what they are doing. Although he expresses fear concerning the external world (where the storms rage), he seems to feel a great deal of confidence about being loved and accepted by his parents. He is sensitive to what goes on in the real world and is in constant contact with the persons around him. Unlike Claire, he does not feel others are unfair or make unreasonable demands. Unlike Stan, he does not avoid realities and withdraw into himself. Things, of course, are far from ideal for him: "out there" is frightening, aggressive, hostile and destructive. He shrinks from going beyond the circumference of the circle of safety, where storms rage and where people wish to harm him. He is safe in his bed (usually) and with his parents. Although his parents are only questionably good helpers against "outside" hostility, they are on his side. He need fear no aggression from them.

How will George make the transition into adulthood? Although he is not capable of functioning independently, he may well be able to manage in an uncomplicated environment in which his activities can be supervised by kind, patient, parental persons. Because he is trusting and ingenuous, people will probably want to care for him; in turn, he will wish to please them and to work for them to the best of his ability.

CONCLUSION

A comparison of Claire, Stan and George reflects the major personality differences and life solutions which can be seen even among those whose "I.Q." is similarly low. As is true of all psychological functions, the organization of abilities and attitudes which we call "intelligence" operates *uniquely* within the total personality. While a low intelligence may limit the degrees of freedom with which a person can create a rich personality organization, low intelligence by itself does not limit freedom to achieve individuality.

Most retarded children have been diagnosed as such by the time they reach adolescence. One rightly wonders why parents bring

their retarded adolescents for examination so late in their development. There can be several reasons. Perhaps the adolescent has
grown up in a setting in which his limited intelligence has created
no special problems (this is particularly true when the limitation is
of a borderline nature). Or the parents have needed to deny their
child's retardation, but they can no longer do so when he reaches
adolescence and is required to deal with more complex life problems. Or the parents have known their child to have limited abilities,
but have nevertheless decided to keep him at home until his developing (real or feared) sexual interests, poorly kept in check by inadequate controls, create difficulties. Or the parents are not as worried
by their child's intellectual limitations as they are by symptomatic
behavior which he develops at the onset of adolescence.

The concept of "mental retardation," as used in this chapter,
is meant in a descriptive sense. GAP Report No. 43 (1959) partly
defines retardation as "a chronic condition present from birth or
early childhood, and characterized by impaired intellectual functioning as measured by standardized tests. It manifests itself in impaired
adaptation to the daily demands of the individual's own social
environment. Commonly these patients show a slow rate of maturation, physical and/or psychological, together with impaired learning
capacity." This definition says nothing about etiology—idiopathic,
"organic," "schizophrenic," "neurotically disturbed" or any other. It
is fairly clear that George's impairment is associated with a rather
severe organic dysfunction. In that sense, he might more properly
belong in the next chapter. Stan's state seems associated with a strong
autistic component. Still, all three adolescents present intellectual
states consistent with the GAP definition.

Where to "put" different adolescent cases raises a major problem
in diagnostic conceptualization. While we all know that individuals
are complex, we must nevertheless try to create some type of sim-
plifying order out of their complexity. Nowhere does the problem
emerge more clearly than in writing a book which deals with clinical
diagnoses, a book which presents persons whose dysfunctions take
many forms. In this chapter, the decision was made to deal with
those adolescents whose limited cognitive equipment lowers the
flexibility with which they can approach adulthood. It is an oversimplification, of course, to focus on only the cognitive equipment,
since cognition cannot be isolated from the total mental functioning
in which it is embedded. Cognitive functions influence and are

influenced, sometimes determined, by affective and motivational ones. To focus on cognition in isolation is arbitrary, but such arbitrariness serves a didactic purpose. Because it is impossible to grasp immense complexity all at once, we can present only a part of it, that way inevitably distorting nature.

Here, then, are three adolescents with impaired intellectual powers, each of whom handles his deficits according to his unique style. Although these young persons share a major problem, the different ways with which they manage it are what is of particular significance in the determination of their life course. Although they have approximately the same verbal abilities, their attitudes toward themselves, toward other people, toward their deficit, toward their future, are not at all the same. These attitudes will mold their views toward, and their ability successfully to grow into, adulthood.

Claire, from the point of view of her chances for a successful development into adulthood, stands between Stan and George. She does not evade reality, but she distorts it significantly and feels pursued by it, vindictively plagued by it, unfairly treated by it. Unless she can change this view, she will grow into chronological, but not into psychological, maturity. She will feel inadequate to deal even with relatively simple life problems. She will feel too badly treated to *want* to deal with everyday affairs. Stan, on the other hand, is often hardly interested in dealing with reality at all. He does not distort it, as Claire does; rather, he creates a reality which suits him. What he creates for himself is not (cannot be) shared with others. Because he does not take cognizance of the real world, he will probably need to be hospitalized, protected from a world he cannot evaluate and hence cannot deal with accurately. George, of course, will also need protection, as would any "little deer" or "seep" need to be protected from marauding lions. But George is able to maintain close touch with real surroundings. While reality often frightens him, he nevertheless has a conviction that those closest to him are kind, do their best to protect him, and wish him well. George has probably the best chance of growing into a relatively satisfying, relatively independent adulthood. His impaired intellectual ability will, of course, set severe limits to his satisfactions. Nevertheless, given the situation with which he is burdened, the important people closest to him have been able to point him in a direction which will permit him to live a life from which, under present conditions, he can derive many realistic gratifications.

3

The Adolescent with Central
Neurological Impairment

The psychological test records of two adolescents with "organic"[1] brain dysfunction are presented and discussed in this chapter. Both Ken and Hal's diagnostic situations are somewhat unusual—Ken's, because the evidence of organic impairment, apparent on the psychological testing, does not appear on physical, neurological or laboratory examinations; Hal's, because the organic dysfunction, so obvious both in his clinical history and on the EEG recording, is not unequivocally apparent on psychological testing, even with hindsight.

In both cases, the "organic" aspects obviously constitute only a fraction of these youths' psychological picture. Actually, an organic dysfunction is not truly psychological in itself—"psychological" is, rather, the *reaction to* it. A person may exaggerate his organic disability, he may react to it realistically, he may deny it, he may project it, or he may use it in any other way which is consistent with his character organization. When the insult-producing trauma occurs relatively late in life (because of illness or accident), the resulting reactions tend to be integrated into existing and relatively set character structures. When, however, the insult occurs to an undeveloped character structure which is still flexible, the resulting disability tends to play a much more significant part in whatever form the final character takes. In both Ken's and Hal's cases it is difficult to say with any degree of sureness how much of their character is

---

[1] Throughout the chapter, patients of this sort will be variously referred to as "organic," "brain damaged," "organically impaired," "neurologically impaired," etc. Although these labels do not accurately describe the conditions to which they refer, they are commonly used and fairly well understood.

a *result of* organic damage and how much the symptoms of the organic damage have been modified and integrated into the pre-existing character structure.

As suggested in the last chapter, it is fallacious to make a sure distinction between "organic" and "functional," primarily because the accurate boundaries of each (if such exist) are not (yet? ever?) known. Distinctions of this type may be scientifically harmful because they assume categories which may not exist (at least, not in the way we have thought).

What is evident in the two cases to be discussed is that "organic" features constitute, at least from the psychological point of view, only one aspect of a complex configuration. Hal's seizures seem to be the result of "organic" (?) problems and are the obvious cause of severe difficulties in his everyday life. Although his psychological development is proceeding poorly, his parents say they would not have brought him for an examination had it not been for his "seizures." Yet the seizures may cause him less objective trouble than the persistent, pseudonaïve denial which leads him to ignore important aspects of his reality. The "organic" difficulty seems no more important than the emotional difficulties that emerge so clearly.

Ken's "organic" difficulties (i.e., graphomotor and conceptual) cannot be minimized, even though, objectively viewed, they seem to constitute a less severe impairment than Hal's seizures. A young man of Ken's general ability is at a major disadvantage, however, when he avoids abstract thought and simple writing because he cannot do either particularly well.

Ken's examinational material follows.

Clinical Summary: Ken

Ken is fourteen years old. He is brought for examination primarily because his parents are concerned about his poor scholastic record.

There was no definite time of onset of Ken's difficulty, but his parents have been increasingly aware of some sort of trouble during the last three years. Actually, Ken has had difficulty with school work from the very beginning, but last year his grades became significantly worse. Although Ken's parents originally placed chief emphasis on his school problems, they are also concerned about the poor relationships he makes with his playmates. They are worried about what they perceive as Ken's general unhappiness, e.g., his feeling he is the "goat" of his class. The parents describe Ken's school problems as his not doing work he dislikes and achieving much less than his "potential." His father characterizes his relationship with Ken as one in which the father uses much constraint and has great difficulty expressing tender feelings toward Ken. He finds Ken somewhat effeminate and infantile, and this makes the father disgusted with his son.

Ken's birth was unplanned. It was a physiologically normal birth, and Ken was a healthy baby who developed normally. When Ken was two, his father entered the service for two years and was away from home most of this time. This was a period in which the family experienced considerable moving around and other turmoil. Both parents feel they were too strict with Ken when he was young and that this has been harmful to him. Ken is still unable to discuss matters with his father. He is submissive toward him and never protests any paternal demands for obedience. Although Ken has always been at ease with adults, he has been much less so with other children and has never been able to defend himself against them very well.

In the first year at school, Ken did not learn to read at all, but since then he has been an avid reader. When he was about eight years old, his poor coordination and lack of ability to play ball were recognized by his parents. This lack of physical ability became a problem to Ken when he was ten, after the family moved. Since then Ken has developed a pattern of associating exclusively with younger children. He has consistently attempted to participate in sports, but he has never been successful and has often felt his schoolmates were making fun of him. At the present time, Ken has almost no friends. His mother is exceedingly concerned about his extreme sloppiness at home. She complains that he rarely does anything well and usually has to be told several times to do it before it gets done. In general, the parents' method of handling Ken's behavior has been to increase their pressure on him to achieve greater social and scholastic success.

Physical and Laboratory Findings: A general physical examination reveals no specific abnormality, although it is noted that Ken is small for his age and has not yet entered puberty. The neurological examination, x-rays, the EEG and routine laboratory work are all within normal limits.

The Psychologist's Description

Ken approaches psychological testing with great tension. He moves restlessly in his chair, and his shallow breathing is often interspersed with deep sighs. More than once he appears on the verge of tears. Frequently blocking causes him not to have immediately available the material he "knows." Although he occasionally teases, his aggressions tend to be self-directed. They take the form of self-depreciation (e.g., "That was certainly a stupid answer."). After he completes the Story Completion Test, he scoots off his chair, laughingly hides behind my desk, and declares he should be fifty miles away. He demonstrates surface acceptance of his parents' and teachers' evaluation of his learning problems—i.e., that he could do better if he "really" wanted to and if he would only study harder. By the end of the examination, however, he tends to think of his school difficulties less in terms of unwillingness to learn and more in terms of inability.

The Wechsler-Bellevue Scale[2]

Name:　Ken　　　　Age:　14-0

	RS	WTS	0 1 2 3 4 5 6 7 8 9 10 11 12 13 14 15 16 17 18 19 20
COMPR.	13-14	11-13	
INFOR.	13	10	
DIG.	14	13	
ARITH.	6-9	7-12	
SIMIL.	18	14	
VOCAB.	25	11	
P. A.	9	8	
P. C.	12	12	
B. D.	28	13	
O. A.	20	12	
D. S.	28	6	

TOT. VERB.　53-60

TOT. PERF.　51

TOT. SCALE　104-11

VERBAL I.Q.:　113-123　　LEVEL:　Bright Normal→Superior

PERFORMANCE I.Q.:　105　　LEVEL:　Average

TOTAL I.Q.:　109-115　　LEVEL:　Average→Bright Normal

2 Wechsler (1941).

[Probably the most remarkable feature of Ken's W-B Scattergram is the extent of his subtest scatter, as it reflects the waxing and waning, the peaks and troughs of his abilities. While his Verbal subscores average approximately 11, he ranges from a low of 7 on Arithmetic to a high of 14 on Similarities. On Arithmetic he achieves an *alternate* score of 12. The distance of five points (between what he achieves at present and what he might potentially achieve) suggests that Arithmetic is an area which may reveal aspects of Ken's difficulties. On the Performance subtests, he ranges between weighted scores of 6 on Digit Symbol and 13 on Block Design. This discrepancy suggests that Ken's difficulty is located primarily in the graphomotor area, rather than in areas involving verbal (high Similarity) or perceptual (high Block Design) conceptualization and organizing skills.]

INFORMATION

No.	Question	Response and Comments	Score
1.	*Who is the President of the United States?*	Eisenhower. ("And before that?") Truman. ("And before that?") Roosevelt. (He seems very tense.)	+
2.	*What is a thermometer?*	.. Uh .. uh .. an instrument by which you measure temperature in degrees. [He wishes to be highly precise.]	+
3.	*What does rubber come from?*	.. Uh .. uh .. it's .. it's .. uh .. it's from a tree. I can't think of the name of it now. [Tension continues to be marked.]	+
4.	*Where is London?*	In .. England .. in Britain. Great Britain.	+
5.	*How many pints make a quart?*	Two.	+
6.	*How many weeks are there in a year?*	Fifty-two.	+
7.	*What is the capital of Italy?*	Paris. ("Are you sure?") Yes, sir. [This inefficiency may be a temporary one, brought about by tension. The "sir" is difficult to evaluate at this time. It may reflect a wish to be, or at least to appear, subservient. It is astonishing how many male adolescents, particularly those in difficulty with the law, use the address of "sir." This mark of ostensible respect usually reflects no respect at all. Often it is merely the mark of having attended military school when the parents could no longer	−

No.	Question	Response and Comments	Score
		control their son at home. Often "sir" is the parody of a respect which mirrors an ill-concealed contempt.]	
8.	What is the capital of Japan?	Uh . . (he snaps his fingers.) I can't remember the name now. (He tries to concentrate and after a while whispers:) I don't know. [Tension brings on another temporary inefficiency. Ken is obviously ashamed of his intellectual lacunae and puts himself at the examiner's mercy.]	−
9.	How tall is the average American woman?	Five feet six inches.	+
10.	Who invented the airplane?	Uh . . the accepted inventors are Orville and Wilbur Wright. [Ken has recovered and again shows his readiness to comply with the examiner's wishes by offering more than the examiner asks for.]	+
11.	Where is Brazil?	South America.	+
12.	How far is it from Paris to New York?	Five thousand miles.	−
13.	What does the heart do?	Circulates the blood.	+
14.	Who wrote Hamlet?	Shakespeare.	+
15.	What is the population of the United States?	Sixty-four million.	−
16.	When is Washington's birthday?	February 21. [This missing of an answer by one digit turns out to be characteristic of Ken. One wonders whether it reflects his need to fail, as an afterthought, and by only a hair. Thus, he fails, but not "really."]	−
17.	Who discovered the North Pole?	I don't know. ("Does any name come to mind?") No.	−
18.	Where is Egypt?	In . . uh . . Africa . . the continent of Africa. [Again, he gives just a little more than is required.]	+
19.	Who wrote Huckleberry Finn?	Uh . . (He snaps his fingers) oh . . I know . . . . (He concentrates.) I can't think of his name right now. Maybe I'll think of it later . . . . . . Mark	+

No.	Question	Response and Comments	Score
		Twain!!! [Is Ken's difficulty with not having information easily available the result of psychic tension or of "organic" interference? Or might some organic condition potentiate tension which already interferes with the availability of information?]	
20.	What is the Vatican?	The what? ("The Vatican.") I don't know.	—
21.	What is the Koran?	I don't know that either.	—
22.	Who wrote Faust?	I don't know. [He appears to have little conflict about admitting lack of knowledge.]	—
23.	What is an Habeas Corpus?	It seems like I heard that someplace, but I can't think. I don't know. ["I can't think" may be an excuse, but it may also be an accurate description of Ken's defective thought processes.]	—

RAW SCORE: 13

WEIGHTED SCORE: 10

COMPREHENSION

No.	Question	Response and Comments	Score
1.	What is the thing to do if you find an envelope in the street, that is sealed, and addressed and has a new stamp?	(He repeats my question.) I believe I'd put it in the mail.	2
2.	What should you do if while sitting in the movies you were the first person to discover a fire (or see smoke and fire)?	Ring the fire alarm.	1
3.	Why should we keep away from bad company?	You get mixed up in the wrong group, and you get in trouble.	1
4.	Why should people pay taxes?	To keep the government going.	2
5.	Why are shoes made of leather?	Cause it stands up well against the weather . . it's good protection against it.	1

No.	Question	Response and Comments	Score
6.	Why does land in the city cost more than land in the country?	Cause in the city, it's scarce. It's harder to get. And you can get more for it. ("How do you mean?") Because of the scarcity: the scarcer it is, the more people are willing to pay to get it. [Although, on first glance, Ken seems to have gotten this answer entirely correct, closer examination reveals the answer is just off the mark. Actually he should get a score of approximately 1½. This characteristic of being "just a little off" is typical of Ken and reflects how his thinking is occasionally just a hair away from being altogether well organized.]	1
7.	If you were lost in a forest (woods) in the daytime, how would you go about finding your way out?	I could look at the sun and find the direction. If I knew what direction I'd come in from. ("How would you tell by the sun?") It appears to rise in the east and set in the west. [His wish to be the obedient, good pupil is evident in the "appears to."]	2
8.	Why are laws necessary?	To keep people from running all over other people. If there weren't laws, people would do just what they wanted to, and it'd be a heck of a world. Nobody'd be safe. [Ken is obviously concerned about the containment of others' aggressions.]	1
9.	Why does the state require people to get a license in order to be married?	I suppose so they know how many married people they have. And it furnishes an income for the government. ("Which answer would you choose?") Uh . . . . for income. [Ken is not able to choose the most relevant in the answers he offers. Is this another example of his "almost-but-not-quite" tendency?]	0-2
10.	Why are people who are born deaf usually unable to talk?	Well, because they never heard anybody talk, and they don't know what it is to talk. A baby hears other people talk and tries to imitate them, but a deaf person can't hear other people talk and can't imitate them. [This is an excellently organized response.]	2

RAW SCORE: 13-15

WEIGHTED SCORE: 11-13

DIGIT SPAN

(Ken correctly repeats eight Digits Forward. When he attempts to repeat nine Digits Forward, he makes three errors. Each error involves repeating a number *one step higher* or *one step lower* than the one given by the examiner. Thus, instead of repeating 275862584, he repeats 276852484.) [Just as one feels more

may be involved than a wild guess when Ken says that Washington's birthday falls on February 21, so one feels something is oddly determined about Ken's failure on Digit Span. He is repeating a much more complexly put together number than the one originally read him. This is not "failure" in the usual sense.]
(He repeats six Digits Backward correctly.)

RAW SCORE:　　14

WEIGHTED SCORE:　　13

ARITHMETIC

No.	Problem	Time	Response and Comments	Score
1.	How much is four dollars and five dollars?	½″	Nine.	1
2.	If a man buys six cents worth of stamps and gives the clerk ten cents, how much change should he get back?	½″	Four.	1
3.	If a man buys eight cents worth of stamps and gives the clerk twenty-five cents, how much change should he get back?	½″	Seventeen . . No! (6″) ("Do you remember the question?") Oh . . eight from twenty-five . . oh no, sixteen! [The phenomenon of Ken's missing an answer by one digit occurs again. This time, however, he "corrects" his answer after he first gives one which is actually right. It seems obvious that Ken needs to change the correct into the just barely incorrect, but it is likely that both his reasons and his techniques for satisfying them are unconscious.]	0-1
4.	How many oranges can you buy for thirty-six cents if one orange costs four cents?	10″	Nine.	1
5.	How many hours will it take a man to walk twenty-four miles at the rate of three miles an hour?	2″	Eight.	1
6.	If a man buys seven two cent	13″	Eighty-six cents. ("How did you do that?") I subtracted fourteen from one-hundred.	0-1

145

No.	Problem	Time	Response and Comments	Score
	stamps and gives the clerk a half dollar, how much change should he get back?		("But I said a half dollar.") Oh! I thought you said a dollar! It would be thirty-six cents. [Is this another temporary disruption created by anxiety or another example of Ken's need to fail, this time by "mishearing"?]	
7.	If seven pounds of sugar cost twenty-five cents, how many pounds can you get for a dollar?	—	Twenty-nine . . No! Twenty-nine . . No! . . yeah! . . Twenty-nine pounds. (After the last Arithmetic problem, I administer this question again, and he correctly answers: "Twenty-eight!") [Once again he misses the correct response by one.]	0
8.	A man bought a second-hand car for two-thirds of what it cost new. He paid $400 for it. How much did it cost new?	1″	Six-hundred. [But Ken is capable of remarkable efficiency.]	1
9.	If a train goes 150 yards in ten seconds, how many feet can it go in one fifth of a second?	—	Eight feet in one-fifth second. (44″) That's going pretty fast. (He gives a tense sigh.) (I ask him to explain how he did the problem, and he explains it correctly. Then, suddenly, he says:) No! That'd be nine feet! [He does it again.]	0-1
10.	Eight men can finish a job in six days. How many men will be needed to finish it in a half day?	42″	One hundred ninety-six. (33″) No. That'd be just plain ninety-six! [He makes another slight mistake, but this time corrects himself spontaneously. The spontaneous self-correction suggests that his drive toward making the tiny—but significant—mistakes is unconsciously powered.]	1

RAW SCORE: 6-9

WEIGHTED SCORE: 7-12

SIMILARITIES

No.	Items	Response and Comments	Score
1.	Orange-banana	Both fruit.	2
2.	Coat-dress	Both clothing.	2
3.	Dog-lion	Both animals.	2
4.	Wagon-bicycle	Both vehicles. They're both on wheels. ("Which would you choose?") Vehicles.	2

No. Items	Response and Comments	Score
5. Daily paper-radio	Both give news.	1
6. Air-water	Both are made up of gases. ("How do you mean?") Oh, like oxygen, hydrogen, carbon dioxide.	1
7. Wood-alcohol	I don't know. ("Can you think of any way?") I think they both come out of trees. I don't know.	0
8. Eye-ear	They're members of the human body . . or any body. [This is a peculiar verbalization. What Ken says is true, but he puts it oddly.]	1
9. Egg-seed	Both reproduce what they come from.	2
10. Poem-statue	A what? (I repeat.) Both are works of art. Both are sometimes in memory of some event or some person. ("Which answer would you choose?") I choose . . they're both art. [This is the second time he is able to make the "best" choice after he states several unequally "good" alternatives. Although his judgment is occasionally impaired by fuzzy thinking, he is often able to rescue himself and avoids becoming lost in an obsessively determined morass of possibilities.]	2
11. Praise-punish-ment	I know, but I can't think of a way to explain it. ("Try the best you can.") They're both meant to help, but that's not a very good explanation. I can't think of any better explanation right now.	1
12. Fly-tree	Both live . . they're both living. [Ken can express excellently organized and clearly formulated verbal conceptualizations. He can function efficiently and logically. This ability to conceptualize abstractly may well be the keystone to well-functioning verbal intelligence. To the extent that this ability is unimpaired, Ken's thought functioning may be considered relatively sound.]	2

RAW SCORE: 18

WEIGHTED SCORE: 14

PICTURE COMPLETION

(Ken correctly finds what is missing on the first eleven items. He misses the next three, but completes No. 15 correctly. On the girl with the missing eyebrow, he says, "Her ear, I guess (18″), although it looks like it would be covered by her hair.") [This response reflects Ken's capacity to correct initially deficient judgment.]

RAW SCORE: 12

WEIGHTED SCORE: 12

PICTURE ARRANGEMENT

No.	Item	Correct Order	Time	Arranged Order	Story and Comments	Score
1.	House	PAT	2″	PAT		2
2.	Holdup	ABCD	7″	ABCD		2
3.	Elevator	LMNO	6″	LMNO		2
4.	Flirt	JANET	25″	JANET	Well, the way I figure it, the King was driving along in his black car. He sees this pretty gal. He tells them to stop and gets out. The next thing you know, this gal has him carrying this load. [Ken distorts the story so that the Little King is no longer the gallant. Instead, he is exploited by the woman. To what extent does Ken generally see women as exploitative?]	3
5.	Taxi	SAMUEL	35″	AMLEUS	Well, this guy got a dummy and hailed a taxi. And he got in there. And the dummy fell down on top of him and made it look like he was smooching around with his girl. So he looked back kind of embarrassed. He didn't want anybody to think that's what was happening. He sets the dummy back, and then it happens again. He gets disgusted and gets out and walks. [Ken's stories to the Flirt and Taxi sequences emphasize his tendency to see women as troublesome and overwhelming.]	0
6.	Fish	EFGHIJ	23″	GFEHIJ	Well, this King, he was fishing. He gets a fair-size fish and pulls it up. And then he puts in his line again and pulls in a bigger size fish. Then he decides it's time to go home, and he yells down, and as it turns out, one of his knights comes up. It must be the knight was down there and putting the fish on his hook. [Ken misinterprets a diving suit as a	0

		Correct		Arranged		
No.	Item	Order	Time	Order	Story and Comments	Score
					knight's armor. Although his story is otherwise without error, his sorting is carelessly done. Or could this be another example of Ken's need to fail by a hair?]	

RAW SCORE:	9
WEIGHTED SCORE:	8

BLOCK DESIGN

(He is very tense. His breathing is shallow.)

No.	Time	Accur.	Description of Behavior and Comments	Score
A.	7″	Yes	(He starts by using only one hand; then he uses both.)	
B.	98″	Yes	(He shows much trial-and-error behavior. He makes a wrong solution, then puts his hand on his hips, with a self-depreciatory sigh.) Jiminy Christmas! (He makes another wrong attempt, which is followed by insight.) It took me long enough to figure that one out. [Ken manifests a significant lapse in smooth efficiency. He is at a loss as he seeks to understand what steps he must take to solve this problem, and it takes a long time before he can extricate himself from his cognitive dead end. Later on, he can solve much more complicated designs correctly. Is Ken's dilemma a reflection of energic waxing and waning, of fading in and out, which often characterizes the performance of the "brain-damaged" person?]	
1.	14″	Yes	(He studies the problem momentarily before tackling it. The length of time he requires for its solution results from motoric fumbling, not from any conceptualization difficulties.)	4
2.	13″	Yes	(Again, he begins by using only one hand.) [Persons taking these tests often wish to demonstrate their apparent casualness in an effort to deny some difficulty or discomfort.]	4
3.	10″	Yes	(He first analyzes and then solves the problem quickly.) [The times required for the successful solutions of the Block Designs	5

No.	Time	Accur.	Description of Behavior and Comments	Score
			have steadily decreased. As Ken feels more at home with the task, his tension apparently lets up and his efficiency becomes greater.]	
4.	25″	Yes	(He makes an excellent analysis of the problem and manifests no trial-and-error behavior in its almost immediate solution.) It had me stumped there for a second. (He smiles.)	4
5.	48″ 67″	Yes	(He is systematic and solves the problem without trial and error. After he is finished:) That took me a long time. (One block is rotated. He notices and corrects his error.) Oh, oh . . I've made a goof!	3
6.	61″	Yes	(He quickly sees how to make the stripes and proceeds systematically, without trial and error. His last block is rotated, but he notices his error and corrects it immediately.)	4
7.	120″	Yes	(He whispers:) Oh, oh, goodness gracious! (He makes an immediate and excellent analysis. He proceeds in an orderly, systematic fashion, and immediately corrects the very few errors he makes. He completes the design without difficulty.) [Just as with verbal concept formation, Ken's perceptual ability to analyze and organize is almost flawless. His better-than-average performance here suggests his essentially sound formal thinking ability. The comment, "Oh, goodness gracious," is rather prissy.]	4

RAW SCORE: 28

WEIGHTED SCORE: 13

OBJECT ASSEMBLY

Item	Time	Accur.	Description of Behavior and Comments	Score
Manikin	23″	Yes	(He is very tense.)	6
Profile	46″	Yes	(Considerable trial and error with the nose and mouth pieces.)	7
Hand	49″	Yes	(He looks puzzled, but after he fits the thumb through trial and error, he has insight.) It took me a while, but I finally figured out what I was making. [Although Ken experiences mild puzzlement through-	7

Item	Time	Accur.	Description of Behavior and Comments	Score
			out this subtest, he proceeds in an essentially planful and coordinated fashion. He does better than average; almost as well as he does on Block Design.]	

RAW SCORE: 20

WEIGHTED SCORE: 12

DIGIT SYMBOL

(Ken is very tense during this subtest. He is never able to develop a rhythm while writing the symbols. Instead, he proceeds arhythmically, now going quickly, now slowly, now losing his place, now suddenly finding his pencil to go in an undesired direction. His symbol drawings reflect the shakiness of his graphomotor control: while his copies are never really wrong, they are blemished by little hooks and wiggles which mark Ken's lack of mastery over his pencil.) [Ken's performance on this test is the first relatively strong sign that he may be suffering from some sort of neurological impairment. It is doubtful that the sudden performance drop is the result primarily of tension or other "functional" factors. Although tension would slow Ken down, it is unlikely that it would slow him to this degree or result in the qualitative distortions which are revealed in this performance.]

RAW SCORE: 28

WEIGHTED SCORE: 6

VOCABULARY

No.	Word	Response and Comments	Score
1.	Apple	A fruit.	1
2.	Donkey	An animal. Is that enough? Do you want me to give some more? ("If you like.") An animal of the horse family. [Evident again is Ken's drive for precision.]	1
3.	Join	What? ("Join.") Connect or meet.	1
4.	Diamond	A rare stone. Very hard.	1
5.	Nuisance	A bother.	1
6.	Fur	Uh . . uh . . hair of an animal.	1
7.	Cushion	Uh . . . . Something soft . . it usually has feathers or foam rubber in it, some material like that.	1
8.	Shilling	Uh . . uh . . coin. A foreign coin.	1
9.	Gamble	Uh . . . . . . hmm . . . . to bet?	1
10.	Bacon	Uh . . a food . . pork.	1
11.	Nail	Uh . . uh . . a piece of steel used to pound in wood, and to hold two pieces together.	1

No.	Word	Response and Comments	Score
12.	Cedar	A tree . . or . . or the wood of which can be fixed so that it's rather expensive. [This definition is formulated in a mildly peculiar fashion. Until now, Ken's definitions have been very much to the point.]	1
13.	Tint	Uh . . I know what it is, but I can't think of how to say it. ("Try to explain it.") You usually use it for . . when you are referring to color. Certain tint of color. That's the best I can think of.	1
14.	Armory	Uh . . a place where arms are kept. I mean, not arms like your arms, but weapons . . and that's the best I can think of right now. [This is another mildly peculiar thought—that the examiner might be confused between the two kinds of "arms."]	1
15.	Fable	A story which is to teach a person a lesson.	1
16.	Brim	The top of something like a cup or a bucket.	½
17.	Guillotine	Uh . . guillotine . . An ancient machine . . not ancient, but a machine that was used for cutting off people's heads.	1
18.	Plural	More than one.	1
19.	Seclude	Kind of hidden away.	1
20.	Nitroglycerine	Uh . . an explosive . . highly explosive material . . liquid.	1
21.	Stanza	Uh . . a verse in a song or poem. [Ken's definitions are again efficiently and parsimoniously worded.]	1
22.	Microscope	. . Uh . . uh . . an instrument used for observing very small particles, such as germs, or viruses. That takes a pretty powerful one.	1
23.	Vesper	I can't think of it.	0
24.	Belfry	Uh . . that's the top tower that bells are kept in, such as church bells.	1
25.	Recede	Uh . . . . . To draw back.	1
26.	Affliction	. . . . Hm . . I know what it is, but I can't think of it. Usually a disease . . physical . . or a hurt.	½
27.	Pewter	Uh . . sort of a dish used for grinding up chemicals.	0
28.	Ballast	I don't know.	0
29.	Catacomb	I don't know.	0
30.	Spangle	I don't know.	0
31.	Espionage	I don't know.	0
32.	Imminent	I don't know.	0

No. Word	Response and Comments	Score
33. *Mantis*	I believe that's kind of an insect.	1

(He is unable to define the remaining words.)

RAW SCORE: 25

WEIGHTED SCORE: 11

STORY RECALL[3]

IMMEDIATE RECALL

+1   +1   +1   −1
December 6. / A small river / overflowed, / and Albany was flooded. Water
        +1   +1   0   +1   0
ran into the streets / and into the houses. Sixteen persons / drowned / and 200
    +1   +1   +1   +1   +1
/ caught cold / because of the dampness / and cold weather. In saving / a boy
        +1   +1   +1
/ caught under a bridge, / a man / cut his hand.

SCORE: 14−1(+4) = 17

DELAYED RECALL

+1   +1   +1   −1
December 6th. / A small river / flooded, / and flooded . . let's see . . Albany. /
    +1   +1   +1   +1
Water ran into the street / and into the houses. / Fourteen persons / drowned /
    +1   +1   +1   +1   +1
and 600 / caught cold / because of the dampness / and cold weather. In saving / a
+1   +1   +1   +1
boy, one man . . / in saving a boy trapped under a bridge, / one man /cut his hand.

SCORE: 16−1 =15

[Of a possible twenty-one memories, Ken retains a decent number. Although
he repeats a mild memory distortion on Delayed Recall, this distortion is insufficient to make one believe that a significant memory impairment exists.]

THE BRL SORTING TEST[4]

PART I

Stimulus	Patient's Sorting	Response and Comments	Score
1. Ken's choice: *Square block of wood with nail in it.*	(Sighs deeply and tensely. Adds: nails; toy hammer; and toy saw.)	The two nails go in here because there is a nail in the block, and the hammer goes because you have to saw a block of wood. Would you want me to put all the rest of the tools because they	Concrete Def.

3 Adapted from Babcock (1930). For administration, scoring and interpretation, see
Rapaport et al. (1945-1946, Vol. I).
4 See Rapaport et al. (1945-1946, Vol. I) for description of this test, for methods of
administration and scoring, and for a discussion of its rationale.

Stimulus	Patient's Sorting	Response and Comments	Score
		are related to the hammer and saw? [Ken's extremely concrete performance is in marked contrast to his good Similarities performance on the Wechsler. The discrepancy of performance underlines the distinction between abilities required for (a) relatively passive verbal concept formation, as on the Similarities subtest, and (b) more active and creative ones, involving a number of concrete items, as on the BRL Sorting Test. On the BRL, the person being examined cannot rely on automatic verbal clichés. Particularly on Part I, where he is required to construct concepts, he is faced with a situation which requires a much more complex response than simply binding together with a verbal category. The BRL Sorting Test is an extremely sensitive instrument for the detection of even slight impairments in the capacity to form concepts. The sudden worsening of Ken's abstraction ability adds to the initial concern about the presence of some sort of brain damage. While the initial item he chooses is a difficult one to form into a concept, the inspection of Ken's further Sorting Test responses will clarify the degree to which a conceptualizing problem can be blamed primarily on the test item and the degree to which it can be seen to lie within Ken.]	
2. Examiner's choice:[5] Fork	(Knife; spoon; toy knife, fork and spoon; corks; sink stopper.)	Well, they're all ordinarily found in a kitchen. [Although Ken originally sorts what he might develop into the abstract concept "silverware," he again	Concrete Def. Syncretistic Def.

[5] This and subsequent stimulus objects on Part I are presented by the examiner. The patient chooses the stimulus object only for the first item on Part I.

Stimulus	Patient's Sorting	Response and Comments	Score
		becomes concrete, explaining the items belong together because they are found in the same place.]	
3. Corncob pipe	(Cigarette.) I don't know whether to put that (rubber cigar) out or not. It's not real; it's a rubber cigar. (rubber cigar; cigar; matches.)	I put the cigarette and the real cigar out there because you smoke them and you smoke the pipe too. I put the matches out there because you need to light it.	Functional Def. Concrete Def.
4. Bicycle bell	(Rubber cigar; ball; eraser; toy hammer and pliers; toy knife, fork and spoon; paper circle; cardboard square.) Could you tell me what that's (cardboard square) supposed to be? ("Whatever it seems like to you.") Chalk. (He wonders whether to add the pipe. Finally he adds it to the other items.)	Well, cause they're all things that a kid might be playing with . . toys. At least, I don't think that corncob pipe is genuine. (He laughs.)	Loose Functional Def.
5. Red paper circle	(Cardboard square; matches; cigarette; cigar; rubber cigar.)	All are either made of paper or have paper on them.	Loose Conceptual Def. Split-Narrow Tendency
6. Toy pliers	(Toy screwdriver; toy hammer; large tools; ball; toy knife, fork and spoon. He is very tense.)	Because they're all toys or real tools. [This is a pathognomonic Chain Response. Ken begins with the concept "toy tools," which he modifies to include all tools. He adds a ball to go with the toy pliers as another "toy,"	Chain Response

Stimulus	Patient's Sorting	Response and Comments	Score
		then he adds the toy silverware. In other words, his concept changes midstream, without his reorganizing the sorting. A Chain Response usually suggests the presence of fairly severe pathology, particularly when the response is given by someone who can achieve a WISC Verbal Score in the Bright Normal to Superior range and whose highest Verbal subtest score is on Similarities.]	
7. *Rubber ball*	(Toy hammer; rubber cigar; toy saw; toy screwdriver; red paper circle; cardboard square; toy silverware; chalk; sink stopper; eraser . . . . . pliers; screwdriver.) This is pretty preposterous, but . . . . (He adds the bell.)	Because . . uh . . they're all toys or rubber, except for the real pliers and screwdriver. I put them in becaue they're related to the toy pliers and screwdriver, and so forth. [This is an even more obvious Chain Response than his preceding one.]	Chain Response

PART II

Examiner's Sorting	Explanation and Comments	Score
1. Red objects	Hm . . Cause they're all red.	Conceptual Def.
2. Metal	They're all made of metal. [Ken is able to give two flawless conceptual definitions in a row. When he is asked to supply the concept for a sorting which has already been made, he is easily able to do so. Although he does not do equally well throughout Part II, he is much more successful here than on Part I. The frequently observed difference between the ability to conceptualize on Part I and Part II, in favor of the latter, reflects how much easier it is to sort "passively." When the person must supply only the name of the concept,	Conceptual Def.

Examiner's Sorting	Explanation and Comments	Score
	after its content has been established, the work required is much less complex than when (as on Part I) he is asked both to create a sorting and designate its name. Because Part II solutions require so much less conceptual effort than those of Part I, pathological forms of thought tend to be in evidence more frequently on Part I than on Part II.]	
3. *Round*	(He gulps somewhat histrionically and investigates the items closely.) I can think of several reasons. These three are red. These three all . . are products of a tree. And these two are toys. (He uses some items more than once.) ("How are they all alike?") . . . . Well, cause they are all found around the house.	Split-Narrow Tendency Syncretistic
4. *Tools*	They're all tools.	Conceptual Def.
5. *Paper*	They're either made of paper or have paper on them.	Conceptual Def. Split-Narrow Tendency
6. *Double*	Because in every pair there's a big one and a little one. Oh! No! (He gives an anxious sigh.) Either there's a big one and a little one, or they're alike.	Failure
7. *White*	They're all white.	Conceptual Def.
8. *Rubber*	They're all made of rubber.	Conceptual Def.
9. *Smoking*	They're all something you either use to smoke or you *act* like you're smoking	Conceptual Def. Split-Narrow Tendency
10. *Silverware*	They're all either kitchen utensils . . or playlike, pretend.	Conceptual Def. Split-Narrow
11. *Toys*	They're all toys.	Conceptual Def.
12. *Square*	. . . . They're all completely . . they come completely . . they come completely from plants . . or else, mostly . . . I imagine that last one was a very stupid one. [Note Ken's sporadic ability to be aware of an inadequate response. He has the important capacity to be self-critical on occasion. Throughout Part II, he vacillates between excellent and poor responses.]	Syncretistic Split-Narrow Tendency

The Story Completion Test[6]

(In connection with this test [see Plate 14] Ken says that his most difficult school subject is writing: "My writing seems to wobble all over." He says his writing never comes out "just right," just as in the sample.

STORY COMPLETION TEST 1

Continue the following story. Describe the situation. Tell what happens, and how it turns out.

He was very angry, and was getting angrier by the minute. *The reason was*

[handwritten] (Tom) had just found out some other boys had his dog and were using it as a sling shot target. So he ran to the place were they had him. He crawled in the bushes and his dog saw him the boys had their backs so he ran up behind all three of them and cracked their heads together this stunned them while he let his dog loose. when their parents found out He keep get a good spanking

[handwritten] Most difficult subject in school is writing. "Seems to wobble all over." Never comes out just right. Same as above.

[handwritten] While I read this story, hides in corner in mock shame. Says he wished he were so miles away while I'm reading it.

PLATE 14

(While I read his story silently to myself, Ken hides in mock shame, in a corner of the office. He says he wishes he were fifty miles away.)

[6] This test was created by W. Kass while he was a staff psychologist in the Children's Service of the Menninger Foundation.

[Although Ken's spelling is only moderately inaccurate, his writing shows the same irregularities, changes in pressure and slovenliness as his Bender drawings. Much more seems to be involved than merely "bad" handwriting. He makes numerous corrections and takes his pencil over letters he has made in order to improve their legibility. The "1" in the word "crawled," in the fourth line of Ken's story, again suggests interference with smooth motor functioning.

[The content of Ken's story is also significant. In the story, Ken is the "outsider," who is unfairly treated and taken advantage of. His age mates, who should be his companions, exploit him. Ken needs to enlist the help of adults to gain proper revenge on his peers. The hero, cracking the boys' heads together and stunning them, reflects Ken's anger with boys his age, as well as his unrealistic fantasies of revenge.]

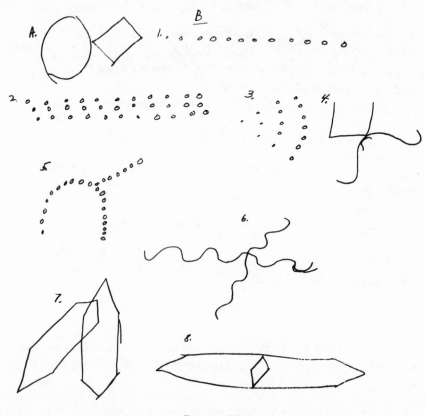

PLATE 15

The Bender Gestalt Test

PART A (PLATE 15, p. 158)

(As he begins to draw Figure A, he says, "I hope these figures don't have to be perfect." He counts portions of the designs and occasionally makes false beginnings, so that he needs to erase. Throughout, he seems tense. On occasion, he sighs deeply.)

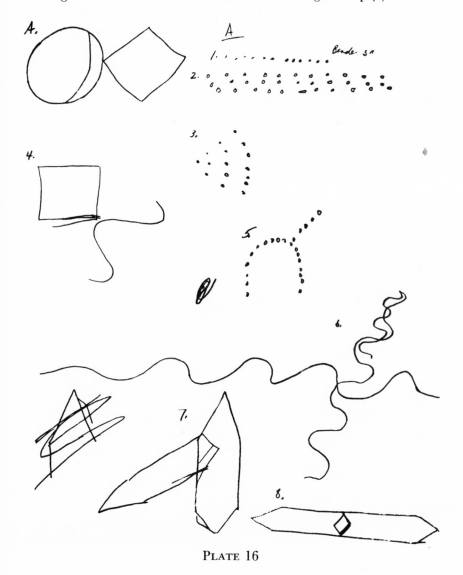

PLATE 16

PART B (PLATE 16, p. 159)

(He frequently counts the dots and tends to outline each design with his finger before he copies it. Again, he exhibits such symptoms of tension as sighing, stomach growling, embarrassed smiling. After he completes Design 4, he says, "It's not very good.") [There is definite improvement as Ken goes from Part A to Part B. Even in Part A, however, he never loses the gestalt of the designs. His problem seems to involve primarily motor execution, rather than gestalt perception. His Part A drawings reflect obvious interferences with smooth motor functioning. The lines are shakily executed, and Ken has a significant problem with directionality. Particularly striking is the problem he experiences as he attempts to re-create the vertical wavy line of Design 6. This line frequently presents difficulty for persons with organic dysfunction of some sort. Notable also is the way Ken's dots tend sporadically to become circles, as well as the way they tend to be irregularly spaced and to vary in size as well as in the pressure used in their execution.

[Ken's performance on Part B is much improved. He is neater and does not need to make so many corrections. Nevertheless, he manifests some of the same problems he shows on Part A. Still, he is able to use information he has gained while doing Part A, and he applies it as he draws Part B. He knows much better, for example, how to organize his page; he does so neatly and well. He demonstrates, in this way, his ability to learn from experience and to apply this learning to future similar experiences.

[It is inescapable by now that something is awry with Ken's motoric, particularly his graphomotor, functioning.]

[With his Rorschach performance, the extent of Ken's emotional disturbance becomes evident. A glance at the Psychogram reveals a number of noteworthy tendencies: Ken has thirty-six responses, a number considerably higher than the average usually given by fourteen-year-olds. Such a relatively greater number may reflect productivity either in the positive, creative, or in the negative, pressured sense. Although the high number of responses may suggest an obsessive thought organization, the location areas do not reflect a concern with arbitrarily delimited and tiny areas. In fact, Ken offers only three Dr responses. Of particular interest is the high percentage of Space responses, demonstrating Ken's need to reverse the usual order, to make figures of what should be ground. A tend-

RORSCHACH TEST

RORSCHACH SCORING SHEET

Number of Responses: 36

Manner of Approach (Location)

W	11
WS	5
D	15
DS	1
Dr	2
Do	1
Drs	1
De	0
Dd	0
Total	36

Location Percentages

W%	44
D%	44
Dr%	6
De%	0
S%	19

Groups of Contents

A	19
Ad	3
H	4
Hd	1
Ghost	1
Obj.	3
At.	0
Ats.	2
Pl.	1
Geol.	2
Total	36

Determinant and Content Percentages

F%	75/94	P%	17
F+%	56/56	At%	6
A%	61	H%	17
Obj.%	8		

Form, Movement, Color and Shading Determinants

F+	11			
F—	8			
F±	4			
F∓	4			
M+	2	M±	1	
FM+	1			
FC	0			
CF	2			
C	0			
F(C)—	1	FC(C)∓	1	
FC′∓	1			
Total	36			

Qualitative Material

Popular	I (IV) V VIII X(2)
Combination	IV VIII IX
Fabulation	8
Confabulation	1
Fabulized Combination	III, V, IX
Masturbatory	5
Castration	10
Autistic	1
Symbolic	1
Aggressive	8
Arbitrary	5
Position	1
Queer	3
Peculiar	1
Confusion	1

EXPERIENCE BALANCE: _3.5/2.5_

ency to set himself in opposition will be apparent in the detailed examination of his protocol; Ken automatically turns each card around the moment he receives it. He needs to put his own stamp on each situation and is reluctant to leave unmodified whatever others may present him with. Highly significant, too, is his poor handling of Rorschach color. He does not incorporate color at all well into his responses. For example, he does not give a single totally satis-factory FC response. Only a little over half his many responses have a form quality which reflects a fairly realistic manner of perceiving. Also particularly striking is the fact that, in ten of his thirty-six responses, Ken makes explicit that "something" is missing. The "Castration" notation given to such responses must not be under-stood too concretely. While the notation may not mean "castration" in its most literal sense, it does reflect Ken's concern with not being whole, with being inadequate, and with being in some ways wanting. Similarly, responses scored "Mast." do not necessarily refer literally to masturbatory conflict, but to Ken's concern with the damaged, the shoddy, the tawdry, the fragmented. Ken sees the world as un-wholesome. His responses reflect an arbitrariness of judgment, a peculiarity of conceptualization and a confusion of interpreting what is going on around him.]

RORSCHACH PROTOCOL

Card #	React. Time	Score	Protocol	Inquiry and Observations
I			May I turn it upside down or something? ∨ ∧	
	34″	WSF∓H Fab. Mast.	1. It looks like a woman with a fancy dress on.	1. ("Tell me about the woman you saw.") Well . . . . the woman was right in the middle and the dress had the holes in it. ("What made it look fancy?") It seemed to be kind of standing out. (The middle section is the woman, and both side D's are the dress.) [Ken has already told us a good deal with this first response. He requires a fairly long time (34″) to organize it. While his initial tendency is to oppose by immediately turning the card around, he can see his first response only after he again turns it in the original direction. He seems to say he must first make a thing his own and reject even normal passivity. Right away, too, he indicates that what may look "fancy" on the sur-

React.			
Card # *Time*	*Score*	*Protocol*	*Inquiry and Observations*

			face actually has holes in it and is, therefore, basically and possibly profoundly, inadequate.]
	WSF+ AP Mast.	2. Or a bat with a bunch of holes in its wings. >	[Again the tattered and torn, with the concomitant emphasis on what should be "ground."]
	WSF−A Fab. Cast. Mast.	3. Or a goose *without a head,* maybe. That takes quite a bit of imagination, though.	3. ("How about the goose?") Right in the middle with its wings . . well, kind of battered. Its wings are all torn up. ("What made it look like a goose?") Well, I don't know. It just all of a sudden seemed to look like it a little bit. [Important here is not only that the goose is headless, but that Ken arbitrarily makes a goose out of an area which to most people looks nothing like a goose. He says, "It just all of a sudden seemed to look like it a little bit," a weak explanation at best. He does not try to demonstrate that portions of the blot have "gooselike" qualities; instead, the area is a goose because it "just all of a sudden seemed to look like it." A better example of the lack of a need to justify an interpretation of reality would be hard to find.]
II		∨ ∧ ∨ > (He sighs deeply and keeps looking at the card in this position.) . . . . ∧ (He grimaces.) ∨	
	60″	WF−A Confab. Aut. Symb. Cast. Agg. Arb.	1. Two goats without a head . . standing on their hind legs. > ∨ (He grimaces.) ∨	1. ("What made it look like goats?") Well, what did I say about goats? (I remind him.) Well, I tell you, at first . . at first, when I saw them . . that splotch at the top made it look like sort of an impact. And

Card #	React. Time	Score	Protocol	Inquiry and Observations

whenever I see an impact like that I think of a goat. And I just happened to think of a goat. [Ken continues to show the arbitrariness with which he responded to Card I; whenever he sees an "impact like that" he thinks of a goat. In this way, Ken shows himself unconstrained by reality and highhanded with objectivity.]

WM±H
Cast.
Agg.

2. Or two people without heads, hitting like that, with their hands straight out. (He demonstrates.) That's all I can see. (He sighs deeply.)

2. ("What kind of people?") Oh, no special kind. Just people. ("Would you describe them?") Well, they were kind of heavy-built. Not skinny, but not real fat . . and . . uh . . they had short legs . . and that's about all. Their legs are kind of out of proportion. [Once more, in addition to headlessness, things are not quite right and out of proportion.]

III

21″
Fab. Comb.

WM+H
Fab.
Agg.
Po.
DF±A

Eek! (He smiles.)

1. Two skeletons pulling something apart . . some small animal . . . .

2. Two skinny people clowning around with a couple of socks. Monkeys are about to fall on 'em. (He holds the card in the air.)

1. and 2. ("What made them look like skeletons?") They were so thin. ("Were the skeletons and the skinny people the same thing?") Well . . . . . no, not really. ("How about the socks?") They just had shapes like socks. [The "skeletons" and "skinny people" seem enough alike in Ken's perception to warrant a single score. Although he laughs when he says "Eek!" the blot nevertheless seems to upset him. He does not attempt to justify the monkeys' falling on the people in that he makes no effort to make sense out of a percept which is determined primarily by the position of its elements.]

Card #	React. Time	Score	Protocol	Inquiry and Observations
		WM+H Agg.?	3. Two people kicking. ∨ ∧ <	3. ("What kind of people are they?") I don't know. They look kind of like Negroes. Their heads remind me of it, I believe. [Responses 1 & 2, on the one hand, and 3, on the other, although similar, are nevertheless different enough to warrant separate scores.]
IV	13″	WFC′≠A Fab. Agg.	1. Well, it looks kind of like a black panther jumping. (He holds the card at eye level and studies it.) ∨ ∧	1. ("Tell me about the panther jumping.") It looks like kinda he's coming down on top of you. (The head of the panther is the top Dr.)
		Comb. ⎰ DF+Obj. (P) ⎱ DoF+Ad	2. & 3. Or two large boots . . with an animal skin in the background. ∨ ∧ > ∧	2. and 3. ("What kind of an animal skin?") Hmm . . fox . . or something. ("What made it look like a fox?") Well . . . . . it had little kind of limbs protruding out of it. (Lower center D.) [It is difficult to see how Ken perceives this combination of "boots" and "animal skin." One cannot pin down his percept precisely, but he seems to see it somewhat unusually.]
		WFM+ Ghost Fab. Agg.	4. Or a big ghost with a tail. That's all I can think of. ∧ ∨∨	4. ("What made it look like a ghost?") The top arms . . it looked kind of like . . (he motions and imitates a frightening ghost). Kind of like a ghost . . it reminds me of one. [The evidence mounts that Ken's world is one in which terrifying forms and shapes stalk, ready to pounce.]
V	7″	WF+AP	1. It looks like a bat. ∨	
		WF+A Fab. Comb.	2. Or a rabbit with wings. ∧ >	2. [This is a fairly common interpretation, but nevertheless an uncritical one. Ken makes no effort to account for the unusual combination of things which he describes.]

Card #	React. Time	Score	Protocol	Inquiry and Observations

Drf—Ad
Agg.

3. Or some alligator.. an alligator's mouth, about ready to snap shut.

3. ("Tell me about the alligator.") The mouth was the main thing, like kinda like that. (He illustrates the jaws opening and shutting with his arms and hands.) [Again, Ken sees this percept in an unusual fashion. He does not see the fairly popular "alligators" often seen near the tips of the "bat's wings." Instead, he sees the "rabbit's feet" as the split tongue of the alligator, and the right and left wing spread of the popular "bat" as the alligator's upper and lower jaws. Thus, Ken continues to perceive and interpret idiosyncratically. One wonders whether a slight contamination might have taken place here. Ken might have seen the popular alligator heads peripherally, and this vague perception may have "caused" the appearance of the "alligator's mouth" in another area. This type of thought organization, which makes one feel that everything needs an over-all tightening, is consistent with Ken's performance on Part I of the Sorting Test.]

VI   ∨ ∧ ∨

7″

WF+Ad
Fab.
Agg.
Arb.
Mast.

1. It looks like an animal skin . . with a tail on fire.

1. ("What kind of an animal?") A bobcat. ("Why a skin?") It looks like skin 'cause . . uh . . it kinda had arms. ("And why a bobcat?") Whenever I think of skins, I think of a bobcat. [Once again, Ken's cavalier attitude toward reality emerges strikingly.] ("What made it look like a skin?") It didn't have any head, and it was spread out. ("And what about the tail being on fire?") There was some-

Card #	React. Time	Score	Protocol	Inquiry and Observations
				thing back there on the tail. It kinda looked like flames.
		DF—A Cast.	2. Some kind of animal with a long neck and no tail. > ∧	2. ("What kind of animal?") I don't know it's kind of an imaginary animal. (Lower D, seen upside down.)
		WF∓A Cast.	3. Or a flying squirrel without a tail.	3. Right in there . . it looked like skin between the legs.
VII			∨ (He sighs deeply and grimaces.) > ∧ ∨	
	30″	WSF—A	1. It looks kinda like a lamb with a big head and no middle.	1. ("What makes it look like a lamb?") . . . . I guess it's just my imagination. [Again, Ken attempts no reality justification. He is probably reacting to the fuzzy shading but is unable to put his reaction into words; this inability does not appear to disturb him particularly. One wonders, of course, to what extent the "big head and no middle" refer to Ken's perception of himself as someone who puts on an appearance without genuine substance.]
			>	
		WF±A Fab.	2. Or two pups trying to push a rock with their heads. That's all I can do.	2. Just a mongrel. [Ken probably sees himself as a "mongrel" who "tries" but goes about things badly and receives little good return for his work.]
VIII	13″		>	
		Comb. { DF+AP DCF geol. Cast.	1. Two animals crawling over colored rocks. Something like coons without tails. (He looks at the card, so that it is level with his eyes.)	(Popular animals.) [Ken's strange manner of examining the Rorschach cards is noteworthy, although it is hard to understand what it might mean.]

Card #	React. Time	Score	Protocol	Inquiry and Observations
		WSF—A Arb. Cast. Mast.	2. Flying squirrel, with holes in itself . . in its skin . . without a head, and no tail. You have to hold it at eye level. (He does so, but he never explains why.) ∨	2. [It is difficult to know precisely what "flying squirrels" mean to Ken. Perhaps he feels affinity to them because their animal status seems equivocal. The squirrels on this card are, in addition, both damaged and incomplete. Again, one cannot escape the conviction that Ken is describing himself.]
IX	26″	∨ > ∨		
		Fab. Comb. { DrSFC(C) ∓Hd DF—geol Arb. Queer	1. It looks like a man's head, surrounded by rocks.	1. Well . . it seems he kinda had holes for eyes. And his nose was covered up. And he had a long red mouth. ("What made it look like rocks?") Well, I had to make them into something. [!] ("Any special kind of rock?") No. (Lower half of central space area, and surrounding area, seen upside down.)
		DSF(C) —A Cast. Pec.	2. Two animals without any legs . . or anything. Around a bunch of rocks.	(Side green areas, seen upside down.) [This time the alterego animals have barely anything to them at all.]
		Comb. { DrF∓A DCF leaves	3. A dragonfly, flying through some leaves.	2. ("What made it look like a dragonfly?") That long body and those big wings . . surrounded by leaves. ("What made it look like leaves?") It was a green pile of something. (Lower pink D—"wings"— lower center Dr—"body"— and side green D—"leaves.")
X			I see some little things, but I can't make the rest into anything. ("Just do what you can.")	
		DF+AP	1. I see a rabbit.	1. (Bottom center D.)
		DF∓Obj.	2. I see the wishbone of a chicken.	2. (The bottom "caterpillars," plus the "rabbit head.")

Card #	React. Time	Score	Protocol	Inquiry and Observations
		DF±Ats Queer	3. I see an esophagus, with a double stomach.	(Topmost gray D.)
		DF—Ats Queer	4. Two pancreases.	4. ("What makes them look like that?") Uh . . . . . well, the pancreas is kind of shaped like a bean, if I'm not mistaken, and that one had kind of little figures on it. (Outermost bottom D.)
		DF+A Fab.	5. And two roaring lions.	5. ("What made them seem roaring?") Because of the way their mouths would be . . it was open. (Yellow "dogs.")
		DF+Obj.	6. And another small wishbone.	6. (The usual "wishbone.")
		DF+AP Cast. Agg.	7. And a spider crab with one claw torn off.	7. [This time it is not only missing; it has been torn off.] (Popular "crab.")
		DF±A Confusion	8. And a cow with ˙ moose's horns. And that's all I can see.	8. (Central blue D.) [The response suggests Ken's activity-passivity confusion.]

THEMATIC APPERCEPTION TEST

Card 1 (A young boy is contemplating a violin which rests on a table in front of him.)

This is Liberace at ten. He saw a violin and went home and asked his mother if he could take violin lessons. She said no, he'd have to take piano lessons because they already had a piano. So that night he talked to his father, and he didn't like it very well, so that night she talked to his father, and his father said that he should take the piano lessons. So he took them, and in about a year, why he was enjoying them, and that's how he got to be such a great man. Ha! ha! ha! [A major theme Ken makes reappear over and over involves things looking bad at first but eventually—apparently—working out for the very best. While this theme appears in somewhat muted and ambivalent form on Card 1, it reappears more overtly and more dramatically in future stories.]

Card 2 (Country scene: in the foreground is a young woman with books in her hand; in the background a man is working in the fields, and an older woman is looking on.)

Jane was a girl of eighteen. Her brother, Samuel, was nineteen. Jane was a schoolteacher at the local school. They lived on a farm with their parents. One day, when Jane went to school, Samuel was staying home and plowing. As he plowed, there suddenly came a flash flood from the river, and they all went home. They were heartbroken because the young plants were just coming up; so they plowed after the flood, reseeded and . . . . about August, they started harvesting. They were awful glad for the flood, for it brought up more fertile ground on the bottom. ("Who's that older lady standing there?") That's the mother. ("And what is she thinking about?") She's thinking how poor the ground is bearing anymore, since it's been all farmed out. ("What part of the story is in the picture right now?") Plowing before the flood. [Both here and elsewhere, Ken expresses a Pollyanna view. Although things may at first look terrible, they end up being very fine. Ken denies "bad" things and stoutly maintains that everything is meant for the eventual best. His tantrums probably occur when denial no longer works.]

Card 3 BM (On the floor against a couch is the huddled form of a boy with his head bowed on his right arm. Beside him on the floor is a revolver.)

This lady has been waiting forty-eight hours for her son, who is on the airplane, to come home. The airplane's late. She has been up all the time. She just now found out that the airplane is grounded in San Diego, 400 miles away, because of engine trouble, and that's where her son is. He's okay, so she just lay down on the floor and went to sleep. ("What's that object, lying next to her on the floor?") I don't know. I can't see it well enough to know. [Ken continues to tell stories in which situations, although they may look bad at the beginning, eventually turn out well.]

Card 6 BM (A short elderly woman stands with her back turned to a tall young man. The latter is looking downward with a perplexed expression.)

This man was visiting his mother, and they saw a car wreck out the window. The man's wondering whether he should run out and try to help, or whether he should stay out off the road. And the mother, she's just so startled, she doesn't know what to think. ("So what does the young man decide?") Well, the ambulance came, and he decided to stay in. ("What did he originally think he might do?") He was a medical doctor in training, and he thought he might be able to help until the doctors came. ("And why do you think he stayed away from there?") Because there were probably other doctors out there anyway. ("Who were the people in the accident?") Just some strangers. ("How did the accident happen?") It was raining outside and this was a blind corner, and the one tried to dash across, and the other one hit him. [Ken probably finds it difficult to commit himself to doing something helpful for others. Although his hero is obviously able to help, he does not give himself the needed push to leave his mother and participate in life.]

Card 7 BM (A gray-haired man is looking at a younger man who is sullenly staring into space.)

The older man was a college professor, and the younger one is a student. The younger one is mad because the college professor just showed him his grade, which is going to be a D. ("So what happens then?") After that, the college student works harder. ("Why did he get a D so far?") Because he hadn't ever studied his lessons. There he acts like me. ("How does the professor feel toward him?") The professor feels like the boy could do better. [Ken shows the degree to which he identifies himself with the adults who tell him his failures are caused by laziness and who try to convince him he could do better if only he "tried."]

Card 10 (A young woman's head against a man's shoulder.)

The boy was pouting because he couldn't go to his friend's house, and his mother whispered a secret to him, and that was that his father was coming home from a long business trip. The boy was still rather unhappy about it, but he stayed without any more pouting, and when his father comes home, he is the first one to greet him. ("Why couldn't he visit his friend?") Because his mother wanted him to be there when his father came home. ("How long had his father been gone?") Three weeks. [Ken deals with this situation in typical style—rather than having his hero continue to pout, he has him undo himself to deny his irritation, so that he greets his father with great warmth, and apparently without anger.]

Card 12 M (A young man is lying on a couch with his eyes closed. Leaning over him is a gaunt form of an elderly man, his hand stretched out above the face of the reclining figure.)

The man standing up, the person, is a kid who got hold of a book that told how to hypnotize people, and he hypnotizes this other boy and got him hypnotized okay, but didn't get him to come back out of it. The family found out about it, and the boy tried every hour for three days, but they couldn't get him out of it. Finally, they got a master hypnotist who couldn't get him out of it. At last, they got him out of it, but the boy never was quite the same again. ("How is that?") Sometimes he'd just fall back into hypnotism. ("And what would happen then?") He'd just stand there and stare. ("Why did the other boy hypnotize him in the first place?") He was just trying it out. ("How did this boy feel when he couldn't get the other one out of hypnosis?") He felt rather guilty. ("And how did the hypnotized boy feel about never really getting out of hypnosis?") He didn't like it so well. ("What effect did all that have on his later life?") He finally grew out of it. [Here seems to be Ken's understanding of what might happen, should he passively submit to someone else. Were he to lose control (as in psychotherapy) he would be helplessly at the mercy of the other person. Ken needs to underplay the hypnotized boy's reaction: "He didn't like it so well." Things eventually work out fairly well.]

Card 16 (Blank card.)

Two friends were walking down the street one time, when a bunch of kids jumped them. They took them to their secret club house, which really wasn't very secret. It was just back in the woods a ways. Everybody knew there was a building there, but they didn't know what it was. So they took them back there and just held them there; didn't do anything to them, tied them up, left them there for about an hour. Then they let them go, and these two friends went walking down the street again and decided they'd better make their own club to protect themselves. So they made them a club, and then they had to decide who was going to be president, and they decided it would be one of these two boys, so they had an election, and one of the boys won, of course, and the other boy got kind of bitter because . . well, he didn't like it very well. He thought he was just as good as this other kid, why couldn't he be president? The other kids tried to tell him that his turn would come, but he was awful mad at them. He just stalked out, and this other bunch of kids got ahold of him again. This time, they climbed up in a tree with him, grabbed hold of him and tied his feet and hands onto the tree, and he couldn't hardly move, and they left him up there for about two or three hours. And then they came up there and untied him and let him go, and he never knew where this tree was exactly because they blindfolded him, and so they let him go, and he never knew who the kids were. He went back to the club house and told them what had happened, so they got awful mad, and a whole bunch of them, they went back to this one club house, the club that . . the other gang's club house and went in there, and there was the whole gang, and they got to see who were there and told their fathers and mothers. And the fathers and mothers complained, and the gang was abolished, and the kids were punished. And the one kid that had wanted to be president decided that it was best to just let the other guy be president, sort of sit still till it was his turn. ("Why were the kids from the other gang picking on this kid?") They didn't have anything to do, and that was just the best thing they could think of. ("How come the other fellow was elected president first?") Well, it wasn't exactly that they liked him better, but somebody had to be president. ("And why did the kids make up this second club?") Well, they just did that so the other gang wouldn't pick on them, because they'd be afraid to jump them if there were more of them. ("After the first club was disbanded, did the second club stay together, or did it dissolve?") They stayed a club. ("And what did they do when they didn't need to use the club for protection anymore?") Oh, they just had fun. [Two themes emerge clearly. One involves the hero's envy and resentment about not being chosen leader—i.e., about not being the best liked. His resentment causes him to withdraw from the peer situation. Another major theme involves the hero's search for companionship as a defensive maneuver. He does not, at least at first, seek friends to have fun with them, but rather to find safety with them. As soon as he leaves that safety he is endangered again. For the sake of relative immunity, he gives up other needs—e.g., the wish to become president. Frequently the stories told to this blank card tend to be consciously autobiographical. The storyteller tends to rely on remembered experience when a blank stimulus is furnished.]

SENTENCE COMPLETION TEST II

He hoped that when he grew up he would be a scientist.

His parents loved him. [This is a rather unusual ending for this stem. More frequently the person comments exclusively about his parents; he does not bring himself in as Ken does. Ken's making a special point of his parents' love for him points up how much Ken is still preoccupied with a concern appropriate for a younger child. This specific mention of what should be a matter of course, makes one wonder whether Ken doubts that his parents truly care about him.]

When he saw what the other kids were doing . . . . he ran and told his mother. ("What did he tell her?") I don't know. (He laughs.) ("Make up something.") Busting a window. [He is still obviously much more parent- than peer-oriented.]

When he compared himself to his friends he was . . scared. ("Why was that?") (He sighs.) I don't know. I can't think of anything. [Perhaps being "scared" of peers is the reason for his reluctance to leave his parents.]

He was sad whenever he thought of his dead aunt.

When he was asked about his aches and pains he said they were terrible.

The person he admired most was a bum. ("How is that?") (He laughs.) Don't ask me. That's your part of the sentence. (He laughs again.) ("Make up something.") I don't know. (He laughs.) [An example of Ken's mixed acceptance-rejection of parental standards?]

His brother was smaller than him, but stronger.

When the girl kissed him he just about went crazy. ("How do you mean?") Well, he just about fainted.

When his father came into the room he was so startled, he broke a glass. [Ken's relationship to his father seems less than optimal.]

When he was with his sister he was always at ease.

At school he had lots of fun. [Since Ken often has a very difficult time in school, this is a further example of his major denial tendency.]

When he looked at the work the other students were doing he was ashamed of his. [Denial is not always used.]

He was very happy when he got an A on his report card.

The thing he found hardest to do was writing. [The last three sentences give a truer account of Ken's feelings about school activities. He can obviously sometimes face his situation more honestly, without having to resort to denial.]

Whenever certain things really bothered him he went off by himself and tried to figure them out. [Often, though, Ken merely withdraws, without trying to "figure them out."]

His dreams were usually nice ones.

When he saw that the man had left the money behind he ran to give it to him.

He thought that his mother was very nice. [Ken needs to present many things as "very nice."]

Whenever he and his family disagreed they always compromised. [In this way, avoiding sharp edges.]

When he was very little he was afraid of the dark. [He was a frightened child and probably still is.]

His best friend had told on him. [This is the first thing that comes to Ken's mind about "his best friend." So far he has spoken of friendship in three contexts: in the first, "friends" are merely allies who offer protection from aggressive peers, but who have few other significant characteristics. In the second, the object of Ken's greatest admiration is "a bum." In the third, his best friend has "told on him." Perhaps Ken feels he needs no friends because he feels so close to his mother.]

He was unhappy with his father when his father said he couldn't go swimming.

When his mother asked about his girl friend he said he didn't have one.

He never thought he would be able to ride a horse.

He always hoped that . . . . his mother wouldn't ask about his girl. [Is he resentful because he feels his mother pushes him into an activity for which he is not ready? He has indicated several times that, although he is excited by girls, he feels helpless around them. Possibly he resents his mother's efforts to push him away from her, into heterosexual adequacy.]

What he liked best about himself was that he could always go to sleep. [This is pride in a pathetic accomplishment.]

His mother was more likely than his father to take him to the movies.

His sister was always lots of fun with him.

When he had nothing else to do he would read a book.

He thought that his intelligence was very high.

What he liked best about school was reading.

When he couldn't see a way out of his problem he asked his parents. [Here is another example of Ken's family orientation—his tendency to solve problems in ways appropriate for a younger child.]

He saw the cockroach on the wall and killed it.

His teacher was awfully mean . . . . sometimes. ("How is that?") She would give him terrifically long assignments. [Ken pulls his punches. His initial strong anger falls victim to undoing, or at least softening, through his use of "sometimes."]

Whenever he got angry he'd go off by himself. [And be caught by the rival gang? Or withdraw?]

He remembered that when he was little he didn't like to get out of his pajamas and into his clothes. [He did not (does not?) like to meet the world.]

When the kids invited him to go with them to the hiding place, he thought . . Oh boy! This is my chance. ("For what?") To get in good with them. [He is thirsting to form a relationship with peers.]

After school he usually rode his bicycle.

He admired his father when he worked out.

When the girl invited him to her party he was very happy.

When he and his brother were together they always had lots of fun.

He thought that his body was rather short.

When he had a lot of homework to do he shut himself up in his room. ("And then?") He did it. [Actually, he probably withdraws.]

What he disliked about school was some of the teachers.

Whenever he spoke about his problems to someone they either laughed or tried to help.

When he entered the haunted house he was awful scared.

When the other fellow offered him a cigarette he told him he never smoked.

He didn't like his mother to . . . . go to a party in the middle of the night. ("How do you mean?") That was just an exaggeration. (He laughs.) ("Does your mother go out at night?") Uh-huh. [Ken may well be tyrannical about his mother's leaving him "in the middle of the night."]

When the baby arrived he was very happy.

When the fellows asked him to join them in a rough game he said "yes!"

Whenever he didn't do what he was told he got a spanking. [Fourteen years is an advanced age to think of being spanked. Ken either thinks of himself as younger, or he is treated as younger, or both.]

What would make him angriest was when somebody teased him about a girl he didn't like. [In one way or another, "girls" offer Ken difficulties.]

In his spare time he built model airplanes.

What troubled him most was his size. [Again.]

When he was alone in his room at night he always had deep thoughts. ("Like what?") Just anything.

What scared him most was when somebody snuck up behind him.

He struck the match and lit the lantern.

He disliked his father when he wouldn't let him do things his own way.

He thought that his looks were okay.

The thing he could do best was read.

He had no respect at all for people that wouldn't do their share of work. [He is probably speaking about himself, again adopting the attitudes of adults who have blamed him for this very thing.]

He always enjoyed playing with the other fellows. [He has told enough to indicate he plays with them very little.]

He had a very uncomfortable feeling when he was among strangers.

He found it easiest to talk to . . . What? (I repeat the stem.) Was his mother or father.

WORD ASSOCIATION TEST[7]

React. Time (In Secs.)	Stimulus	Response	Recall[8]	Recall Time (In Secs.)[9]	Inquiry[10] and Comments
1	1. *hat*	(He sighs.) dress	coat √		
1	2. *lamp*	shade	√	3	

[7] For information regarding the administration, scoring and rationale of this test, see Rapaport et al. (1945-1946, Vol. II).

[8] A check mark indicates the person is able to give the same word on Recall as originally, in accordance with instructions.

[9] Recall reaction times are indicated only when they are two seconds or longer.

[10] Inquiry follows Recall of *all* 60 test words.

React. Time (In Secs.)	Stimulus	Response	Recall	Recall Time (In Secs.)	Inquiry and Comments
12	3. *love*	(He snaps his fingers.) kiss (He laughs.)	√	3	3. ("Why did it take such a long time at first?") I don't know. I just couldn't think of anything. No word came, and I just had to think hard. [It is not surprising that the word *love* mildly disorganizes Ken. Although he says he was unable to think of a word, there may be a number of additional reasons to account for the 12″ delay.]
1½	4. *book*	read	√		
½	5. *father*	mother	√		
1½	6. *paper*	pencil	√		
4½	7. *breast*	arm (He laughs.)	√	5	[It is usual for sexual or sexually toned words to be associated with longer delays. The presence of some sort of pathological process is suspected only when long associative delays occur after relatively "tame" words.]
3	8. *curtains*	shade	√	3½	[Frequently a difficult (i.e., affectively toned) word sets up a "reverberation," so that reaction times of the word or words which immediately follow are also (or instead) affected. Ken's strong reaction to *breast* apparently reverberates to *curtains* and *trunk*.
4	9. *trunk*	suitcase	√	3½	9. ("What happened on 'trunk'?") I thought . . at first I thought I didn't know whether you meant elephant trunk or suitcase trunk. I puzzled that out. [Obsessions of this type sometimes cause a delay in reaction time. To what extent does Ken need to resort to obsessive rumination still to defend against the impact of the word *breast*? To what

React. Time (In Secs.)	Stimulus	Response	Recall	Recall Time (In Secs.)	Inquiry and Comments
					extent is the "elephant's trunk" reminiscent of phallic protuberances?]
1½	10. *drink*	eat	√	3	10. [Although one can find specific "reasons" for Ken's associative delays—a clinician is never at a loss for specific reasons—it is beginning to look as if Ken's delays are reflective of a more generalized disturbance. Delays to objectively innocuous stimuli, caused by unexplainable factors, are more worrisome than are delays following probable conflictual areas. Ken's thinking process does not function smoothly; he manifests occasional pauses and other blockages which attest to the presence of mildly disorganizing factors. Although Ken's Word Association performance does not reflect nearly so much pathology as his Rorschach, it nevertheless suggests a mild disorder of the formal processes of thinking, in the way of holes, gaps and inadequate thought cogwheelings.]
4½	11. *party*	fun	√	2½	11. ("Why did 'party' take longer?") I don't remember what I said (he smiles). ("Do you like parties?") I've never been to one. ("You've never been to a party?") I went to a skating party once. They're okay. ("How about a birthday party?") I've had one quite a few years ago. Oh, I've been to birthday parties. I went to one, one or two years ago. [It is difficult to believe Ken has never been to a party. As he thinks about it more, he remembers having been to a few. Appar-

React. Time (In Secs.)	Stimulus	Response	Recall	Recall Time (In Secs.)	Inquiry and Comments
					ently he wishes to convey the impoverishment of his social-peer contacts, but one certainly feels by now that Ken is exceedingly reluctant to exchange family for peer contact.]
2½	12. *spring*	fall	√	3	12. [Again the unaccountable delay, suggesting that some intrusive process is interfering with optimal efficiency. Or can the delay be accounted for by the preceding *party?*]
6	13. *bowel movement*	toilet	√		13. [Delay on a "difficult" item is to be expected. It cannot be put in the same category as Ken's delays on apparently innocuous words.]
1½	14. *rug*	carpet	√		
1½	15. *boy friend*	girl friend	√		
1	16. *chair*	table	√		
1½	17. *screen*	door	√		17. [Ken is hitting an efficient stride now.]
3½	18. *penis*	testicles	√		
4½	19. *radiator*	engine	motor	2	19. [The delay is probably caused by *penis*.]
1½	20. *frame*	picture	√	4	20. [Why 4"?]
1½	21. *suicide*	kill	√		
2	22. *mountain*	hill	√		
2	23. *snake*	bird	animal	6½	23. ("What happened on 'snake'?") I don't know. I don't remember what I said. ("You said 'bird.'") I heard the other day something about a bird coming down to a snake because the snake had caught its eye. ("How do you mean?") I mean, hypnotized it. [Something grossly disturbing seems

React. Time (In Secs.)	Stimulus	Response	Recall	Recall Time (In Secs.)	Inquiry and Comments
					to have occurred to Ken here. He shows one of his longest reaction times on Recall and is unable to remember the word he gave originally. One assumes that *snake*, possibly because of its symbolic meanings, has been a source of disorganization.]
1½	24. *house*	home	√		
—	25. *vagina*	What? ("Vagina.") I don't know!	(Not repeated)		25. ("What about 'vagina'?") I never heard of it before! [One wonders about a fourteen-year-old boy never having heard the word *vagina*, when he uses the word "testicles."]
1	26. *tobacco*	spit	√		26. ("What were you thinking about with 'tobacco'?") My grandfather always chews tobacco, and he spits it. He used to chew it. He doesn't anymore. [A private association.]
1½	27. *mouth*	nose	eat	2	
1	28. *horse*	cow	√		
—	29. *masturbation*	Hmm . . I don't know!	√	—	29. ("How about 'masturbation'?") I didn't know what that meant. [Again, one wonders about a fairly alert fourteen-year-old boy not knowing this word.] (He sighs deeply as I turn the page of the test.)
1	30. *wife*	husband	√	7	30. (He does not know why he paused so long on Recall.) [If Ken's delay is caused by his inability to recall the original response, then this would indicate fairly significant disorganization, since Ken's original "husband" is the popular association to *wife*. It is more likely, however, that his 7″ reaction time is caused by the reverberation of the word *masturbation*.]

React. Time (In Secs.)	Stimulus	Response	Recall	Recall Time (In Secs.)	Inquiry and Comments
½	31. *table*	chair	√		
3	32. *fight*	make up	√		32. ("What were you thinking about with 'fight'?") I just thought what you did after a fight. What you sometimes did. ("What do you do?") I don't think I fight too much more than the other kids. ("Tell me about it.") When I fight, it's usually words. ("What'll get you mad?") I never thought about it before . . . . People tease me because I'm so little. I don't know. I got a terrible temper. [This is at least the third time Ken directly expresses unhappiness about his size. Although he never manifested instances of his "terrible temper" during testing, his parents say Ken's "terrible temper" presents a serious problem at home.]
2½	33. *beef*	pork	Ah .. √	6	33. [Is the 6″ Recall delay on beef caused by the preceding *fight?*]
3½	34. *stomach*	intestines	√	2½	
8	35. *farm*	What? (!) farmer	√	2½	35. [A major poorly accountable delay. Maybe *stomach* is the culprit? Maybe there is no specific culprit.]
1	36. *man*	woman	√		
2½	37. *taxes*	government	√		
2	38. *nipple*	bottle	√	2	
1	39. *doctor*	nurse	√	5	39. [Even if the long pauses are accounted for by the explanation of their being delayed reactions, this explanation would emphasize the ease with which Ken becomes disorganized. Were he psychologically put together more effi-

React. Time (In Secs.)	Stimulus	Response	Recall	Recall Time (In Secs.)	Inquiry and Comments
					ciently, he would be able to recover much more easily.]
2½	40. *dirt*	earth	√		
2	41. *cut*	heal	√		
3½	42. *movies*	Movies? ("That's right.") shows	pictures	2	
1½	43. *cock-roach*	bug	√		
1½	44. *bite*	eat	√	2½	
1½	45. *dog*	cat	√	2	
2½	46. *dance*	stand	√	2	46. ("Why did you say 'stand' when I said 'dance'?") I don't know. That's just the first thing I thought of. ("How would you explain that thought?") Cause you're moving when you're dancing and not when you're standing. ("Do you dance?") Me? No. Not hardly. ("Do you like dancing?") Oh, I don't know. I don't have any use for it now. I might in a couple of years, but now I don't care for it. ["Stand" is a distant, unusual association. It is typical of Ken's thinking to be able to go along appropriately and efficiently until a certain point when he unexpectedly comes up with an unusual response. His saying he is too young to dance further underlines his wish not to leave the home and begin to enter adulthood.]
2	47. *gun*	bullet	What? ("Gun.") I don't know what I said.		47. [Aggression tends to lead to disorganization.]

React. Time (In Secs.)	Stimulus	Response	Recall	Recall Time (In Secs.)	Inquiry and Comments
3½	48. *water*	sand	√	6½	48. ("What do you think happened with 'water'?") I don't know.
1	49. *husband*	wife	√		
3	50. *mud*	dirt	√		
1	51. *woman*	man	√	2	
2	52. *fire*	cold	√	3	
7	53. *suck*	drink	√	5	53. [This is a word after which one expects a delay.]
2½	54. *money*	rich	√		
1	55. *mother*	father	√		
2	56. *hospital*	sick	√		
1	57. *girl friend*	boy friend	√		
1	58. *taxi*	car	√		
3	59. *intercourse*	I don't know.	—		59. ("What happened on 'intercourse'?") I don't know what it meant. [Ken denies knowledge of all sexual words, other than *penis* and *testicles*. Is his sexual naïveté genuine? Defensive? Parentally fostered?]
3½	60. *hunger*	thirsty	√	2½	60. [One suspects Ken knows the meaning of *intercourse*, and that this may be the reason for his initial delay on *hunger*.] ("Did you have any images?") Yes. ("Which ones do you remember?") I saw a taxi in my mind's eye. ("Do you remember any others?") Hmm . . boy friend.

THE PSYCHOLOGIST'S REPORT

Ken functions intellectually at an Average to Superior level, achieving an extra value Intelligence Quotient of 109-115 (Verbal Quotient 113-123; Performance Quotient 105). His subtest scores range erratically, from a low score of 6 on Digit Symbol to a high of 14 on Similarities. Such a heterogeneous distribution suggests considerable interference with efficient intellectual functioning, an interference which can most clearly be seen on the Arithmetic, where Ken's alternate score is five points higher than the one he eventually obtains. Typically, he tends to miss the correct answer by one digit. He apparently cannot permit himself either clear-cut failure or success. He needs barely to fail, while at the same time making clear that he could actually succeed. Sometimes he gives an incorrect response after first giving a correct one, so that his unconscious drive to avoid success, for whatever reason, stands forth clearly. Ken's "failures" may in part express his need to oppose and negate in a passive way, a need which is also reflected in his tendency, on the Rorschach, to turn each card upside down as quickly as he receives it in his hand. But his rather intense anger is never expressed overtly during testing. On Sentence Completion, for example, Ken explains that whenever he and his family disagree, they compromise. Yet we know that Ken is given to rather explosive temper outbursts at home. Either extrafamilial situations call forth less extreme reactions in Ken, or he is able to exert some control over his aggressive outbursts when the occasion seems to require it.

Ken demonstrates an excellent capacity to use words appropriately, sharply and nonobsessively. He is able to speak in a playful, sometimes rather sophisticated, manner. Thus, when presented with the blank Thematic Apperception Test card, he grins and says that it would be simple to create a story to such a "well-defined" picture. His concept formation on the verbal level is also excellent, and it is on Similarities that he achieves his highest Wechsler-Bellevue score.

A graphomotor incapacity is suggested by Ken's poor performance on the Digit Symbol subtest, where he demonstrates low speed, hesitancy, an arhythmical approach and some errors. He encounters similar difficulties on all other graphomotor tests. On the Bender Gestalt 5″ Exposure, for example, he has difficulty drawing even a simple circle. Other Bender figures tend to be drawn in a messy, inaccurate, inexact and wobbly fashion. Ken's graphomotor difficulties are most strikingly evident in his writing, which he says is his most difficult school activity. He complains that his pencil won't go where he wants and that "it wobbles all over." He makes many writing errors, which he attempts to correct. Thus, when he wishes to make *p,* he makes *d,* and often when he intends to go up, his pencil goes down. His writing demonstrates significant arhythmia, and some letters are much larger than others. Sometimes wide spaces develop between letters; other times, the letters are practically on top of each other. Such motor-executive problems suggest impairment of motor center functioning. It may be that a portion of Ken's hyperactivity reflects not only his psychic tension but certain "organic," spasticlike characteristics.

Ken's behavior on structured tests appears to be no more than neurotic. As he begins to work on less structured items, however, much more severe pathology becomes evident. On the BRL Sorting Test, for example, he shows a significant loosening of thinking. When he is asked to create his own concepts, he gives two pathognomonic chain responses; i.e., when told to put with a red rubber ball whatever he thinks should go, he adds: the toy tools, rubber cigar, red paper circle, red cardboard square, toy red plastic silverware, chalk, red rubber sink stopper, eraser, pliers, screwdriver, and bell. He explains, "They're all toys or rubber, except for the real pliers and screwdriver, and I just put them in because they're related to the toy pliers and screwdriver, and so on." Such a sorting shows how, in Ken's thinking, several different things can be alike at the same time, for different reasons.

Ken's Rorschach performance further suggests the seriousness of his disturbance. Only a little more than half his thirty-six responses are of acceptable form level. He organizes his percepts arbitrarily; even Popular responses must be inquired into, since they tend to be idiosyncratically organized. He tends to emphasize the decayed and battered (e.g., "a bat with a bunch of holes in its wings"; "a goose with its wings all torn up"). In this way, he conveys his damaged, empty, incomplete self-concept. Thirty percent of Ken's responses reflect a significant amount of castration anxiety: he is concerned about missing heads, tails and other limbs. He describes an animal with "no arms, no legs, no nothing." On Card VII, he sees a lamb "whose insides are missing." Such descriptions as "dogs trying to push something" reflect Ken's feeling of paralysis in the face of obstacles he has a hard time overcoming. The arbitrary nature of Ken's thinking is sometimes startling. He sees Card II as two goats butting their heads together. He explains "That splotch at the top (a red detail) made it look like some sort of an impact, and whenever I see an impact like that, I think of a goat." Card IX is "a man's head, surrounded by rocks." Asked about the rocks, he smiles and says, "I had to make them into something." Ken's difficulty in modulating affect is suggested by his inability successfully to integrate color into the formal aspects of his percepts.

His Rorschach content contains much that is fearsome and aggressive. In addition to the responses already described, he sees "two skeletons pulling some small animal apart"; "a black cat that's jumping . . looking like he's coming down on top of you"; "an alligator's mouth about ready to snap shut"; "a spotted crab with one claw torn off." An area looks like a "big ghost with a tail. It's holding out its arms, as if ready to attack." The arbitrary, idiosyncratic and fearful-aggressive nature of Ken's Rorschach suggests that his disorganization is serious enough to indicate a process of decompensation.

As far as his self-image is concerned, Ken sees himself as short, scared, and terrible-tempered. He agrees with his parents and teachers that he is not living up to his good intelligence. He feels a great gap between himself and other children and ambivalently longs to belong. He finds it impossible, however, because other children are tough, disagreeable, delinquent and aggressive. Their main purpose seems to be to tease him and otherwise to make his life miserable. But most important, he does not yet feel ready to leave the young position in the midst of his family. He cannot yet give up his early objects and establish new relations with his peers. His story to the blank TAT card indicates that his main reason for entering into a relationship with other children involves a wish to have them protect him. Whatever other satisfactions a group might provide are secondary to this. Ken is unable to stand up to the aggressions of other children, and he enlists the help of his parents, particularly his mother, to handle the peers who treat him aggressively. Parental and community authority are highly important to Ken—they are guardians of law and order; without them "people would run all over other people. It would be a heck of a world. Nobody'd be safe."

Not even one's best friends are trustworthy. Ken tells a TAT story of a friendship which breaks up because the two friends compete for the presidency of a club. Another story deals with two friends who fight over a loan. On Sentence Completion, he says, *His best friend had* "told on him." On Word Association, he blocks on the word *party* and explains that he has never been to one. Later, he recalls some parties which he has attended, but the picture of isolation is nevertheless striking. Whenever he is hurt, unhappy or angry, he is tempted to go away by himself. On Sentence Completion, he states, *What he liked best about himself* "was that he could always go to sleep" (i.e., withdraw). Ken's difficulty in taking part in a life situation is epitomized by his TAT story of the young doctor who sees an accident on the street and wonders whether to go outside and help; eventually, he decides to stay inside, with his mother.

Ken's projective stories further reflect his major dependence on his parents. He requires their approval before he commits himself to any course of action. Parental word is law; Ken's only defense against it is silent pouting. Ken's ambivalently valued closeness to his mother is suggested by a TAT story in which a mother is distraught because her son fails to return from a trip on time, but then she finds out his plane has been grounded. Ken thinks of his father as a rather unavailable person who goes on long trips. When the father is around, he tends to criticize his son's poor scholarship. On Sentence Completion, a father's entering a room causes his son to drop a glass. Ken perceives women (mothers?) as exploiting men and as imposing on them. For example, he explains the outcome of the Picture Arrangement *Flirt* sequence not as the Little King's offering to carry the woman's bundle, but as "next thing you know, this gal has him carrying her load."

Young dependency relations at Ken's age are perceived by him as bringing rather severe problems with them. His anxiety regarding such relationships in which he finds himself enmeshed is suggested by his story to the TAT "Hypnosis" card. He tells of one boy's being hypnotized by another. The youthful hypnotist is unable to wake his subject, even when he tries "every hour for three days . . . . . Finally they get a master hypnotist who couldn't get him out of it. At last, they got him out of it, but the boy never was quite the same again . . . He'd just stand there and stare."

Although Ken seems, on the surface, to be fairly well integrated, his performance on less well-structured items suggests quite severe basic pathology. While the "organic" manifestations appear to be secondary to emotional conflicts, they must nevertheless be taken into account. Ken's parents and teachers might be helped to understand how Ken's writing difficulty, for example, stems from inability rather than from lack of will. They might be encouraged to stop pressuring him in areas he can handle only with difficulty. Tutoring is probably better given outside the home, in view of Ken's complex intrafamilial situation.

DISCUSSION

Ken's test protocol suggests that he has a fairly mild, well-contained, central neurological impairment which interferes particularly with graphomotor and complex conceptual functioning. It is difficult to say to what extent the "organic disability" alone affects school performance, to what extent the significant emotional factors are additionally responsible, and to what extent both "organic" and emotional factors play interacting, destructive roles. It is impossible to disentangle the causes and the effects in such an instance (or in most clinical instances, for that matter). Are Ken's emotional difficulties exacerbated by the "organic" ones? Is it the other way around? Do the emotional and the "organic" constantly interact and reinforce each other?

In any case, it is once again apparent that a patient need not be *either* brain damaged *or* emotionally disturbed. Certainly, most persons who are unable to perform adequately in certain areas because of "organicity" react to this feature of their lives in some way. It is rare to see organically caused disability by itself, without emotional factors playing a complicating role.

Ken is unable to take the adolescent step of appropriately freeing himself from his home, and it is probable that the task of achieving freedom is made more difficult because of his organic problems. His impairments create a certain helplessness which, in turn, plays into both his need to remain young and his mother's apparent need to keep him so.

Ken has use for his age mates only as they protect him. He hardly goes to parties, and thoughts of heterosexual contacts tend to disorganize him. He cannot trust the one friend he has because "he tells on" him. In other words, in many ways it is best to stay at home, to stay a preadolescent child.

It is difficult to evaluate the significance of Ken's thought dis-organization. Adolescence is usually a period during which much internal reorganization takes place. Because there is so much inner flux, one frequently sees what superficially seems to be fairly severe disorganization. As the adolescent steers himself into adulthood, however, processes that were loosely, roughly and inefficiently organized become more tightly, smoothly and efficiently integrated. It is difficult to say what the limits of "normal adolescent peculiarity" are. Probably it is most helpful simply to suggest that adolescent peculiarities be weighted differently from peculiarities found at earlier or later ages, since they may well disappear as the adolescent becomes older. Is Ken beyond the limits of what can "normally" be expected? With what we know at this time, we must content our-selves with waiting and seeing.

In evaluating the significance of Ken's unusual thinking, his "organic" involvement must be taken into account. That there is an organic involvement seems fairly certain, even though it is apparent only on psychological testing. The organic impairment may have subtle, far-reaching effects beyond what is seen on psychological testing.

While Ken serves as an example of an adolescent whose organic impairment appears only on psychological testing, Hal, whose case follows, serves as another kind of example: the adolescent who suffers from clinically and neurologically apparent impairment ("epi-leptic seizures"), but who demonstrates little on psychological testing which leads one to suspect organic involvement. At the same time, as was true of Ken, Hal has rather severe emotional problems associ-ated with his "organicity."

CLINICAL SUMMARY: Hal

Hal is fifteen years old and was brought to the examination after he began to develop successive grand mal epileptic seizures. He has an older brother and sister and a younger brother.

Apart from his seizures, Hal has always had difficulty in school. In the seventh to ninth grades he received low grades, and his teachers felt he could have done much better. They report that he seems to be a nervous child. He is a disciplinary problem at school and at home and is much less able to take responsibility than his siblings are. He has always had difficulty in getting along with his peers and prefers to be with older or younger people. Hal's parents feel, however, that they would not have considered his problems serious enough to bring him for examination if it had not been for his seizures.

According to his mother, her pregnancy with Hal and his delivery were completely without incident. His development seemed normal, except for his continuing night wetting until he was eleven or twelve years old. At the age of four, he fell and had to have two stitches in a cut on his head, but he did not lose consciousness.

A significant factor in Hal's immaturity seems to involve his mother's inability to permit him to grow up. During the neurological examination, for example, she would not let him answer his own questions, but interrupted him whenever he tried.

Physical and Laboratory Findings: The physical examination was essentially normal, as were the laboratory studies. The x-rays were within normal limits.

The EEG was abnormal, with diffuse paroxysmal dysrhythmia, spike wave type. This record is entirely consistent with what is often seen in so-called idiopathic convulsive disorders. The neurological examination was entirely normal.

THE PSYCHOLOGIST'S DESCRIPTION

Hal is a pleasant, friendly boy who looks at the world with almost constant wonderment and surprise. Although he achieves an Intelligence Quotient in the Bright Normal range, his persistent questioning is reminiscent of a child with a dull intelligence. His questions are naïve and artless, both in form and content. His ingenuous comments sometimes verge on the tactless, but he seems unaware of this tendency.

He is anxious not to offend and needs very much to please. He takes pains, for example, to help me put test items back into their boxes. He finds it important to keep his personal relations free of friction and must immediately deny any even mildly aggressive impulse that slips through his rigid guard. He has a sanguine attitude toward his seizures. Following his laboratory appointment, during which he was told the results of his EEG, he mentioned having heard that his type of brain wave could be obtained from a person suffering bad headaches—this, even though he had had several serious seizures recently. He has obviously been unable to face the significance of his illness. The extent to which his reality testing is based on wish fulfillment is apparent. Superficially, Hal appears nonreflective and nonintrospective, even though he is exceedingly sensitive to the ways in which things do or might possibly fit together, sometimes almost hyperalert and suspicious. In his alertness, he occasionally attends to the relatively insignificant and misses the obvious.

THE WECHSLER-BELLEVUE SCALE

Name: Hal   Age: 15-11

	RS	WTS	0 1 2 3 4 5 6 7 8 9 10 11 12 13 14 15 16 17 18 19 20
COMPR.	12-14	11-12	× (≈14)
INFOR.	13	10	× (≈12)
DIG.	9-10	6-7	× (≈6)
ARITH.	10	13	(≈13)
SIMIL.	9-12	8-10	× (≈10)
VOCAB.	21½	10	(≈10)
P. A.	16	14	(≈14)
P. C.	10-11	9-10	× (≈9)
B. D.	30	14	(≈14)
O. A.	18-22	10-13	× (≈12)
D. S.	41	10	(≈10)

TOT. VERB.	52-55
TOT. PERF.	57-61
TOT. SCALE	109-116

VERBAL I.Q.:   109-113   LEVEL: Average—Bright Normal

PERFORMANCE I.Q.:   111-117   LEVEL: Bright Normal

TOTAL I.Q.:   111-117   LEVEL: Bright Normal

[The W-B Scattergram reflects the sweep of Hal's abilities, which range from a low of 6 on Digit Span to a high of 14 on Picture Arrangement and Block Design. Such a wide score discrepancy, although it often indicates the presence of disturbance, is quite commonly seen among "normal" adolescents and reflects their not yet completed effort to stabilize what is preferably not yet stable. Such an extreme test scatter in the record of an older person would rightly be cause for concern. In an adolescent, however, one almost hopes for such a pattern of high and low abilities, since such a lack of integration assures the absence of a premature internal equilibrium. Where one finds too much stability (e.g., too much uniformity of subscores) in adolescence, one is concerned that the adolescent may be giving himself insufficient opportunity to experiment with the world, that possibly he is trying to shut off his adolescent development too soon. Hal's low Digit Span score suggests the probability that he is dealing with intense anxiety, again a state of affairs almost to be hoped for, certainly to be expected, in adolescence. His high Picture Arrangement score suggests his alertness to the social forces that surround him, an alertness that is clinically apparent. His high Arithmetic and Block Design subscores reflect Hal's general alertness, his brightness and his capacity for perceptual organization. His somewhat higher Performance than Verbal level suggests he may be more at ease "acting on" rather than "thinking about" matters. A tendency to find solutions through action is further suggested by the higher score on Block Design than on Similarities; both tests involve the requirement to form concepts, the former on a perceptual-motor (i.e., action), the latter on a verbal, level. A higher Comprehension than Information score is often seen among persons organized in terms of "appropriate," "good" and "acceptable" behavior; that is, among those who tend uncritically to accept the norms of the culture. Such a view of how the world does or should function is, of course, frequently seen in persons who have a "hysterical" character formation.]

INFORMATION

No.	Question	Response and Comments	Score
1.	Who is the President of the United States?	President Eisenhower. ("Who was President before that?") Truman. ("And before that?") . . . . . . Oh, I know, but I can't think . . Roosevelt! [This test was given in 1955, when President Roosevelt's name was much more in the air. Hal's comment, "I know, but I can't think," raises the question of repressive defenses.]	+
2.	What is a thermometer?	To check the temperature.	+
3.	What does rubber come from?	Rubber tree.	+
4.	Where is London?	England.	+
5.	How many pints make a quart?	Two.	+

No.	Question	Response and Comments	Score
6.	How many weeks are there in a year?	Fifty-two.	+
7.	What is the capital of Italy?	Rome. [Hal gives his responses clearly and easily, without wordy obsessiveness.]	+
8.	What is the capital of Japan?	. . . . That I don't know. ("Could you make a guess?") I have no idea. ("Can you think of any Japanese city?") Sing Pu is one. [The suspicion that Hal may have a repressive orientation is somewhat strengthened. Persons who rely on repressive defenses know notoriously little about world geography, and Hal has no idea about the name of any Japanese city. He blandly creates a Japanese-sounding name, which might have come from *The Mikado* or from some other musical.]	−
9.	How tall is the average American woman?	About five feet seven inches to five feet eight inches. ("Which do you think is nearer?") About five feet seven inches.	−
10.	Who invented the airplane?	Wright brothers.	+
11.	Where is Brazil?	. . . Brazil? . . . . Brazil. I keep thinking Brazil is just a country by itself. ("Where would it be?") South America. But Brazil is considered a country, isn't it? [Although Hal achieves credit on this response, his naïve way of handling the question is notable. Again, he becomes vague when asked to think beyond his immediate environment.]	+
12.	How far is it from Paris to New York?	It would be about . . 20,000. [More of the same.]	−
13.	What does the heart do?	Well, it functions to make the blood . . it pumps the blood to make it streaming through your body.	+
14.	Who wrote Hamlet?	Shakespeare.	+
15.	What is the population of the United States?	. . . . . Oh . . I don't know. ("Would you make a guess?") Oh . . 150 billion. I think that's way off. [As with geography, numbers have a way of throwing "hysterical" patients into vagueness. Numbers involve still another situation where they must function precisely. Precision requires a state of mind contrary to the preference of the person who typically relies on repression.]	−

No.	Question	Response and Comments	Score
16.	When is Washington's birthday?	The twenty-second . . the twenty-first. ("Of?") February. You know how I know that? It's the day after it today . . wait, it's the twenty-second. Look at your calendar over there. [The day was, indeed, the twenty-third of February.]	+
17.	Who discovered the North Pole?	Byrd . . North Pole . . Wait! . . Byrd discovered the South Pole, didn't he? ("What do you think?") I don't know . . the North Pole, I wouldn't know who did, but Byrd discovered the South Pole.	−
18.	Where is Egypt?	. . . . . . Egypt is in . . . . over by . . . . I know, but I just can't say it. ("Could you guess?") No. I couldn't. The movies take a lot of stories off of it. ("On what continent might it be?") That's what I'm trying to think. Over by France, I think, but I just can't remember to think of it today. What would your teacher do if she saw you write like that? (Referring to the fact that I have to write in the margin.) [Geography is once more Hal's downfall, and he comes up with an answer as wrong as it is naïve. His overconcern with propriety, with what "the teacher" might say if she saw me writing in the margin, is typical of the hysterical person's concern with the proprieties expected by authority and, of course, the "concern" also represents a not-too-subtle criticism of the examiner.]	−
19.	Who wrote Huckleberry Finn?	He wrote Tom Sawyer . . I just got through reading that last week . . Mark Twain. [The tendency to personalize—"I just got through," etc.—is frequently found among hysterical persons.]	+
20.	What is the Vatican?	I don't know. ("Have you heard of it?") No.	−

(Hal is unable to answer the remaining questions. He wonders whether *Habeas Corpus* wasn't "used in biology a little bit.")

RAW SCORE: 13

WEIGHTED SCORE: 10

COMPREHENSION

No.	Question	Response and Comments	Score
1.	What is the thing to do if you find an envelope in the street, that is sealed, and addressed and has a new stamp?	Well, I'd probably take it to the nearest mailbox and drop it in.	2

No.	Question	Response and Comments	Score
2.	*What should you do if while sitting in the movies you were the first person to discover a fire (or see smoke and fire)?*	I'd go up and, so that it wouldn't alarm everyone else, tell the manager, and so that it wouldn't alarm everybody before the manager knew about it. [Hal's emphasis on not alarming anyone suggests he is at least unconsciously struggling with a temptation to react impulsively. Apparently he seeks to control this tendency.]	2
3.	*Why should we keep away from bad company?*	Well . . the people see who you're running around with and judge you, and they might put your family down lower. [Hal is apparently less concerned with what a person is than with what he appears to be.]	1
4.	*Why should people pay taxes?*	Well, the country would go broke and . . . One way, if we didn't we wouldn't have a good government . . The country wouldn't be able to protect theirselves by arms or any other way.	1
5.	*Why are shoes made of leather?*	Well, leather shines up better than any other stuff, and probably it's the warmest stuff you can get, and probably you can wear it longer. ("Which of those answers would you choose?") I think the warmest would be the best. I never thought of it like that, but I don't think they make shoes out of any other stuff, hardly. [Although Hal is able to give correct answers, he is unable to choose the most correct one. The answer of leather being the "warmest" is not well thought through. His idea that leather "shines up better" again emphasizes his concern with the way things appear to others.]	0-1
6.	*Why does land in the city cost more than land in the country?*	Well, in the city you're living in a residential district, and in the city you're expected to keep it up more . . and there're more houses around, and you have to pay taxes. In the country, you can just dump anything on it. ("And why does land in the city cost more?") In a residential district your houses are built better, and usually paved streets are in front, and usually you've got your sewer taxes, too. [Again, Hal shows his preoccupation with the way things look—city land has to be "kept up." His sporadic passes and failures—on the next item he obtains full credit—underscore his satisfaction with the superficial, his readiness to accept whatever comes to mind, without thinking about it further or judging its appropriateness.]	0
7.	*If you were lost in a forest (woods) in the daytime,*	Well, your moss is on your north side of the tree . . and . . . you usually follow it, so you could find somewhere . . a road or something. [Hal's response	2

No.	Question	Response and Comments	Score

*how would you
go about finding
your way out?*

is about as vaguely put as it is possible to do and
still achieve full credit.]

8. *Why are laws
necessary?*

Well, if you didn't have laws, people would be
doing everything wrong and destroying other
people's property, and we just couldn't keep
anything looking pretty. [Hal expresses himself
naïvely—e.g., "doing everything wrong." He again
shows his concern with appearances.]

Score: 1

9. *Why does the
state require
people to get a
license in order
to be married?*

Well, that way they would have a record of who
got married . . and how many in the country and
state are married . . and just so that not anyone . .
was under age . . could go out and get married. (I
repeat the question.) Well, it's better to prevent
people who are under age from getting married.
Look at me, I'm going to school, but a lot of
people would get married if they had the chance.
You probably knew some like like that, too. [Hal
resorts to self-reference to justify his belief.]

Score: 1-2

10. *Why are people
who are born
deaf usually
unable to talk?*

Well, we got a boy up in our room like that. He
hasn't ever heard anyone talk . . No one could
train him to talk or anything. (I repeat the question.) They've just never heard anyone else talk
. . they've just never been able to hear 'em, to
try to train 'em. [Once again, the self-reference.]

Score: 2

RAW SCORE: ___12-14___

WEIGHTED SCORE: ___11-12___

DIGIT SPAN

(Hal repeats five Digits Forward on his second try. Although given three opportunities, he is unable to repeat six digits. He can repeat four Digits Backward,
and five on a third try.) [Hal's low score here suggests a high degree of anxiety
and emphasizes his low anxiety tolerance.]

RAW SCORE: ___9-10___

WEIGHTED SCORE: ___6-7___

ARITHMETIC

(Hal solves all problems except the ninth. It takes him ten seconds to do the
last problem, and he does the others in one-half to one second each. He loses
credit on the ninth problem, primarily because he rushes to his solution impulsively and makes several thoughtless errors.) [Hal's Arithmetic performance reflects
his basically efficient thought organization, marred by an impulsive tendency. He
could easily have achieved the top obtainable score, were it not for his headlong
rushing with its resulting carelessness.]

RAW SCORE: ___10___

WEIGHTED SCORE: ___13___

SIMILARITIES

No.	Items	Response and Comments	Score
1.	*Orange-banana*	Both fruit.	2
2.	*Coat-dress*	Both garments that you wear.	2
3.	*Dog-lion*	Both animals.	2
4.	*Wagon-bicycle*	Both on wheels and you can ride them . . they can be ridden on. [He changes to an apparently preferred functional orientation.]	1
5.	*Daily paper-radio*	Both . . you can hear news and what's happening.	1
6.	*Air-water*	Both a substance. ("Could you tell me a little more?") Well . . both of them . . both got oxygen and different articles of matter in 'em. [Note Hal's somewhat pretentious but basically careless way of expressing himself.]	0-1
7.	*Wood-alcohol*	Both got uh . . uh . . both . . Wood's got sap and alcohol a running deal, but I don't know how they both go together. Do you teach anything at the university? It's a pretty nice college. Have you ever been to K. State or K.U.? ["A running deal" is a fine example of Hal's rather careless expression. His shifting the task to ask instead of being asked suggests that he is beginning to sense difficulty.]	0
8.	*Eye-ear*	Both part of the body.	1
9.	*Egg-seed*	Well, both . . uh . . I don't . . Egg and a seed . . Well, they both go into some sort of food . . like a wheat seed and an egg . . both go into food.	0-1
10.	*Poem-statue*	A poem tells about something and a statue shows you. ("How would they be alike?") Well, on some statues there's a poem underneath them, telling what the guy did.	0
11.	*Praise-punishment*	Well, praise is when you do your job good, and punishment is when you flub it up. So, if you do a good job, you'll be praised, and when a good one . . I mean, a bad one, you'll be punished. ("And how are they alike?") I couldn't tell you . . except, when a guy robs a bank he's praised, but when he's caught, he's punished. I can't ever figure what makes them do that! Do you think it'll be all right to get a job? (He expresses concern about his ability to hold a job. With his "attacks," what will others think of him? Must he tell them? How long will his seizure condition last?) [Ever since Hal has experienced more difficulty answering questions, he has tended to go	0

No. Items	Response and Comments	Score

further afield in his answers and to ask about or say things that, on the surface, appear irrelevant. *Praise-punishment* triggers off thoughts of bank robbery, as well as concerns about ability to find work. One wonders whether, unconsciously, Hal equates "bank robbery" with his "attacks." To what extent do both represent "punishment?"]

12. *Fly-tree* Both are from . . both live outdoors . . and . . tree? 0-1
. . They both grow, but I don't see hardly how a fly grows . . but I guess they do. ("Which answer would you choose?") They both live outdoors. [Hal does less well on Similarities than on some other subtests. It is possible that the organic insult which is causing the seizures is also somewhat limiting his capacity to think abstractly. At the same time, it must be kept in mind that Hal is not a thoughtful, theoretically inclined person. He appears not to enjoy thinking abstractly and prefers instead a "functional," action approach. Originally one wonders if he could think abstractly were he required to, as he can with Arithmetic. Even with pressure, however, he does not seem able to unify some of the superficially discrepant Similarities items with an adequate abstraction.]

RAW SCORE: 9-12

WEIGHTED SCORE: 8-10

PICTURE COMPLETION

(Hal achieves full credit on ten Picture Completion items. On *Face,* he says, "Part of the nose is missing in this one, too. Oh . . half the mustache is missing (he laughs). On *Card,* he points to the corner numbers, one of which reads 9, while the other appears to read 6. He says, "Well, one of the numbers is wrong." He misses the *Mirror, Bulb* and *Girl* items. He works speedily, so that many of his responses—both right and wrong—are given in one to two seconds.) [Frequently Hal works quickly and efficiently. Almost as often, however, his nonreflectiveness produces not only speed, but error as well. Were he to give himself a little more time to contemplate what he does, he might be more accurate. A number of his errors are careless and, like his speech, the result of being satisfied with approximations.]

RAW SCORE: 10-11

WEIGHTED SCORE: 9-10

PICTURE ARRANGEMENT

(Hal sorts all items correctly and speedily, except for the third Arrangement which he sorts LMON. He tells the following story to this item: "About the King coming up the elevator . . and . . and coming down." He achieves extra time credit on the last two items.) [Again, Hal's thoughtless, headlong rushing penalizes him. Although he receives a very high score on this subtest, he could achieve an even higher one, were he less impulsive.]

RAW SCORE: 16

WEIGHTED SCORE: 14

BLOCK DESIGN

(Hal proceeds rapidly and efficiently, and achieves credit on every item, frequently with time credits. Strangely, he experiences his major difficulty on Sample B. He makes a totally erroneous design, sees his error and spontaneously corrects it. Still, he requires 28″ for all this.) [One often expects persons with "organic brain damage" to have difficulty on this subtest. Hal, however, performs exceedingly well on it. He shows an excellent capacity for analyzing the designs into their component parts and is almost never at a loss about how to proceed. His difficulty with Sample B is puzzling, but it seems probable that his difficulty is the result of the same old unreflective rush into action.]

RAW SCORE: 30

WEIGHTED SCORE: 14

OBJECT ASSEMBLY

(Characteristically, Hal proceeds rapidly and efficiently, although he makes impulsive little errors which he corrects when his attention is drawn to them. Thus, for example, he is able to complete the *Profile* item in 15″. The ear, however, is upside down. When I draw his attention to the profile and ask whether it is completely accurate, he sees his error and corrects it. The whole assembly, therefore, requires 10″ longer.)

RAW SCORE: 18-22

WEIGHTED SCORE: 10-13

DIGIT SYMBOL

(Although Hal does not demonstrate much speed, his symbols are drawn neatly and without error.)

RAW SCORE: 41

WEIGHTED SCORE: 10

VOCABULARY

(Hal again shows his tendency to give somewhat shabbily conceptualized and carelessly thought through responses. In defining *join,* for example, he says, "To go up with somebody else. ('How do you mean?') No . . to join . . uh . . to go with them." To *diamond,* he says, "Uh . . a jewel that is harder than any other subject, that will cut steel." He defines *shilling* as "a term of money." Of *guillotine* he says, "Oh! A device used in olden times . . to kill people with . . it consists of a sharp axe-type of deal.")

RAW SCORE: 21½

WEIGHTED SCORE: 10

STORY RECALL

IMMEDIATE RECALL

0   +1   +1   +1   +1

A week ago / in a small town / ten miles / from Albany / . . a flood went

0   +1   +1   −1   +1

into the city. Many persons / caught cold. / A man / cut his head / while sav-

+1   +1

ing / a boy / under a bridge. [Hal achieves an adequate score on this test. Apart from the fact he distorts *hand* into "head," his performance is not remarkable. It may well be that his distortion results from a hearing misperception rather than constituting a memory distortion.]

SCORE: 9−1+4 = 12

DELAYED RECALL

+1   0   +1   0

December 6, / a week ago, / a flood went over the banks / and ran into cities /

+1   0   0   0   +1

and into houses. Many people / were hurt, / and many / caught cold, / and a

+1   +1   +1   +1

man / cut his hand / saving a boy / by a bridge. That sort of makes the first one look bad (referring to what he feels is his much better performance on Delayed than on Immediate Recall.) (He wonders how long I had to go to school before I could do the work I am doing now.) [Even though Hal's score of 8 is rather poor, his memory seems fairly intact, although he manifests occasional distortions (e.g., "by" instead of "under" a bridge) and omissions. He does not show the type of fragmentation one often finds in brain-damaged persons. Evident again is his unconcern with precision—e.g., "many people were hurt and many caught cold," instead of *"fourteen persons were drowned and 600 persons caught cold."*]

SCORE: 8

THE BRL SORTING TEST

PART I

Stimulus	Patient's Sorting	Response and Comments	Score
1. Hal's choice: *Lock*	(After a long pause:) Well, I don't think there is anything that would go with it.	[This is the first strong indication of something being rather seriously amiss with Hal's concept formation, although it is possible that he penalizes himself by initially choosing one of the more difficult items for which to create a category. Hal's subsequent responses suggest, however, that his conceptual impairment is a genuine one.]	Failure

Stimulus	Patient's Sorting	Response and Comments	Score
2. Fork	(Knife; spoon; toy fork, knife and spoon; sugar.) These are supposed to be sugar, aren't they?	Well, a knife, fork and spoon are always used together, and sugar is usually dipped by a fork. ("How do you mean?") When it is in the sugar bowl . . to get it out. [The pattern of Hal's concrete thinking is becoming clearer. It is still not altogether certain, however, whether his concreteness is the result of inability or preference.]	Loose Concrete Def. Peculiar
3. Corncob pipe	(Cigar; matches; cigarette; rubber cigar.) Did that use to be a trick or something? (Referring to the rubber cigar.)	They're all smoked.	Functional Def.
4. Bell	Nothing goes with that one, either.	[Another somewhat difficult item. Still . . .]	Failure
5. Red paper circle	(Cardboard square; file card.)	They're all a shape . . As far as that's concerned, almost everything there (all remaining objects) would go together. ("And why do these that you've sorted go together?") They're all made of paper. [Hal first demonstrates his noncritical way of thinking; then, however, he pulls himself together sufficiently to offer a good concept.]	Syncretism; Conceptual Def. (Narrow)
6. Toy pliers	(Pliers; screwdriver; toy tools; nails.)	They're all tools . . to work on something with. (He helps return the items to the pile of objects.)	Conceptual Def. Functional Def.
7. Ball	Nothing else would go with that.	[This is Hal's third failure on Part I. Once again, he leaves unclear to what extent he fails because he does not wish to invest the time and effort, and to what extent he fails because he is not able to do better.]	Failure

PART II

Examiner's Sorting	Explanation and Comments	Score
1. Red objects	They're all a shape. (He is given the same grouping after he completes Part II:) They're all one color.	Syncretistic Conceptual Def.
2. Metal	(He first looks questioningly, to see whether he should add the screwdriver. I shake my head as I continue to put out more items. As I am putting them before him, he adds several metal items.) They're all metal. I caught on to that as soon as. . . .	Conceptual Def.
3. Round	They're all one shape . . and they're all used for something. ("Which would you choose?") They all got round.	Syncretistic Conceptual Def.
4. Tools	They're all used for tools.	Functional Def. Conceptual Def.
5. Paper	They're all made out of paper.	Conceptual Def.
6. Double	(Toward the end, he again has caught on to the intended concept and helps put out items. He begins to put out the cigarette and chalk as a pair, but changes his mind and replaces them.) They're all pairs.	Conceptual Def.
7. White	They're all one color.	Conceptual Def.
8. Rubber	They're all made out of rubber.	Conceptual Def.
9. Smoking	They're all used for somebody who smokes. That one (pipe) has never been used, has it? [Although Hal leans in a somewhat concrete direction on this response, he has until now been giving excellent Conceptual Definitions. He is able to conceptualize abstractly, if necessary. It is not certain whether he can do this *only* in the passive situation, where he is supplied with the required conceptual elements, or whether he can do it whenever he feels sufficiently motivated. Although his performance on Part II helps to answer the question whether his previous concreteness is determined by preference or disability, the question is still not answered fully;	Concrete Tendency Conceptual Def.

Examiner's Sorting	Explanation and Comments	Score
	it has, in fact, become more complex. To the dimensions of *abstract-functional preference versus ability* have been added those of *active-passive inclination*.]	
10. *Silver*	(He looks around for items to add.) They're all used for eating.	Functional Def.
11. *Toys*	They're all used for playing around . . by little kids.	Functional Def.
12. *Square*	Well . . they're all . . they use the same lines. What I mean is . . these (cardboard square and square block of wood) go together, and these go together . . They all have straight lines.	Conceptual Def. Split-Narrow Tendency
	[Probably Hal is able to think conceptually if he is required to. By and large, however, he prefers to think in terms of active "doing," rather than in terms of more static abstraction.]	

THE BENDER GESTALT TEST

PART A (PLATES 17 AND 18)

(Hal makes his first drawing—A—so large, and he places it so in the center of the page, that he wonders whether he should use new sheets for subsequent designs. He decides, however, to continue on the same sheet. He draws very quickly, almost without resting his hand on the paper.

(He begins Design 3, dislikes what he has made, but lets it be and begins again on a final version, counting softly to himself.

(On Design 5, he draws the rounded figure with dashes instead of dots. After he has completed the design, he changes many dashes to dots.

(He draws Design 6 on a new sheet of paper, after he has filled up the first page. He leaves too little room for other drawings he might need to make.

(He draws Design 7 without hesitation, as if drawing seems to present no difficulty whatever.)

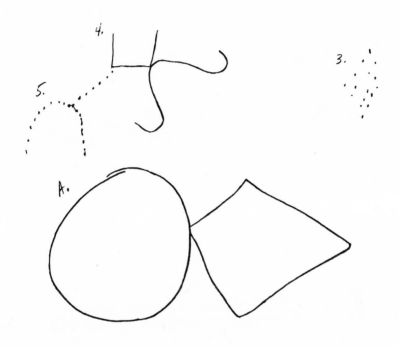

PLATE 17

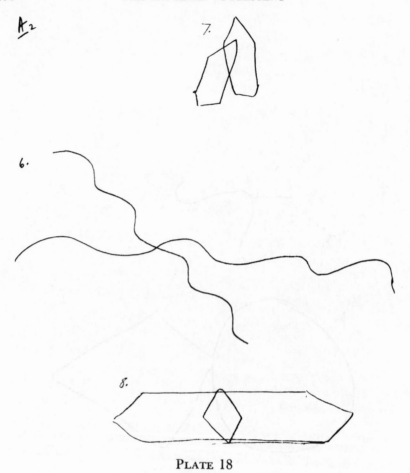

PLATE 18

PART B (PLATES 19 AND 20)

(These drawings are less hastily executed and are drawn nearer their original size. Hal does a good deal of counting of dots and circles. After he checks his count on Design 2, he says:) That has a lot to do with it, doesn't it? ("What does?") How many there is.

(After Design 3, he says:) I think I got this one right. I'm not sure, but I think I did.

(He asks:) You do this most of the day, don't you? [The implication is clear.]

[Although his Part A figures are less neat and precise than those of Part B, Hal's inaccuracies seem to be primarily the result of hurried execution. He does strikingly well when he copies the designs; if he is troubled by perceptual-motor dysfunctions, they certainly are not evident in his Bender drawings. If his seizures do have other psychological expression, it seems to be in the conceptual area (if even there). So far, Hal's ability has been significantly less than appropriate for his age only on Digit Span, on the active sorting of the BRL, and possibly on Similarities. His lowered Digit Span performance can best be attributed to poorly bound anxiety. And as has been said, it is difficult to know whether a conceptual limitation really exists or whether Hal's performance on this type of task

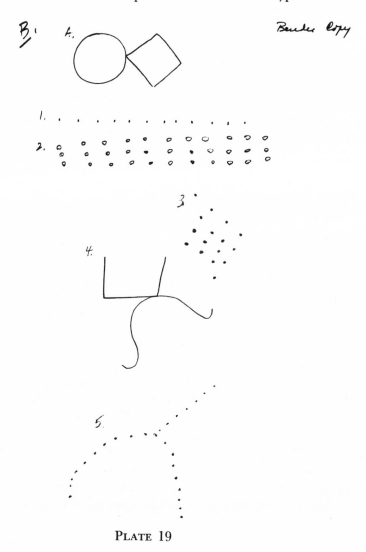

PLATE 19

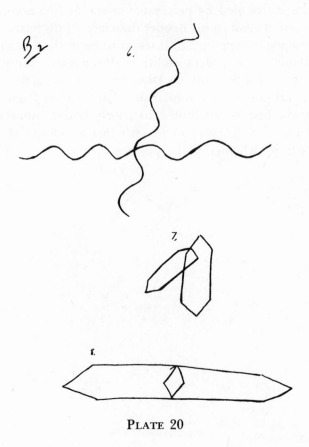

PLATE 20

reflects his preference for more functional, more passive functioning.

Significantly, Hal's drawings are poorly contained. He again demonstrates his impulsivity and splatters the drawings in the middle of a page, without regard for possible future needs for space. When he begins on another page, he shows the same poor planning. On Part B, however, he has apparently been able to use his experience sufficiently to organize more effectively for what is ahead. Although he requires almost as much area for his drawings as in Part A, the Part B drawings are placed in a much more orderly sequence.

[From the way Hal handles these drawings, and from the way he handled earlier material, it is apparent that he tends planlessly to plunge into activity, sometimes aware of possible consequences only after it is too late.]

THE TACTUAL FORM TEST

(On this test Hal shows well-functioning perceptual-motor ability. He is able to gain an accurate conception of forms through the tactual modality. His visual copies are reproduced with great accuracy.) [As on the Bender Gestalt Test, Hal shows no apparent impairment of formal perception.]

THE DRAW A PERSON TEST

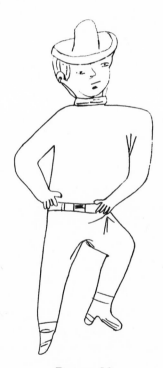

PLATE 21

PART I (PLATE 21)

(He draws quickly and effortlessly. Before he begins, he asks:) Could it be a cartoon?

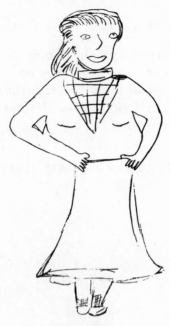

PLATE 22

PART II (PLATE 22)

(As he draws, he says:) The face don't matter too much, does it? (He asks what is the matter with an adolescent girl who shares the waiting room with him while both wait for their appointments.) Does she come in here? She's nice. She's smart.

[On Part I, Hal draws the kind of young man he wants to be (and which, in part, he probably is)—a devil-may-care cowboy who casually lounges with apparent ease, and who epitomizes action orientation. The figure probably represents Hal's almost conscious ego ideal. But while his drawing of a man seems entirely consistent with the picture of himself he has presented so far (action oriented, impulsive, nonreflective, dramatic and primarily self-oriented), the girl or young woman on Part II, by contrast, lacks the casualness, effortlessness and easy carelessness of the male. Hal requires many more obsessively executed lines to achieve a much less successful end product. Judging by this awkward, almost misshapen (certainly in contrast to Part I) drawing, one can infer the discomfort Hal probably experiences with girls. Although he has tried to make his young woman look feminine, he has made her appear aggressively masculine. She is stiff and unbending, in great contrast to the effortlessly disposed young man of drawing I.]

RORSCHACH TEST

RORSCHACH SCORING SHEET

Number of Responses: 21

Manner of Approach (Location)		*Groups of Contents*	
W	8	A	12
D	11	H	4
Dr	2	Obj.	1
De	0	Pl.	1
Total	21	Geol.	2
		Volcano	1

Location Percentages

W%	38			
D%	52	*Determinant and Content Percentages*		
Dr%	10	F%	67/95	Obj.%	5
De%	0	F+%	86/90	P%	57
		A%	57		

Form, Movement, Color and Shading Determinants

H% 19

F+	11
F—	0
F±	1	*Qualitative Material*
F∓	2	Popular	I II III IV V VII
M+	4		VIII IX X (4)
		Combination	VIII
FC+	2	Fabulation	3
(C)F	1	Vague	3
Total	21	Castration	2

EXPERIENCE BALANCE: 4.0/1.0

[Hal's Rorschach Psychogram does not present many surprises. He performs very much as one would expect, with his W and D emphasis, his high percentage of Popular responses, his tendency toward vagueness, his emphasis on easy content and his high F+ level. But what is surprising is his high number of Movement responses. A detailed study of these, however, reveals that, although of good form quality, they are nevertheless not well articulated and emerge as a result of quick, "easy" construction. Although a number of the Movement responses are Populars, one is struck by the vague, fluid fashion in which they are formulated and described. Hal continues to convey the impression of someone who has considerable basic intelligence and capability which, however, he does not take the effort to develop.]

RORSCHACH PROTOCOL

Card #	React. Time	Score	Protocol	Inquiry and Observations
I	2″	WF+AP	1. A bat. ("Anything else?") Can I turn it upside down? ("Sure.") ∨ ∧ > I sure can't see anything else in it. Oh . . wait! . . . I can't see anything else in it. ("Anything at all?")	
		WM±H Fab. Vague	2. Just here for a moment, I thought I saw something running away . . girls or boys . . and something holding them in the middle. But I don't know.	2. ("You saw something holding them?") I don't know. ("Tell me what it seemed like.") Just seemed like . . I don't know. ("Did they seem to be girls or boys?") Boys. [Hal sets the scene for vagueness. Things appear to him momentarily, only to disappear again. His lack of thinking things through is exemplified by such phrases as "something holding them" and "it just seemed like . . I don't know."]
II	4″	WFC+A	∨ 1. Well, it looks like a butterfly.	1. ("Tell me about the butterfly.") Well, it had tentacles going down . . and red and . . Oh, just like any regular one. [More vagueness.]
		WM+H(P) Cast. Fab.	∧ 2. Then it looks like two persons clapping hands . . with their hands in the middle, and their legs going down. That's about all I can see.	2. ("And the persons clapping hands?") Well, it looked like they had long, pointed heads, and then their feet was off or something . . or like they continued someplace else. ("What makes it look like that?") Just jagged at the bottom.

(As I write his name on top of the next page he says:) By the time I get out of here, you should know my name, at least. [Will he not let me know much else?] |

Card #	React. Time	Score	Protocol	Inquiry and Observations
III	4"	WM+HP	1. Well, it looks like two persons taking something out of a basket.	1. ("What kind of persons?") Women. ("What makes it look like that?") Well, they had on .. well, just the features, and they had on long heels. [He does not mention the bosom —which most obviously makes them resemble women.]
		Vague	And it looks like something in the background, but I don't know what it is.	("Tell me about the 'something in the background.' ") Just two little spots up there (red D's), but I wouldn't know what it would be.
IV	29"	DF+Obj(P)	∨ (16") .... ∧ 1. Well, I see a pair of boots. > And ..... that's about it.	
V	12"	WF+AP	1. That looks more like a butterfly than the other one did. That's all I can see in it.	
		DF+A	2. Oh, and another thing. Right here in the middle, it looks something like a rabbit .. but that other stuff doesn't look like it ... I don't know where I ever got that at.	[Hal seems surprised—"I don't know where I ever got that at" —by one of his mental products. He wonders about quite an ordinary, frequently given percept and seems objectively to disown responsibility for his mental contents.]
VI			∨ ∧ (After 17", he says, "Hm.") (After 30" of studying the card, he says:) I can't see anything in it. ("See if you can't see something.") Well .... (He gives a long yawn.)	

Card #	React. Time	Score	Protocol	Inquiry and Observations
	75″	WF∓A Fab. Vague Cast.	1. Well, it looks like some sort of a bush, with something looking out on each side . . maybe a fox, or a bear, or something.	1. ("Tell me a little about it.") I don't know . . . . just like maybe a tree starting to grow again, after the stump had been hacked . . . . with just twigs coming out of it. ("And what about 'something looking out on each side'?") Well, you couldn't see the full body of whatever it was, so something had to be in front of it, so I just thought it had to be a bush or something. [The poignant expression of inadequacy at first seems at variance with Hal's drawing of a man. A closer look at the drawing, however, shows that it resembles a boy much more than a man. It is significant that this theme of impotence emerges on a card with such a strong phallic component and after such a lengthy initial delay.]
VII	3″	DM+H(P)	1. Well, I see a little Indian, with its feathers going up there, and then its arrows on the back. ∨ ∧ And that's about all I can see.	1. ("Tell me about the little Indian.") Well, it was just with an arrow pack on its back and a feather on its head. It had sort of a square head. ("Can you tell me any more about it?") It was just sort of standing there.
VIII	10″	DF+AP	1. Well, I see some sort of animal. There's its four legs, and climbing. ∨ ∧	1. ("What kind of animal?") I don't know. Just a four-footed animal.
	Comb.	DrF±pl.	2. And a big tree. There goes its bark . .	2. and 3. ("Tell me a little about the tree.") I don't know. It was just straight down and just out from nowhere. And then it looked like a mountain behind it. [Within the vagueness, Hal might well be talking about himself.]
		DrF∓geol.	3. It seems to be growing out of a bunch of rocks.	

Card #	React. Time	Score	Protocol	Inquiry and Observations
		D(C)F geol.	4. W a i t , t h i s could be a mountain . . this is a cliff . . and then, rocks down at the bottom.	4. ("Would you describe the mountain?") It was round, sort of, with a shadow on 'em . . . . ("How do you mean?") Just like the sun casting on one side and the other side was dark. [This is a sensitively organized response, one which is more carefully constructed than the others. It suggests that Hal is capable of a sensitivity which emerges in special circumstances, possibly in spite of himself.]
IX			∨ I sure can't see nothing in this! (He laughs.) Oh, wait a minute.	
	40″	WFC+Volc. (P)	1. Here comes your mountain up here . . and your volcano, with the smoke coming out of it, and the lava coming down the side.	1. ("Tell me about the lava.") Just that smoke above it, and the top of the mountain apart like that. So it looks like it was erupting. ("Could you see the lava?") Yeah, the orange that was coming down. ("And the smoke?") Just a blue smoke. (I show him the card.) I mean, it was orange.
X			∨ (Immedi- ∧ ately.)	
	4″	DF+AP	1. Well, here's two crabs.	
		DF+A	2. And here's two little gophers.	2. ("What makes them look like gophers?") Well, sort of . just sort of the shape of a gopher. (Bottom side sepia D's.)
		DF+AP	3. Two dogs.	3. ("What kind of dogs did they seem to be?") Collies. (Yellow D's.)
		DF+AP	4. And here's a little face. It looks like a rabbit's face. And it looks like . . . . . (laughs) . . > ∧ > <	

Card #	React. Time	Score	Protocol	Inquiry and Observations
		DF+AP	5. And this looks like two little animals. I don't know exactly what they'd be. It looks like they're climbing up a piece of a tree.	(Top center D.)
		DF+A	∨ 6. And here's two . . uh . . sea horses.	6. ("Tell me about the sea horses.") Well, it just . . their head came down like this . . usually like you see in the show or something. (Bottom center green D's.)

THEMATIC APPERCEPTION TEST, WORD ASSOCIATION TEST AND SENTENCE COMPLETION TEST

[Hal reveals extremely little on the Thematic Apperception, Word Association and Sentence Completion Tests.]

(A typical Thematic Apperception Test story is the following told to Card 3 BM:) Well, it's about someone who's just heard some tragic news and just went off crying or something, and I don't know what to think about it. It's pretty sad. ("What is the tragic news?") I wouldn't know. Maybe her husband or boy friend was lost overseas on a mission, or something. ("And how does it all work out?") Well, in the end he comes back, and they're happy. (Hal's other TAT stories are similarly vague and unrevealing.) [Repressive defenses seem so strong that Hal keeps himself entirely unaware of conflict. As has been obvious on his other test responses, he permits himself only limited awareness about the content of his thoughts. Although Hal's TAT stories tend to be brief and nonrevealing, they reflect his feeling that a warm, close bond exists between him and the rest of his immediate family.

[Typical of his defending himself against "knowing" is his reaction to all sexual words on the Word Association Test.] (To the word *penis*, he responds, "What's that?" I repeat the word. "I couldn't think that right there." On Recall, he waits 6″, and then says "I can't remember what I said." Questioned, he says, "I didn't know what the word meant." ["What do you think it means?"] "It's part of the body, isn't it?" ["Do you have any idea what part it might be?"] "Not right offhand." To the word *vagina*, he responds, "mound," after 3″. He adds, "I've heard it somewhere." On inquiry, he explains, "Well, I didn't know what it meant. I was thinking for a minute it was some sort of sickness. I don't know quite what it means." ["Do you have any idea?"] "I was trying to remember what it was. I've heard it on . . I've heard it on *Medic,* I think before. It would be used on that, wouldn't it?" To the word *masturbation,* he responds "Biology," after 9″, and adds, "I was trying to think what that meant." To the word *intercourse,* he says, "College," after 4″. On inquiry, he explains, "I couldn't quite place it. There's an intercourse in college, isn't there?" ["What is that?"] "Well, a more advanced subject.") [It is apparent that Hal "knows," although his conscious conception of these words is undifferentiated. He appears busily to repress more explicitly differentiated meanings, but he is not altogether successful in his endeavor.

[Hal's reaction to Sentence Completion is similar to his reaction to the other two tests. His endings are bland and unrevealing. He says little that would encourage another person to want to know him better. He permits almost no personal information to slip through his repressive (suppressive?) barricade. He gives very little information which would make others aware there was more to him than appeared on the surface.]

The Psychologist's Report

Hal's Wechsler-Bellevue Intelligence Quotient is in the Bright Normal range (Total Quotient 111-117; Verbal 109-113; Performance 111-117). His general manner, however, appears much duller because he needs to play down the alertness and sensitivity which are potentially available to him. He often appears naïve and bland, and he uses repression to a great degree. Thus his thinking tends to be superficial and imprecise; he expresses his knowledge vaguely and approximately; his judgments, decisions and solutions tend to be thoughtlessly, impulsively and poorly thought through. His problem solving is nonreflective so that he makes numerous careless errors. He plans poorly because he cannot wait and because he needs to do things "right now," regardless of consequences. He is concerned with the appearance of things, rather than with their intrinsic worth. He frequently uses his own experiences to justify what he should decide on an objective basis, even though he experiences distance from his own mental products. Thus, he is occasionally surprised at thoughts which occur to him, and he may refuse to take responsibility for them. All these characteristics, together with a high anxiety level, organize themselves into a diagnosis of a hysterical character.

It is surprising, in a person so repressively oriented, to find the high number of Movement responses which he is able to organize on the Rorschach. Two things are apparent, however. Hal's Movement responses are not sharply defined and require a great deal of inquiry to emerge clearly. Second, Hal does not utilize the abilities he has. His good Intelligence Quotient and his high number of Movement responses both suggest that he is capable of much more alertness, sensitivity and capacity for delay than he wishes to exert.

Hal's self-concept is expectedly vague; he does not appear to think about himself very much. He wants to be a casual, devil-may-care doer of deeds, but it is doubtful that he comes as near to this ideal as he wishes.

It is difficult to say to what extent the impairments that cause Hal's seizures affect his other psychological abilities. He does excellently on such Performance items as the Block Design subtest. At the same time, he seems to experience some interference with the capacity to form adequate conceptualizations. Still, it is almost impossible to determine to what extent Hal's somewhat lowered performance on such tests as Similarities and the BRL Sorting Test may be attributed to a lessened ability on the one hand, or to a preference for thinking in terms of action rather than more static abstractions on the other. On the passive sorting of the BRL, for example, he is able to solve many problems on an abstract conceptual level. Does he do better here because the task is easier, or because he prefers a more passive position, which requires less energy expenditure of him? Maybe he conceptualizes abstractly when this is the only way open; possibly he can function more abstractly when some of the work is done for him.

There is a suggestion that Hal finds himself uncomfortable in heterosexual situations, that he feels that girls and women exploit men and make them psychologically impotent. Although he sometimes expresses considerable aggression toward women (e.g., his TAT story of the husband who kills the wife), he ordinarily denies this sort of destructive feeling along with others. Thus, in Hal's

TAT wife-murder story, he explains that the wife really does not die at all. Repression is particularly marked in the sexual realm. Hal denies knowledge of all sexual words on the Word Association Test, although his marked blocking on these words and the content of his associations make clear he has at least preconscious familiarity with them.

Considerable warmth seems to exist within Hal's family. Hal reflects his parents' values regarding right and wrong behavior. He indicates, for example, that he would abstain from certain behavior because his mother would find it displeasing. Two TAT stories in which father and son listen to a story together, and another in which father and son go to work together, suggest the closeness between Hal and his father.

In summary, Hal is a boy of high average intelligence whose personality is organized along strongly repressive and impulsive lines. His marked use of denial prevents him from accepting the severity of his illness; without help, it is quite possible that he may ignore the potential danger to himself and others of activities in which he wishes to engage. A relatively brief series of therapeutic sessions is recommended. Their purpose would be to clarify Hal's illness to him, to help him face and accept its implications and to help him with a realistic plan for the future.

Discussion

Hal emerges as an almost sixteen-year-old adolescent who needs to appear uninteresting and uncomplicated. He depends enormously on his repressive defenses and appears to go harmlessly through life, not hurting anyone and seemingly not aware of hurts which the world may inflict.

Adolescence poses two major problems for him: The first involves his serious convulsive disorder, the second his major repressive reaction, both specifically to the disorder, and, more generally, to his inner and outer world. He chooses to ignore an aspect of reality (i.e., his seizures) which may potentially complicate his life enormously, all the more so if the denial continues. Although he asks whether he will be able to take on a job or drive a car, he seems to wonder about these matters primarily in terms of gaining permission from authority, rather than in terms of possible problems and dangers involved for himself and others. Hal, in other words, approaches adulthood unrealistically. He can not continue to ignore potential problems which will arise in connection with his "epilepsy." Although others may admire him for being "brave" in the face of his severe disability, Hal's "courage" may well get him into trouble. The seizures involve only one of the reality features (probably the most troublesome) Hal chooses repressively to ignore. To the degree that he needs to continue to perceive inner and outer reality vaguely and fuzzily, he will not be able to deal with it effectively.

Conclusion

Two adolescents suffering from so-called "organic brain damage" have been discussed in this chapter. Hopefully, a number of truisms have been illustrated: (1) persons react individually to brain damage; (2) altogether different functions may be involved in the condition; (3) "organic" difficulties are not invariably picked up on psychological testing or neurological examination; (4) "brain damage" always occurs within a context of personality organization. As was already apparent with the retarded adolescents discussed in the preceding chapter, impairments noted in these conditions have their primary meaning given them by the person afflicted with them. He may ignore his disabilities, compensate for them, recognize them, try to overcome them, suffer with them, gain courage from them, derive secondary satisfaction from them and so forth. A disability obviously does not have the same impairment meaning in different people. Whatever meanings it achieves are those attributed by the person who has the impairment.

So far, we have dealt with conditions which affect primarily the cognitive area of functioning. Starting with the next chapter, we will deal with adolescents suffering from so-called "schizophrenic" disorders which, in different ratios, affect both cognitive and affective areas.

4

The Disorganized Adolescent

Al and Bill, the two adolescents whose test protocols follow, seem to have almost nothing in common but a diagnosis of "schizophrenia." Al is at the mercy of poorly differentiated, grossly biologically determined impulses, over which at times he has no control and which often flood his entire consciousness. Bill seems polished where Al is gross; restrained where Al gives in to impulse; "correct" where Al appears vulgar. Bill functions socially much more effectively than Al—he is more able, more sensitive, more differentiated and has many more facets to him. Yet, with present-day nomenclature, both are considered to have essentially the same diagnosis. What characteristics connect the psychological organizations of these adolescent boys so they can be given almost identical labels? Does the diagnosis capture a significant similarity or does it actually muddy major differences?

CLINICAL SUMMARY: Al

Al is thirteen years old and has a sister who is ten. He has suffered with severe psychological problems all his life and has been referred to agencies for diagnosis and treatment since the age of two. He has been variously diagnosed as mongoloid, schizophrenic and brain damaged. He has had major difficulties in school and has always gotten along very badly with both children and adults. His behavior has never been anything but strange and disruptive, and recently has become acutely disturbed and disturbing.

Al's mother resented her pregnancy with Al, her first, because it forced her to stop working. She had many difficulties during pregnancy, including pus in her urine, severe bleeding in the third month, persistent low back pains and many colds and chills during the seventh month. Delivery was uncomplicated, but Al was breast fed for only one month because his mother developed mastitis. She

221

continued to work while he was from one to sixteen months old. At that time, she returned home because the people who were supposed to care for Al were, for one reason or another, entirely unsatisfactory.

The parents were extremely rigid in their upbringing of Al—they rarely picked him up, and left him to himself most of the time. In order to prevent thumb-sucking, they forcibly removed his thumb from his mouth. They required him always to use his right hand. When he was still not toilet trained at the age of three years, the father spent several days with him, reminding him constantly to go to the toilet. The mother threatened to make Al eat his feces if he continued to soil himself; once she actually put feces on his mouth.

Though Al's early motor development was normal, his later development was slower. He spoke a few words at eighteen months, but then he stopped speaking and did not start again until after he was four years old. He has had asthma and hay fever since the age of four, but these conditions seem to have become less severe lately.

As an infant, Al cared very little for people. He had severe screaming spells until the age of three, and from the age of two to five he was in the habit of wandering around the house at night, finally climbing into bed with his mother. He began repetitive and almost constant rocking at twelve months, and he seemed to ignore others while doing this. He had fears of large buildings, darkness, ghosts and frightening animals. He is still fearful of being hurt, develops frequent preoccupations with crime and punishment and avidly reads newspaper accounts of crimes. Since a very early age, he has been scratching and biting himself, his mother, and, more recently, girls his own age.

At the age of three and a half he was seen in psychiatric consultations, and a diagnosis of a possible organic defect was advanced. At the age of four, he achieved a Stanford-Binet I.Q. of 57 and a Merrill-Palmer Quotient of 68. At that time a diagnosis of "Retardation with dyslexia" was made. At the age of ten, he was studied once more and given a diagnosis of "Childhood schizophrenia, with undetermined organic substrate." He had two months of treatment at that time, but the treatment was abruptly terminated by the parents because of their vacation. Another diagnosis of "Autism with retardation" was made a little later. He now achieved a Stanford-Binet I.Q. of 103, and his performance was marked by wide scatter. After some time in private schools, he was placed in a public school, where he was reported to be disruptive and provocative. A psychiatrist recommended that he be removed from school and placed in a residential treatment center. He spent the last year in a private school, but made very little academic progress, and his behavior was extremely disturbing to his fellow students and teachers.

Lately, Al has become acutely disturbed, has masturbated publicly, exposed himself, touched various girls and women in public, run away from school, burned matches and made constant sexual approaches to his mother. He has recently been hospitalized elsewhere and has been given a diagnosis of "Schizophrenia with some organic substrate."

Physical and Neurological Data: The physical examination is within normal limits. The neurological consultant found evidence of relatively mild developmental motor aphasia, accompanied by mild motor incoordination and mild dysarthria. None of these problems seem to require further neurological investigation or treatment at this time. Laboratory data were within normal limits.

THE PSYCHOLOGIST'S DESCRIPTION

Al's most immediately arresting characteristic is his flat, loud, penetrating voice. His facial expression, too, does not undergo affective change, even when he expresses thoughts which are ordinarily accompanied by intense feeling. Instead of modulated emotional expression, he seems capable only of making a grimace—a frozen, mirthless smile, sometimes accompanied by a nervous, unpleasant giggle.

Particularly after we first meet, Al shows an intense need to maintain control. Each time I wonder whether I might ask the first test question, he says he has not quite finished what he has to tell me. It is necessary almost literally to push through Al's obsessive, fearful defensiveness, since otherwise no testing might ever be begun.

Compulsively, and in great detail, he tells about the hospital from which he just came, about other patients, nurses, doctors and particularly about "bad treatment" he feels he received there. His hospital stories are concerned almost exclusively with how "nice" or "mean" the other people there were. He expresses particular anger about having been placed in physical restraints and talks a great deal about old men, fellow patients, whose symptoms had been ignored and who had been humiliated and left to die. He asks many questions about how we would treat disturbed children here and wonders if we would lose our tempers with them and become angry or "fresh."

During the last testing hour, Al was almost entirely preoccupied with outright sexual, anal and urethral thoughts, as well as with thoughts concerning vomit, death and diarrhea. When observed as he was tested in the one-way vision room, he masturbated through his clothing, and toward the end of the hour he was about to expose himself, but he was able to stop when told to. During a previous hour, Al was concerned that he would not be able to urinate for his laboratory examination. For this reason, he compulsively drank liquid and said that, if he needed to go to the bathroom, I had better take him to the lab immediately, since otherwise he would have to urinate in his Coke bottle. During the time we were together, he laughingly passed flatus, belched loudly, spat on the floor and ate Kleenex.

THE WECHSLER-BELLEVUE SCALE

Name: __Al__   Age: __13-9__

	RS	WTS	0 1 2 3 4 5 6 7 8 9 10 11 12 13 14 15 16 17 18 19 20
COMPR.	6	5	
INFOR.	9-10	7-8	
DIG.	8	4	
ARITH.	3-4	3-4	
SIMIL.	8	7	
VOCAB.	16	7	
P. A.	6	6	
P. C.	5-6	3-4	
B. D.	3-6	3-4	
O. A.	10	4	
D. S.	20	5	

TOT. VERB.	29-31
TOT. PERF.	21-23
TOT. SCALE	50-54

VERBAL I.Q.: __78-81__   LEVEL: __Borderline→Dull Normal__

PERFORMANCE I.Q.: __61-64__   LEVEL: __Defective__

TOTAL I.Q.: __66-69__   LEVEL: __Borderline__

[Since the appearance of the WISC, one would probably administer the WISC instead of the Wechsler-Bellevue to Al. At the time Al was tested, however, it was thought that the Wechsler would reflect his abilities most accurately. Al's present Intelligence Quotient of 66-69 is similar to the ones he achieved at the age of four (Stanford-Binet I.Q. 57; Merrill-Palmer I.Q. 68), but much lower than the Stanford-Binet I.Q. of 103 which he achieved at the age of ten. Either Al has again become much more disorganized during the last three or four years, or the W-B is more sensitive to his disabilities than the Stanford-Binet. Had there been more testing time available, it would have been important to readminister the Stanford-Binet. Al's subtest abilities scatter somewhat (from 3 to 7), but not remarkably; one will want to check whether these final scores result from rather divergent within-subtest passes and failures (as it turns out they do). From the Scattergram alone one can determine little more than that Al functions primarily in the Borderline range of intelligence. Later on, in the actual test protocol, the reader can almost immediately see the extent not only of Al's *sub*organization, but of his *dis*organization.]

(Before he can permit himself to be asked any test questions, Al tells innumerable stories and makes it very difficult for the examiner to get a word in edgewise. Al keeps saying, "Let me finish my story," as he tells of doctors he has had who were "strict," or "nice," or "mean." In a highly pressured way, he gives the dates of his previous hospitalizations, tells about hospital "punishments" he has received and goes into limitless detail about his past behavior. He frequently rocks in his chair or walks around the room. Many of his stories have to do with how he has needed to giggle in the past, and after he is told he may giggle, he occasionally stops pacing and storytelling in order to giggle self-consciously.)

INFORMATION

No.	Question	Response and Comments	Score
		("Can I start asking you questions now?") Not quite yet. I have to finish my story. (He continues with a long, rambling, rather incoherent tale, and it becomes increasingly obvious how afraid he is to let me start asking him test questions.)	
1.	*Who is the President of the United States?*	Eisenhower. ("And who was president before him?") Truman! ("And before him?") Roosevelt.	+

No. Question	Response and Comments	Score
2. *What is a thermometer?*	Something that you take a temperature with.	+
3. *What does rubber come from?*	A tree.	+
4. *Where is London?*	England. [So far, Al's responses have been correct and appropriate.]	+
5. *How many pints make a quart?*	Sixteen. ("Are you sure?") I don't know exactly. [Here it starts.]	–
6. *How many weeks are there in a year?*	I don't know. ("Make a guess.") Sixteen? [For the moment at least, "sixteen" covers up not knowing the correct answer.]	–
7. *What is the capital of Italy?*	Rome.	+
8. *What is the capital of Japan?*	Uh . . I don't know that. ("Make a guess.") . . Hong Kong.	–
9. *How tall is the average American woman?*	This tall. (He demonstrates a height with his hands.) ("How tall is that?") Four feet. [This is an exceedingly childish way of estimating a dimension. It is reminiscent of the four-year-old who shows a number of fingers to tell his age.]	–
10. *Who invented the airplane?*	. . . . . . Uh . . Who invented the airplane? . . The Wright brothers. I'm cooperating. You're better doctors than those at A_____.[1] They once laughed at a boy. (He talks about an old man vomiting and having diarrhea, and he goes on and on about this.) [The strange sequence of passes and failures (e.g., knowing who invented the airplane but not how many weeks are in a year) is typical of persons with Al's particular type of severe disorganization. While a person who is primarily "retarded" tends to fail *all* items as they become more difficult, someone with major *cognitive and affective disorganization* passes and fails sporadically, as Al continues to do. Al's autobiographical storytelling, although it intrudes somewhat, does not take over as it will later, when his anxiety mounts even more. One of Al's primary wishes is to show how hard he tries and how, therefore, the accusations of others are unfair.]	+

[1] The previous hospital at which he stayed.

No.	Question	Response and Comments	Score
11.	*Where is Brazil?*	. . . . . . (He talks in a pressured way, on and on, about his past experience.) (I repeat the question.) South America.	+
12.	*How far is it from Paris to New York?*	One thousand.	−
13.	*What does the heart do?*	It beats. ("Could you tell me some more about it?") For your blood. ("How do you mean?") It pumps blood through your system.	+
14.	*Who wrote Hamlet?*	Uh . . . . I don't know. ("Does any name come to mind?") Edward . . Edward Thompson. [This name, which appears in modified form later on, may have a private meaning of some sort.]	−
15.	*What is the population of the United States?*	Uh . . Population of the United States . . A million people. [Numbers offer Al a particular problem. So far, he has failed all questions that require his answering with a specific number.]	−
16.	*When is Washington's birthday?*	March.	−
17.	*Who discovered the North Pole?*	Thomas Peary. [Might this be Edward *Thompson,* in modified form?]	− +
18.	*Where is Egypt?*	In . . Africa. [!]	+
19.	*Who wrote Huckleberry Finn?*	*Tom Sawyer.*	−
20.	*What is the Vatican?*	I don't know. ("Have you heard of it?") Never.	−

(He cannot answer the remaining questions.)
[Not only do Al's preceding responses demonstrate peculiar, arbitrary tendencies, as well as major obsessive concerns regarding his prior hospitalizations, but the erratic pattern of successes and failures suggests that there are islands of effective functioning in the midst of areas that function poorly or not at all.]

RAW SCORE: 9-10

WEIGHTED SCORE: 7-8

COMPREHENSION

No.	Question	Response and Comments	Score
1.	*What is the thing to do if you find an envelope in the street, that is sealed, and addressed and has a new stamp?*	Call the police. ("Why would you do that?") Because I don't know who it belongs to . . and the police are smart guys, and they can help find out. [This response reflects both the degree to which Al's problem solving is occasionally naïvely dissociated from practicality and "common sense," and the extent to which he depends on authority to solve relatively simple problems for him. It apparently does not occur to him to act autonomously in this situation.]	0

No.	Question	Response and Comments	Score
2.	*What should you do if while sitting in the movies you were the first person to discover a fire (or see smoke and fire)?*	I was asked that question before. Warn everybody. I'd yell, "I see a fire!!" [Al's reaction points up both his sense of continuity with the past—"I was asked that question before"—and his tendency to act impulsively, regardless of consequence.]	0
3.	*Why should we keep away from bad company?*	I don't avoid bad company. Because they get you in trouble. I enjoy bad company . . you mean like bad kids? I enjoy it. I went with them. I had a burning feeling in my penis because of yellow urine, and that also could have caused it. (He asks questions about the inpatient department.) This school sounds like a good school. (He asks many questions about discipline.) [Significant is Al's apparent lack of shame. He undoubtedly likes "bad company," but one is taken aback by the openness with which he admits this preference for the "bad" and by his lack of apparent defensiveness about it.]	1
4.	*Why should people pay taxes?*	To pay the government. ("How do you mean?") I don't know.	1
5.	*Why are shoes made of leather?*	Because . . I don't know that. ("Make a guess.") Because they're warm for your feet. ("Can you think of any other reasons?") They're . . . . . . comfortable.	1
6.	*Why does land in the city cost more than land in the country?*	Cause ther're more people. ("Why would that make it more expensive?") I don't know. ("Can you think of any reason?") No. [Al teeters on the edge of an answer that would give him full credit, but he is not quite able to give it.]	1
7.	*If you were lost in a forest (woods) in the daytime, how would you go about finding your way out?*	I don't know. ("Can you think of any way?") Look for signs, perhaps. ("How do you mean?") Signs to help find my way out. (He walks around the room and sits in a chair well removed from my desk.) I'd like to go to one of these psychiatric schools. I think they're nice. [One can see how Al needs to leave the field, literally and figuratively, as the intellectual going gets rougher.]	0
8.	*Why are laws necessary?*	To protect yourself and other people.	1
9.	*Why does the state require people to get a license in order to be married?*	I don't know. ("Can you think of any reason?") So . . to pay a tax.	0

No. Question	Response and Comments	Score
10. *Why are people who are born deaf usually unable to talk?*	Because they can't hear. ("And how would that work?") I feel jittery and have to rush back and forth. (He does.) I like to rock and can't stop. (He does.) I heard something on the radio that gives me a jittery feeling down my leg and penis. Once I was going to kill father and mother, but my grandmother stopped me by squeezing my hand so hard I had to drop the knife (etc., etc.). [Even on such a well-structured test as the Wechsler-Bellevue, Al's obsessive concerns and memories intrude. He is excessively preoccupied with himself and feels everyone must or should be equally caught up in his peculiarities. In part, of course, Al's recounting of his symptoms is somewhat appropriate, since he considers it the examiner's job to find out as much as he can in order to be of maximum help. Al finds it so easy to talk about his symptoms, however, and experiences so little apparent conflict about describing them, one feels he must almost constantly indulge himself in this way. Do the preoccupations compulsively issue forth because Al finds the test material increasingly hard to handle, or is the material hard to handle because the obsessions take over almost all of Al's consciousness, leaving almost no primary ego autonomy available for a task Al does not consider at all central to his welfare?]	1

RAW SCORE: ___6___

WEIGHTED SCORE: ___5___

DIGIT SPAN

(Al repeats five Digits Forward correctly. When he tries six, he consistently exchanges the sequence of two numbers. He repeats three Digits Backward correctly, but he becomes confused with four. At one point he says:) I want to do it because I want to get to the bottom of my problems. (He tells a story about how cruel the police have been to him.) [It is difficult to evaluate Al's sincerity when he says he wants to get to the bottom of his problems, or when he makes similar comments. He undoubtedly wishes to suffer less and to have his situation eased. It seems, however, that he tries to conform to what he thinks are the wishes of the significant adults (i.e., that he act "better," try "harder," give in less to his illness). One cannot avoid feeling that, in a highly intellectualized way, Al says things that he thinks are expected, but that he has no real conviction about getting to the bottom of his problems, nor much understanding of what "getting to the bottom" might entail.]

RAW SCORE: ___8___

WEIGHTED SCORE: ___4___

ARITHMETIC

No. Problem	Time	Response and Comments	Score
1. How much is four dollars and five dollars?	1½"	Nine.	1
2. If a man buys six cents worth of stamps and gives the clerk ten cents, how much change should he get back?	21"	What did you say? (18") (I repeat the problem.) Ten, take away six, is three . . is four. (21") One nurse at A_____ was real nice. She had blond hair.	0-1
3. If a man buys eight cents worth of stamps and gives the clerk twenty-five cents, how much change should he get back?	—	What did you say? (18") Eight and sixteen is twenty-four . . take away something . . and add seven, is fifteen. I don't know. I just don't know. Also, there was one fat nurse there who was nice. I couldn't sleep at all last night. [Al's need to present himself as extremely disturbed is apparent. He repeats the behavior he showed in response to Problem 2, i.e., not hearing the question because of intrusive thoughts. On Problem 2, the absent-mindedness seems genuine, but when he again asks, "What did you say?" after letting exactly the same amount of time pass, the absent-mindedness seems more consciously motivated, as though Al were putting on an appearance of distraction to make the degree of his disturbance obvious to the examiner.]	0
4. How many oranges can you buy for thirty-six cents if one orange costs four cents?	2"	Nine. [When the examiner nevertheless continues to ask questions, i.e., when Al sees he cannot basically modify the course of testing, he solves the next problem easily.]	1
5. How many hours will it take a man to walk twenty-four miles at the rate of three miles an hour?	11"	Forty-five miles? ("What's the question?") Eight! [Again it is hard to know how much Al's original answer is determined by disorganization and how much by the wish to appear disorganized.]	1
6. If a man buys seven two cents stamps and gives the clerk a half dollar, how much change should he get back?	—	(He rocks back and forth.) Two cents by seven equals fourteen. So twenty-five take away fourteen. (He begins to do the problem out loud but is not successful.) . . . . There's . . uh . . they were too rough with me at L_____.[2] My parents don't	0

2 A residential school Al formerly attended.

No. Problem	Time	Response and Comments	Score
		want me to go back there because of bad company. (He talks about the mutual sex play at the school.)	
7. *If seven pounds of sugar cost twenty-five cents, how many pounds can you get for a dollar?*	—	(This item was begun the following day. Before I had a chance to ask Al the problem, he immediately began to speak about maltreatment he experienced at the last hospital.) (I repeat the problem.) I don't know. ("How would you do it?") Divide or multiply. ("Which?") A hundred times twenty-five. (Since Al seems to have no conception how to do this and future, even more complicated, problems, the Arithmetic questions were discontinued at this point.)	0

RAW SCORE: 3-4

WEIGHTED SCORE: 3-4

SIMILARITIES

No. Items	Response and Comments	Score
1. *Orange-banana*	They grow in Florida. [This type of concrete over-specificity is typical of a much younger child's thinking.]	1
2. *Coat-dress*	You wear them.	1
3. *Dog-lion*	They roar. [Al's concrete orientation is strikingly apparent.]	0
4. *Wagon-bicycle*	Uh . . you ride them. A lion and a dog look alike, don't they? (He spits on the floor; then he spits in the wastepaper basket.) [Al's returning to the preceding question partially reflects his wish to answer adequately, a wish which competes with a desire to demonstrate *in*adequacy. The return to a previous question also indicates Al's need obsessively to "hold on," not to "let go." His spitting on the floor reflects not only his apparent unawareness of what is appropriate, but probably also his wish to test the limits of the examiner's patience. The behavior again raises the questions, to what extent does he "know better," to what extent does he realize his behavior is asocial, and to what extent does he consciously use this type of behavior to demonstrate how "disturbed" he is?]	1
5. *Daily paper-radio*	They give news.	1

No.	Items	Response and Comments	Score
6.	Air-water	You need them to live. [After a total failure and some only partial successes, suddenly the first completely successful abstraction!]	2
7.	Wood-alcohol	You get alcohol from wood. ("And how might they be alike?") Fish get oxygen in water, and people get oxygen in the air. [Again, he returns to the preceding question when he feels unsure of his handling of the present one. Significant once more is the erratic manner in which successes and failures are distributed. Instead of a gradual lessening of ability as the questions become harder, Al's scores get higher and lower without an obvious pattern.]	0
8.	Eye-ear	You see with the eye and you hear with the ear. ("How are they alike?") They're organs.	1
9.	Egg-seed	Life comes from them. [A good abstraction, even though it is officially given only partial credit.]	1
10.	Poem-statue	I don't know. ("Can you think of any way?") I can't think of any way.	0
11.	Praise-punishment	Praise is . . you give praise when they're good, and you give them jija punishment when they're bad. ("What's jija?") It's a word I picked up. It's one of my problems. It means anything I don't like. [Al's use of such a neologism reflects the seriousness, as well as the probable chronicity, of his condition.]	0
12.	Fly-tree	A fly goes in the air, and so does a tree.	0

RAW SCORE: __8__

WEIGHTED SCORE: __7__

PICTURE COMPLETION

No.	Item	Time	Missing	Response and Comments	Score
1.	Girl	3″	nose	The bo . . the chest and stomach and the arms. ("What's missing in the picture itself?") The ears, and part of the nose. [On this subtest, indicating as missing what the artist never intended to be present (i.e., in this facial profile, the portion below the neck), is always an alerting, serious sign, reflecting an impairment of "normal expectation." Al's Picture Completion performance is presented in its entirety, since, once again, it dramatically illustrates the	0

No.	Item	Time	Missing	Response and Comments	Score
				erratic pattern of his successes and failures, which distinguishes his test performance from that ordinarily obtained from someone who suffers from an uncomplicated "mental retardation."]	
2.	Face	1″	mustache	Do you bawl bad boys out? (I cover the item while he asks the question and show it again after he has finished.) Part of the mustache and part of the body. ("Which would you choose?") The body. [Again, he shows his inability to distinguish what is from what is not salient.]	0-1
3.	Profile	3″	ear	Ears . . and the body. (He goes on and on, telling about his previous hospitalization. He speaks about how they should try to understand him as being "nervous.") ("Which answer would you choose?") Ear.	1
4.	Card	15″	diamond	I don't know. ("What do you think?") The king. ("Where should that be?") In the middle.	0
5.	Crab	3″	leg	The third leg (points correctly).	1
6.	Pig	3″	tail	I don't know what's missing. An eye perhaps. (He talks compulsively about how he was treated by the personnel at the last hospital.) [The reader notes by now how matter-of-factly the examiner responds to Al's efforts to sway the examination away from its relatively limited goals. To deal with Al otherwise would make the completion of the test battery impossible in the time available. Further, to follow Al's conversational lead consistently would increase his anxiety because he would fear that the examiner had lost control.]	0
7.	Boat	3″	stacks	The cloud. ("Anything else?") I don't know.	0
8.	Door	2″	knob	The floor. ("Anything else?") Nothing else. (He tells more stories about how he was treated.)	0

No.	Item	Time	Missing	Response and Comments	Score
9.	Watch	10″	hand	Nothing's missing. (4″) ("Are you sure?") No. Yeah, the second hand.	1
10.	Pitcher	1″	water	The water pouring. [Noteworthy is not only the erratic pattern of successes and failures but also the speed with which he is sometimes able to give his correct response.]	1
11.	Mirror	8″	reflection of arm	Hairbrush.	0
12.	Man	½″	tie	The tie.	1
13.	Bulb	3″	thread (or prong)	The light. Old men can die, especially when they're senile and in restraints. It makes me giggle.	0
14.	Girl	2″	eyebrow	The ears. (He continues to speak about old men who are mistreated.)	0
15.	Sun	—	shadow of man	Nothing's missing there. (He talks about people being called "fresh.")	0

RAW SCORE: 5-6

WEIGHTED SCORE: 3-4

(Al says he is becoming nervous, so we take a brief time out while he drinks a Coke.)

PICTURE ARRANGEMENT

No.	Item	Correct Order	Time	Arranged Order	Story and Comments	Score
1.	House	PAT	3″	PAT	I gotta have a bowel movement after I finish the Coke. What do you do when kids have a tummy ache?	2
2.	Holdup	ABCD	8″	ABCD		2
3.	Elevator	LMNO	10″	LMNO		2
4.	Flirt	JANET	15″	TNAEJ	I don't know how to rearrange this. ("Do the best you can.") (He passes flatus.)	0
5.	Taxi	SAMUEL	20″	ALUMES	Some people were getting married. They rode, and I don't know the rest. [These items are becoming obviously too difficult for Al. He has only the vaguest idea of what is going on and can no longer	0

No.	Item	Correct Order	Time	Arranged Order	Story and Comments	Score
					even begin to order the cards correctly. On this test, Al's performance, along one dimension, is reminiscent of "simple retardation": he solves the "easy" items easily and correctly, but as they become more complex, he experiences increasing difficulty.]	
6.	*Fish*	EFGHIJ	18″	EJIFHG	A king went fishing. He caught a fish. Then he met a diver. The diver yelled at him. (Al belches and rocks.) . . . . . He pulled hard at a fish, and he probably lost it. I couldn't get interested after I got out of restraints, and I still can't get interested. [Al seeks to excuse his lack of ability by pleading lack of interest.]	0

RAW SCORE: ___6___

WEIGHTED SCORE: ___6___

(Between subtests, Al says:) Maybe I should urinate in the Coke bottle because I might not be able to urinate in the laboratory.

BLOCK DESIGN

(Al solves Sample A accurately, after 17″. He is unable to construct Sample B and says:) I can't make it. No. ("Try a little longer.") I did try. I just can't seem to make it. (The examiner demonstrates how to do the design, but Al still cannot copy from the model.) No, I can't do it.

(At 12″ he has Design 1 correct, except that he has turned all blocks to blue when they should be red. Nevertheless, he maintains that his design is exactly like the sample. When I ask if his blocks and the model are the same color, he says:) No. I thought I'd use blue instead of red. It doesn't make much difference. (He then changes the blocks to show the correct colors. He does the second design correctly, although he is slow and uncertain. He cannot construct any more designs correctly within the time limit. He gives up easily and frequently asks for my help. After he unsuccessfully tries to do Design 4, he stops and says:) Let's talk a little. (He completes Design 5, but only at 3′ 15″, and after first complaining he has an insufficient number of blocks. His initial construction is correct, except for two rotated corners. He corrects these slowly, after I say his design is not an exact copy.)

RAW SCORE: ___3-6___

WEIGHTED SCORE: ___3-4___

OBJECT ASSEMBLY

(Al achieves full credit only on the first, *Manikin*, item. Even here, however, he first places one arm so that its reverse side shows. As he does the *Manikin*, he says:) This is better than restraints. [Probably not much, though.] (He obtains only partial credit on the *Profile*. After 50″, he indicates he has completed the *Hand*. Although he has created a gross hand shape, he has completely reversed the order, so that no pieces are accurately placed.)

RAW SCORE: 10

WEIGHTED SCORE: 4

DIGIT SYMBOL

(Al's symbols are relatively neatly and accurately drawn, although he has obvious difficulty in joining lines at right angles and in keeping his efforts within the required boundaries. He works slowly, painfully and his symbol drawings reflect marked changes in pressure.)

RAW SCORE: 20

WEIGHTED SCORE: 5

VOCABULARY

No.	Word	Response and Comments	Score
1.	Apple	It's a fruit you eat.	1
2.	Donkey	It's an animal you ride.	1
3.	Join	To put together.	1
4.	Diamond	A jewel. (He belches.)	1
5.	Nuisance	A pest.	1
6.	Fur	Something you put around your neck. ("Could you tell me a little more about it?") It's made from a fox.	½
7.	Cushion	Something you sit on. ("Could you tell me a little more about it?") It's a pillow.	1
8.	Shilling	I don't know.	0
9.	Gamble	Somebody plays a game for money.	1
10.	Bacon	Meat. ("Could you tell me a little more?") It comes off a pig.	1
11.	Nail	Something you have to dig the nurses if they restrain you. These (points correctly). [Over and over one observes how difficult Al finds it to maintain an objective, nonself-inclusive orientation.]	1
12.	Cedar	Wood.	1
13.	Tint	I don't know.	0

No.	Word	Response and Comments	Score
14.	*Armory*	A place . . an Army hospital.	0
15.	*Fable*	A story.	1
16.	*Brim*	I don't know. ("Have you heard of it?") I think so, but I don't know what it means.	0
17.	*Guillotine*	Knife. ("Could you tell me something more about it?") It's used to cut off bad people's heads. It makes me giggle nervously. [Al is trying again to create interest in his symptoms. The examiner hopes that the symptom of "talking about symptoms" will become attenuated as he takes no interest in it.]	1
18.	*Plural*	I don't know. ("Any idea?") It's . . uh . . when you put an "s" at the end of a word.	½
19.	*Seclude*	I don't know.	0
20.	*Nitroglycerine*	Acid. ("Do you know any more about it?") No. [Although Al does not get this word fully correct, it is surprising to see the sophisticated concept, "acid," available to him, while he denies knowledge of such words as *shilling* and *brim*.]	½
21.	*Stanza*	A song . . a line of a song.	½
22.	*Microscope*	Something you look at things through. ("How is that?") They have . . . . . a . . uh . . . . slide that goes through. ("And what do you see?") Germs . . germs and stool and drops of urine. [Al's concern with various bodily excretions once more reflects the degree and nature of his self-preoccupation, the inadequacy of his sublimation and his unabashedness about saying things which other adolescents or latency children would not mention to a relatively strange adult.]	1
23.	*Vesper*	I don't know. (See the item immediately following.)	½
24.	*Belfry*	A belfry is a bell. ("Could you say some more about it?") A Christmas service. A vesper is a service. [Al's last three sentences, in which he goes from *belfry* to *vesper* seem to involve a contaminatory process.]	0
25.	*Recede*	Something you pay with money. ("How do you mean?") I don't know. [He apparently has "receipt" in mind.]	0
26.	*Affliction*	When you're sick, and you shake all over.	½

No.	Word	Response and Comments	Score
27.	*Pewter*	Puke. [An obvious clang association, again reflecting Al's preoccupation with the things which come from his body.]	0
28.	*Ballast*	I don't know.	0
29.	*Catacomb*	I don't know.	0
30.	*Spangle*	A jewel or piece of colored sugar. ("Where would you find it?") In a jar, like little sugar candies. I've eaten a whole dish of spangles.	0
31.	*Espionage*	Sponge. [Another apparent clang association.]	0

(Al does not know the remaining word meanings.)

RAW SCORE: 16

WEIGHTED SCORE: 7

THE BENDER GESTALT TEST

PART B (PLATE 23)

(Only the Bender Copy is administered because Al might find the 5″ Exposure so difficult to complete that his self-esteem would suffer greatly. On Design 2, he loses track of even the small number of circles in each column; i.e., in a column requiring three circles, he first draws four, and then corrects himself. While drawing Design 3, he says:) I'll dig them if they restrain anybody in the hospital where I go. (He looks into space then but is able to finish the drawing when I encourage him.) [Al's drawings are relatively accurate, in the sense that he maintains the essential gestalt of each design. At the same time, one notes Al's lack of rhythm and regularity. His drawings lack smoothness of execution because of his poor motor control. His lines are jagged and have corners where curves should be. Design elements evidence sudden, unplanned changes in size. Pressure is very heavy, reflecting the absence of sensitivity to counterpressures; i.e., there is no interaction between Al and his sheet of paper—he does not flexibly respond to the pressures of table, paper or pencil. Such a lack of responsiveness may well indicate some sort of "organic" factor. Psychically based immaturity, confusion and fragmentation alone probably do not account for all the graphic distortions. The suggestion of "organic dysfunction" opens up the Pandora's box of the degree to which "autistic" or "atypical" or

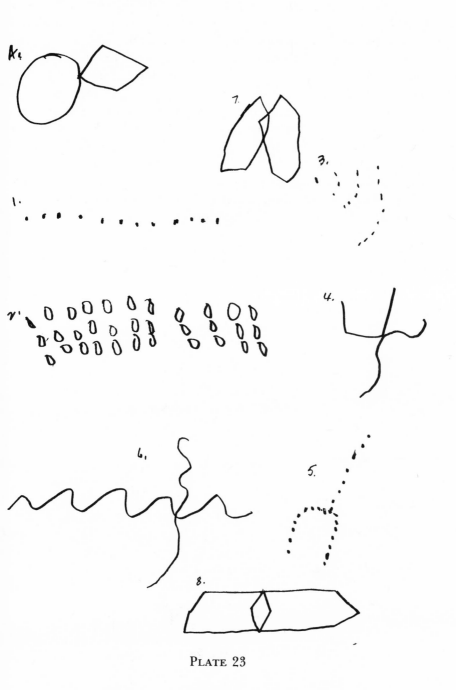

PLATE 23

"schizophrenic" conditions are of exclusively "functional" etiology. One is struck, again and again, by the fact that the intrafamily situations usually blamed for the psychological disorganization of these children often does not seem destructive enough to have produced such a profound degree of disorganization. One is left with the (emotionally based?) conviction that "organic," possibly constitutionally determined, features play a significant role in the development of these grave childhood conditions. It may be most useful to think of an "organic readiness" either to develop or not to develop a disorganization of this kind. For a child with such readiness, it may take little (if, indeed, anything beyond the expectable stresses of growing up) to develop such severe psychic malfunction. It is at least questionable that parents can do much to prevent the development of such disorganization, once the organic (?), innate (?), constitutional (?) basis has been laid down.]

THE DRAW A PERSON TEST

PART I (PLATE 24)

(After the instructions, he says:) I'll draw my grandfather.

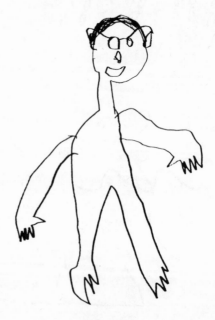

PLATE 24

PART II (PLATE 25)

(After the instructions, he says:) I'll draw my grandmother.

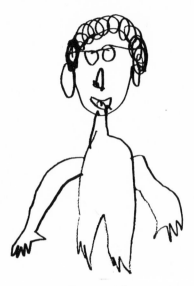

PLATE 25

[These drawings of persons demonstrate Al's chaotic ego organization. His drawings are poorly differentiated, immaturely conceived, primitively constructed. His "man" is somewhat better drawn than his "woman," who is particularly poorly put together. One of her hands has four fingers, the other five; both feet have three toes; the legs and body together occupy only a little more space than the head.

[In both the man and the woman the face is by far the most differentiated feature. One surmises that the face and its expressions are exceedingly important interpersonal aspects to Al: whether people look "mean," "nice," "fresh," and so on.

[The two drawings point up even more strongly the type of dysfunction apparent in Al's Bender drawings. One sees here not only his motor inadequacies, but his conceptual primitivity as well. In some respects, Al's drawings are much nearer those of a four- or five-year-old than a thirteen-year-old.]

[The scoring sheet gives only a very rough summary of Al's detailed Rorschach performance. His perceptions and the descriptions he gives of them are extremely vague; allotting them scores results in spurious precision. The actual Rorschach is so arbitrary,

Rorschach Test

RORSCHACH SCORING SHEET

Number of Responses: 27

Manner of Approach (Location)

W	8
WS	1
D	14
Dd	0
Do	3
Dr	1
De	0
Total	27

Location Percentages

W%	33
D%	56
DR%	15
De%	0

Form, Movement, Color and Shading Determinants

F+	9
F−	11
F±	1
F∓	2
MC′+	1
FC	0
CF	3
Total	27

Groups of Contents

A	10
Ad	4
H	2
Hd	1
Obj.	1
At.	0
Ats.	1
Pl.	5
Gremlin	1
Cloud	1
Anus	1
Total	27

Determinant and Content Percentages

F%	85/89	Obj.%	4
F+%	43/46	P%	22
H%	11(15)	At%	4(7)
A%	52		

Qualitative Material

Popular	III (III) IV V VI VIII
Combination	III
Fabulation	8
Vague	5
Confusion	1
Color Denom- ination	1

EXPERIENCE BALANCE: 1/3.0

so confused, so vaguely perceived and described, so consistently inadequately differentiated, that a Psychogram offers little more than formal verification of what is obvious without it.

[In the midst of the signs of Al's major disorganization are two indices of some mental order which generate the mildest hope that Al might be helped at least a little out of his psychological quagmire. The most significant index of this sort is the relative frequency with which Al sees Popular responses, indicating his ability to share most people's way of perceiving the environment. Further, Al's W/D ratio of about ½ is what one might "normally" expect. These two indicators unfortunately stand alone on the "positive" side of Al's Rorschach reactions.]

RORSCHACH PROTOCOL

Card #	React. Time	Score	Protocol	Inquiry and Observations
I	2″	WsF+ Gremlin face Fab. Vague	1. A gremlin. ("Anything else?")	1. The top of the . . . . it looked like a gremlin. ("What made it seem like that?") The jija eyes. ("What's that?") Just a nervous reaction put that word in my mind. ("What do they look like?") They look like this. (He demonstrates with his fingers.) ("And what about it made it look like a gremlin?") Cause it was ugly. ("How much of the blot seemed like a gremlin?") Half. ("Just how did you see it?") The face. If I have to go to the bathroom, you better take me to the lab to piss. Because you won't have my urine to make, and I got to go to the lab. Don't be like Mrs. K. (a nurse at the previous hospital), or else I'll have to piss in the Coke bottle. ("Is there something about the blot that's upsetting?") The ugliness. (As I give him the card later, so that he can show me more specifically what he has in mind, he vaguely points to parts of the entire blot, in the way much younger children do.) [Al's way of handling this unusual percept—his vagueness, arbitrariness, and the triggering off of concern about urinating successfully, set the scene for the kind of Rorschach to come.]
		DoF+Ad Vague	2. A cat.	2. ("What made it look like a cat?") The ears. ("Anything else?") Nothing else. [The use of a highly peripheral aspect (the "ears") to give meaning to a much more inclusive area is typical of the fragmentation of Al's thinking. Undoubtedly the entire blot, with its eyes,

Card #	React. Time	Score	Protocol	Inquiry and Observations
				mouth, cheeks and ears, gives him the impression of a cat. He is unable to analyze his perception, however, so he is aware only that the "ears" make it look like a cat.]
		DoF—Ad Vague	3. Sting ray fish . . . . ("Anything else?") Nothing else.	3. The body. (He points only to the very small Dr section jutting out the bottom and calls it the "tail.") [This is a repetition of the partializing tendency noted in Al's preceding response.]
II	3″	WF—A Fab. Vague	1. Sting ray fish. ("Anything else?") (The Coke makes him belch. He makes no effort to subdue it and lets it emerge at full volume.)	1. A body. ("What does it look like?") I don't know. ("Tell me as best as you can remember.") I just don't know. (The only portion he can point out is the "stinger" of the fish— the upper central Dd section.) [He perseveratively falls back on the last response of the previous card—a response which, incidentally, preceded the card's being removed.]
		WF—Hd Fab.	2. Uh . . A man. ("Anything else?") Uh . . I don't know. (He makes peculiar mouth motions, as though he might spit out his Coke.)	2. He's ugly. ("How do you mean?") Not too handsome. ("What makes him look that way?") The way the picture was drawn. ("How's that?") He had a long chin. ("And what else?") I don't know. (He is extremely vague when he is shown the card and asked to point to the different sections. The "head" is the upper central Dd section, the "face" the central S section and the "chin" the bottom red D section. He blows his nose into his fingers and wipes the fingers on his sleeve. When I give him a Kleenex, he takes it and mentions that one of the nurses at the previous hospital was real mean-looking; then he chews on the Kleenex.) [Not only is Al's overt be-

React.			
Card #	Time Score	Protocol	*Inquiry and Observations*

Inquiry and Observations

havior odd and often repellant; his disorganization can be seen to invade wide areas of functioning. His perceptual process is exceedingly vague, fragmented and arbitrary. It not only becomes difficult for an outsider to put himself in Al's place so as to be able to see things the same way as Al; it is difficult for Al himself to empathize with his own state of a few moments before. Al's major stability appears to rest on (probably distorted) memories of ways he and others were treated previously—everything else is evanescent.]

III   4″   WMC′   1. Two men.
        +HP
        Fab.
        Comb.

1. They were ugly. ("What made them that way?") The way the picture was drawn. ("What about the picture?") I don't know. ("What do you recall?") They were black. They were Negroes. [Many things appear "ugly" to Al. This ugliness has no "real" basis; things simply look that way to him.]

DF+AP   2. And a butterfly.

2. It was ugly. ("How was that?") The way the picture was drawn. ("What way was that?") I don't know. ("Could you tell me whatever you remember—anything about it?") No. (Central red D.) [It is hard to know to what extent "ugly" has become a perseverative answer, like Claire's "bugs" in Chapter II. Al sees that the examiner seems to take an interest in what Al means by "ugly," so he begins to call everything "ugly," even though it might appear quite ordinary to him.]

DF−Obj.   3. And pipes.
Fab.

3. Ugly pipes.

Card #	React. Time	Score	Protocol	Inquiry and Observations
		DF∓A Fab. (Comb.)	4. And they're holding crabs.	4. (The "crabs," constituted by the lower central D, are being held by the "men" of Response 1.)
IV	3″	WF+AP Fab.	1. A bat. (He looks away from the card.) ("Anything else?") Nothin' else.	1. It was ugly . . Do they have Coke-flavored candy? ("What did the bat seem to be doing?") Flying. [Although an examiner would ordinarily not ask such a leading question (i.e., "What is the bat doing?"), Al's perception is so amorphous that he seems to require this type of structuring.]
V	½″	WF+AP	1. Another bat . . or a bird. Nothin' else.	1. ("How was this bat different from the one before?") I don't know. How do you know they won't holler if you take your urine in a bottle? (He expresses concern that people might yell at him.) [It is clear that, by now, Al can involve himself in the test only partially. He cannot shut out the worrisome laboratory examination to which he will go right after the present appointment.]
VI	3″	WF+AdP	1. A bear skin.	1. It was flat. ("Could it have been another animal, too?") A cat's.
		WF−A Confus.	2. A cat. (He studies the card.) It seems like no urine is piling up. I won't have no urine.	2. ("What reminded you of a cat?") The head. ("What about the head?") I don't know. ("Can you tell me what made it look like a cat rather than, say, a dog?") Uh-uh. It looks more like a dog . . the mouth. (He rests his head on the table.) [Al obviously has hardly any commitment to his responses. It can be a dog as easily as a cat, a cat's skin as easily as a bear's—anything, simply to keep the examiner from asking questions about his Rorschach responses when

Card #	React. Time	Score	Protocol	Inquiry and Observations
				a much more important situation—the visit to the lab—is imminent.]
VII	4″	DoF—Ad	1. Legs, and	1. ("What kind?") A dog's. (The "dog's legs" include the upper two-thirds of the blot—the usual "Indians.")
		DF—Anus	2. A hind end. That big colored man, he threatened to take me over his knee! (At the last hospital.) ("Do you see anything else?") M'hm. ("What do you see?") Nothing else. And the Spanish man who was with him (he goes on and on) . . He said, "All the time, you're running around the hospital showing your penis, so you asked for it."	2. ("What kind of hind end?") A person's. ("What did you see?") I saw an anus. You better get some more water so I'll have urine. [Al's poor ability conceptually to compartmentalize is demonstrated by the ease with which his perception of a "hind end" leads to a great storehouse of rather distantly related memories.]
VIII	3″	WF—Ats Vague	1. A brain. (He looks away.) ("Anything else?")	1. ("What made it look like a brain?") The way it's fixed up. ("Can you tell me any more?") No, I can't.
		DF+AP	2. Animals climbing up. (He looks away.) ("Anything else?") I don't know.	2. ("What kind of animals?") Bears.
IX	3″	DrF∓A	1. Beetles.	1. (The usual "head" and "antler" areas of the upper orange D.) (It is impossible to find out the determinants of Al's percepts. He gives "beetles," "bears" and "babies" quickly; then he eats his Kleenex. Our discussion of how he might be trying to affect me by doing things of this sort takes enough time to cause him to "lose" the percepts he has given. He is no longer able to answer questions about his

Card #	React. Time	Score	Protocol	Inquiry and Observations
				beetles, bears and babies by the time I inquire about them.)
		DF—A	2. Bears, and	2. [Depending on how he sees the bears, this response might have acceptable form level— but he can no longer show what he saw. The percept has vanished.]
		DF+H	3. Babies. (He begins to eat his Kleenex again, and I tell him that this does not "upset" me. He tells how it used to upset a nurse at his last hospital. I wonder whether he would like it if I were to become upset, but he says he would not.) Mary (the receptionist) is a very pretty girl, isn't she? She's really nice and kind, too. I bet other kids think she's pretty. [Is this last a transference comment and, if so, what does it mean?]	3. (Bottom pink D.)
X	3″	DF±A	1. Crabs.	1. (Upper gray central D "bugs.")
		DF—Pl	2. A tree.	2. (Top central elongated gray D.)
		DCF Cl	3. Clouds.	3. ("What made them seem like clouds?") They were pink.
		DF—Pl Fab.	4. Flowers.	4. ("Tell me about the flowers.") They were ugly. ("What made them ugly?") The drawing. ("Could you tell me what kind of flowers they were?") Nah! (He laughs.) I think that's a funny word. (Central blue D's.)

Card #	React. Time	Score	Protocol	Inquiry and Observations
		DF+Pl	5. & 6. And green.	5. & 6. (The green D's.) [Al's
		DCF Pl	("Green what?")	pointing to and outlining of
Color naming		DCF Pl	Leaves.	areas becomes so haphazard

that the examiner is left to judge as best he can how adequately Al has perceived the items he mentions. Since Al frequently helps only very little during inquiry, so that the examiner often needs to resort to educated guesses, there are bound to be a number of scoring errors throughout Al's Rorschach protocol. Al's worry about the imminent lab visit and his limited tension tolerance (as well as, by now, that of the examiner), make the last several test cards little more than tasks to be completed, rather than the source of new and revealing information. The examiner feels that the Rorschach is consistent with the initial diagnostic picture which became rather clear early in the first meeting with Al. The examiner is by now particularly eager to find out what degree of organization Al is able to muster, since the degree of his *dis*organization is painfully apparent, both clinically and on tests. The tests may be helpful in showing what areas are relatively integrated, what areas are not constantly responding to destructive, disorganized and disorganizing forces.]

THEMATIC APPERCEPTION TEST

(Only a few of Al's stories are given here.)
Card 2 (Country scene: in the foreground is a young woman with books in her hand; in the background a man is working in the fields, and an older woman is looking on.)

There's some people working out on the farm. There's supposed to be a tornado coming . . . . and the lady is standing, holding a book, and another one is standing by a tree, and a man is walking his horse . . . . ("What about the tornado?") It does all damage. It kills people . . . . ("Does it harm any of the ones here?") No. They hide in a storm cellar . . . . ("Who are they to each other?") Relatives. ("What kind?") Blood relatives. ("I mean how are they related to each other exactly?") I don't know. ("Could you make up something?") I don't know. ("What are they thinking about?") The tornado . . . . ("What about the tornado?") That it's going to come and kill them . . . . ("What's the girl in front thinking about?") I don't know . . about what she read. ("How about the man with the horse?") The weather. That boy downstairs who's nervous, does he go to school? (Referring to a young patient who greeted me in the waiting room.) [The most striking thing about this story is its fragmentation—its separation of one character from another; of action from motive; of one story element from the next. Al cannot tell a story, largely, perhaps, because he lacks the cognitive capacity for it. Judging by the remaining stories, however, his lack of creativity is not exclusively the result of the emptiness of his fantasy but also of inhibition resulting from his fear that, once he lets go, almost anything may emerge—as, indeed, it does in later stories.]

Card 3 BM (On the floor against a couch is the huddled form of a boy with his head bowed on his right arm. Beside him on the floor is a revolver.)

Somebody is sick. They're leaning on the bench, and they're going to die. ("What happens?") He dies . . . . ("What was wrong?") He had an ulcer or heart attack . . . . ("How old is he?") twenty-one . . . . ("Does anyone care?") Nobody cares. ("How about his folks?") They don't care. ("Why is that?") Because they don't like him . . . . ("Why don't they?") I don't know. ("What's wrong with him?") He's sick mentally . . . ("Is that why they don't like him?") M'hm. Why is it when you get an ulcer people don't care? ("How do you mean?") Those nurses didn't care when the old man had an ulcer. Didn't they like him or something? [Al enlarges on his responses only when they involve one of his major preoccupations. This TAT story is included not only because it again illustrates the poverty of Al's imagination and the strength of his obsessions, but because it points out vividly how aware he is of the dilemma he offers his parents and how puzzled and heartbroken he is about the realization that others find him unlikable.]

Card 16 (Blank card.)

Well, there's an old man. He is working, and a bunch of kids are bothering him. He is getting grouchy and saying, "You asked for it!" (Said in a threatening voice.) ("What happens then?") He goes senile. ("What does that mean?") He doesn't know anything. He thinks everyone is somebody else, and he thinks something is something else. ("Anything more?") He was . . after a week of being in the hospital he was diagnosed. And treatment was to send him home and have his relatives and a nurse watch him. (He puts his head on the table.) And after a year, he died. [Al obviously identifies himself with these sick, senile old men—primarily with their helplessness and their having been forgotten by those closest to them. The story's ending reflects the hopelessness he feels about his own future.]

Sentence Completion Test II

He hoped that when he grew up he would be a doctor.

When he saw what the other kids were doing he did it. Were they being fresh? [Al finds it almost impossible to be independent of others. He has almost no capacity to hold himself apart from them. He must do whatever they do, not only because it is "fun" but because separation brings with it intense feelings of isolation and helplessness.]

When he compared himself to his friends he scratched his balls. (He talks about eating semen.) [This test triggers off fantasies, memories and impulses which take over and eventually leave Al almost no "self-control." He eventually becomes the helpless victim of internal forces which he cannot direct.]

He was sad whenever he thought of nobody liking him.

When he was asked about his aches and pains he said I'm gonna puke.

The person he admired most . . . . was Carey Miller. ("Who's that?") In my church, she's so pretty. She makes my jigger stick out. I'm kinda scared to pull out my jigger.

His brother . . . . His brother . . uh . . liked the girls in this church.

When his father came into the room . . . . he said, "Come on, let's go to the hospital."

When he was with his sister he punched her.

At school . . At home . . (I repeat the stem.) Uh . . I . . uh . . an old man was puking all over the floor.

When he looked at the work the others were doing he pulled his jigger out.

He was very happy when . . when they felt each other's balls.

The thing he found hardest to do was say "fuck you."

Whenever certain things really bothered him he cussed and he pissed and made stool . . made shit all over the floor.

His dreams were of people pissing and making shit all over the floor. I'm helping you get to the bottom of my problem, to show you how bad I can talk. [A modicum of control is demonstrated by Al's wish to have me "use" his lack of control, so that I will "understand" him better.]

He liked hillbilly.

When he saw that the man had left the money behind he stole it.

He thought that his mother was shit.

Whenever he and his family disagreed he said, "shit." (In an effort to see how much control Al can exert at this point, I ask that he try not to use any "bad talk.")

When he was very little he went to L——school.

His best friend was Edward.

He was unhappy when his father died.

He never thought he would be able to . . . . uh . . stand restraints. They're mean to put you in restraints.

He always hoped that . . . . . (he laughs) . . . . he could see an old man.

His parents liked him.

What he liked best about himself was that he shit. [After a brief period of control, apparently helped somewhat by my suggestion, Al once more becomes the victim of his impulses.]

His mother was more likely than his father to shit (he laughs). (I make another attempt to stop Al from using "shocking" words.)

When he had nothing else to do uh . . he read comics.

He thought that his intelligence was shit (he laughs). [The respite is even briefer this time.]

What he liked best about school was the kids who talked about fuck, shit, piss and puke (he giggles).

(Continuing with this test causes Al more and more to lose control. It is apparent that he can no longer pull himself together sufficiently to give "appropriate" answers. For this reason, the test is discontinued.) [Al's ability to control is seen to be progressively more limited.]

WORD ASSOCIATION TEST

React. Time (In Secs.)	Stimulus	Response	Inquiry and Comments
1	1. *Hat*	Something you put on. (I explain again that I want him to say only one word.)	[The ability to give only *one word* requires a type of abstraction capacity almost invariably absent in young children. Al shows this kind of abstraction difficulty. After two false attempts, however, he is able to give a one-word association.]
1	2. *Lamp*	You light.	
2½	3. *Love*	Uh . . like.	
2	4. *Book*	Read.	
1½	5. *Father*	Man.	
2½	6. *Paper*	Read . . write! I've got sexual feelings about Mary (the receptionist).	[Until this point, Al is able to prevent fantasies from intruding into the task and to organize himself sufficiently to prevent "sexual" thoughts from spilling over. Gradually, however, the freedom encouraged by the lack of firm structure in free associating makes it difficult for him to avoid being inundated by his various biological preoccupations.]
2	7. *Breast*	(He laughs.) Girls.	
3½	8. *Curtains*	Uh . . shades.	

React. Time (In Secs.)	Stimulus	Response	Inquiry and Comments
2½	9. *Trunk*	Uh .. closet. (He speaks about having sexual feelings about his cousins.)	
1½	10. *Drink*	Soda. I have sexual feelings about my sister.	
1½	11. *Party*	Dance. Dancing gives me sexual feelings.	
3	12. *Spring*	Ssss .. May.	
3	13. *Bowel movement*	S .. P ..... *SHIT!*	[This stimulus word has caused the low dam of inhibition to break down momentarily.]
2	14. *Rug*	Carpet.	
2	15. *Boy friend*	Boy .. girl .. boy.	
2½	16. *Chair*	Seat. I used to have sexual feelings (etc., etc.), but they've turned to hate, and now I feel like socking.	[As was apparent in previous instances, Al has "learned" to rattle off interpretations, and he uses them to intellectualize.]
2	17. *Screen*	Window.	
	18. *Penis* (omitted)		[Using such frankly sexual words would be too stimulating for Al; they are omitted for that reason. The

React. *Time (In* *Secs.)*	*Stimulus*	*Response*	*Inquiry and Comments*
			examiner's effort is still to see how well Al can remain organized, since it is clear how severely *dis*organized he easily becomes.]
2½	19. *Radiator*	Pipes.	
3	20. *Frame*	Wood.	
1	21. *Suicide*	Kill . . kill yourself.	
6	22. *Mountain*	Ant . . hill.	[The 6″ delay may well be the result of the preceding *suicide*.]
3	23. *Snake*	Rep . . tile.	
4½	24. *House*	Building.	[Is the 4½″ delay caused by the symbolism of the preceding *snake?*]
	25. *Vagina* (omitted)		
7	26. *Tobacco*	Leaf.	[The long delay might possibly be related to secret smoking.]
4	27. *Mouth*	This (points to his own mouth) hole in your face.	
1½	28. *Horse*	Animal.	
	29. *Mastur-* *bation* (omitted)		
1	30. *Wife*	Lady.	
17	31. *Table*	I don't know . . . I don't know . . . . Something with four legs.	("Why did that take so long?") It reminded me of when mother made me eat shit. [This word triggers off an apparently genuine memory.]
1	32. *Fight*	Beat.	

React. Time (In Secs.)	Stimulus	Response	Inquiry and Comments
2	33. *Beef*	Meat. I stepped in dog shit once.	
4	34. *Stomach*	Organ.	
1½	35. *Farm*	Prairie.	
5	36. *Man*	Person. There are many pretty girls who go to the same church on Sundays (etc., etc.). (He speaks about the erections he has during church services.) (The test is discontinued at this point. The remaining twenty-four stimulus words and the entire Recall portion are omitted.)	[Again, the examiner considers this (Word Association) procedure to be too stimulating and disorganizing. He has satisfactorily answered his question regarding Al's capacity to fend off disorganizing influences. It is again apparent that Al becomes the almost helpless victim of thoughts which flood consciousness and which often lead to almost immediate action. It becomes more and more apparent how little strength Al has to fight the intrusions of his disorganization and that almost any word, no matter how apparently objectively distant its meaning, quickly leads Al to private, intimate associations.]

The Psychologist's Report

Much of Al's behavior seems to have as one of its main goals the arousal of anger, pity and disgust in the adult who happens to be with him at the time. When I wonder whether he is checking to see how well I can control my feelings, he may laughingly reply he does not want me to become angry, but following this type of discussion, he usually stops his "offensive" behavior, at least for a while. During the last testing hour, after his tension has been building up over a number of days and as he experiences little limitation to self-expression, he finds it almost impossible to stop using obscene words and "shocking" expressions. On Sentence Completion, for example, his endings become increasingly filled with such words as "puke," "piss," "shit" and "fuck." Earnestly, he explains that he uses these words to show me one of his problems. When I tell him I understand this particular problem now and ask him to stop using the words, he gives more usual endings to the next few stems but then gigglingly reverts to obscene ones. Although he uses "dirty" words and behavior for their shock value, this way of speaking also has a compulsive, uncontrollable quality. Judging by his tests and clinical behavior, it is apparent that Al's world is one of decay and deterioration, that it is never good, never wholesome, that it is composed of offal and other excretions.

Although Al practices much aggressive teasing, he says that he would like me to get "to the bottom" of his problems, and he frequently wonders if I completely understand him yet. He becomes extremely disturbed when, in response to his question, I admit I have not yet seen the "home movies" which the family has brought along. Angrily and mournfully, he says I simply *have* to see them; otherwise I will never understand his problems.

In his intellectual functioning, Al not only shows the severe disturbance of effective organization caused by the intrusion of inappropriate, often irrelevant material; he shows a limited basic cognitive capacity as well. In other words, his thinking frequently reflects both a *distortion* and a *lack,* an inability to deal with intellectual problems age-adequately. On the Wechsler-Bellevue Scale, he achieves an Intelligence Quotient of 66-69. His Verbal Quotient is 78-81 and his Performance Quotient 61-64. His weighted scores range from 3 to 7, and he never achieves a level which suggests a significantly greater potential ability. Disorganization, rather than lack, is suggested by his pattern of within-subtest successes and failures. These do not appear in an orderly, expectable fashion, in that Al occasionally misses quite easy questions (often because of the intrusion of obsessive concerns) and later successfully deals with much more difficult ones. Occasionally, particularly on the Thematic Apperception Test, he misperceives in a rather striking fashion. He misinterprets, for example, a man pictured as standing in a graveyard. Al sees the man standing on top of a tall building. Occasionally he uses the neologism "jija" which, he explains, has to do with his feeling "nervous" (it may also have to do with "jigger," Al's term for penis).

Al's odd, unusual, often inappropriate and frequently bizarre views emerge easily, often blandly, without apparent conflict or other barrier. For example, without a moment's hesitation he explains that "Edward Thompson" wrote *Hamlet*. Asked why people should avoid bad company, he says, "I don't avoid bad company. Because they get you in trouble. I enjoy bad company. You mean, like bad kids? I enjoy it. I have went with them. I had a burning feeling in my penis because of yellow urine, and that also could have caused my trouble." On Picture Completion, shown a door with a knob missing, he explains the floor is gone. He organizes, describes and elaborates his Rorschach percepts very inadequately. Once he no longer sees the blot before him, it seems almost no longer to exist. After the card is removed from sight, he usually does not remember it well enough to describe any significant features. Even as he looks, his percept seems to fluctuate, so that boundaries and contents shift and merge. His Rorschach responses are of poor form quality and are lacking in creative imagination. The same imaginative lack is evident on Al's Thematic Apperception Test stories. Although Al ordinarily spends an immense degree of time "in fantasy," the fantasy is a poor, meager thing, concerned almost totally with bodily products of some sort, or with the behavior and attitudes of others toward him. He fears they will hurt, attack, punish and, eventually, probably destroy him.

Since Al tends to interpret everything in egocentric terms, he has great difficulty evaluating the external world in an objective fashion. He characterizes it almost exclusively in affective terms; the only objects worth even noting are the people charged with his care, who are either "nice," "mean," or who stimulate him sexually. He is also aware of other patients, particularly old men.

One of Al's major problems involves his inability to control sexual and aggressive impulses, whose ideational derivatives are forever intruding themselves into his awareness. There are only few moments when he is not consciously preoccupied with the temptation to act out sexually or aggressively. Blandly, for example, he explains, "Once I was going to kill my father and mother. My grandmother stopped me by squeezing my hand so hard I had to drop the knife." Al seems much more concerned about his grandmother's "cruel" treatment than about his having had the impulse to kill his parents. The ordinarily inhibiting affect of shame seems not at all developed in Al. Judgment is so poor, reality so distorted, shame so underdeveloped and general control so ineffective, that it does not seem at all unlikely that Al might at one time or another perform a grotesque, bizarre, terribly destructive act, attenuated neither by unconscious conflict nor by conscious inhibition.

A minimal degree of control is available to Al through hyper-developed obsessive defenses and through intellectualization. While these defenses modify the directness of his impulsive expression somewhat, they obviously cannot do an effective job of it.

Al's condition has previously been diagnosed as "Schizophrenia, with an undetermined amount of organic substrate." His perform-ance, particularly in the perceptual-motor area, suggests that some kind of organic involvement is present. He is able to solve correctly only one of the Block Designs; on Object Assembly, he has difficulty putting together even the simplest item (*Manikin*); his drawings are grossly constructed, exceedingly poorly differentiated, and in many ways made as one might expect of a four-and-a-half- to five-year-old. Although it is difficult to separate from Al's severe "emotional" illness, it seems highly likely that an "organic" factor accounts for some of his impoverishment.

Al is aware of being out of tune with the world. On the Thematic Apperception Test, for example, while describing the behavior of senile men, with whom he strongly identifies himself, he says, "They act in ways that don't make sense, and they think of things that don't make sense, and they behave in ways that don't make sense." As Al interprets this kind of situation, the world is out of step with the old men and should adapt itself to their needs. But although Al pro-jects almost all the blame for this lack of harmony between himself and the world, he nevertheless achieves occasional glimpses of the fact that part of the problem lies within himself. The following story, told to the blank Thematic Apperception Test card, partly demon-strates such awareness—it reflects, too, Al's hopelessness about the possibility that he will ever receive significant help:

> Well, there's an old man. He is working, and a bunch of kids are bothering him. He is getting grouchy and saying, "You asked for it!" (Said in a threatening voice.) ("What happens then?") He goes senile. ("What does that mean?") He doesn't know anything. He thinks everyone is somebody else, and he thinks something is something else. ("Anything more?") He was . . after a week of

being in the hospital he was diagnosed. And treatment was to send him home and have his relatives and a nurse watch him. (He puts his head on the table.) And after a year, he died. [Al obviously identifies himself with these sick, senile old men—primarily with their helplessness and their having been forgotten by those closest to them. The story's ending reflects the hopelessness he feels about his own future.]

In summary, Al is a very severely disorganized adolescent with limited and distorting intellectual abilities. Although he uses obsessive and intellectualizing defenses in an effort to control impulses that are forever erupting into action, these defenses are not adequate. Al needs external help to control himself, but often even such help does nothing. He needs constantly to test others, to see what their threshold of anger and disgust is and to make sure they are willing to accept him, in spite of his repellant behavior. While he constantly tries to upset others, he is secretly afraid he may be successful. His fantasy is exceedingly pedestrian and uncreative, obsessively concerned with gross bodily functions and gratifications, with decay and with horror. What most others would find disgusting, Al makes a point of appearing to find gratifying. Thoughts about sex, elimination, illness, old age and general disintegration flood Al's consciousness and make it impossible for him to view the world objectively. Some symptomatic behavior appears to be under at least some conscious control and its expression has the partial purpose of making others aware of his plight.

Discussion

To speak of both Al and Bill (whose tests follow next) as "schizophrenic," i.e., to put them in the same diagnostic category, points out the major inadequacies of present-day labeling systems. Both boys, it is true, demonstrate characteristics of thinking which are mildly similar and which vaguely correspond to the abstraction designated "schizophrenia." But it is apparent that the two adolescents are extraordinarily different in most respects: Al is organized on a simple, poorly differentiated, primitively gross level. He has few structures to mediate between impulse arousal and impulse expression; impulse hardly ever becomes transformed into anything but the most immediate reflection, in thought and action, of the arousing force. He has limited outside interests, few abilities and little capacity to transcend his intense self-preoccupation.

Bill, on the other hand, although his thinking is at times peculiar, loosely organized and based on private logic, and although he is to some extent also preoccupied with "decayed" ideas, is nevertheless a very different sort of person from Al. Bill has many more facets, which not only make possible a more varied spectrum of expression, but also are the basis for a much more differentiated impulsive-defense organization—i.e., impulse is rarely immediately and grossly expressed. It is likely, in fact, that Bill defends too much against impulse, that defensive barriers inhibit expression where it would be appropriate.

CLINICAL SUMMARY: Bill

Bill is sixteen years old and has a brother aged thirteen. The referral followed an incident in which Bill terrorized his younger brother by locking him out of the house and threatening to kill him.

Bill has had lifelong problems of not getting along with other children and not taking sufficient responsibility for himself in such matters as dressing and feeding. Throughout his schooling he has been reported to be a dreamer and has had difficulty with his academic work, despite his apparently good intelligence.

Although Bill's early development is described as having been quite normal, he has frequent tonsillitis, which was usually accompanied by high fever, and, on one occasion, by some jerking movements. He has always been afraid of pain, and, when he was very young, it was difficult to take him to the doctor or dentist because of this fear. It was not until the age of twelve that he was able to tolerate medical care. At the age of three, following a visit to his paternal relatives, he developed a panic about going to the bathroom, and this fear continued for about three months. Contradictory passive-active trends during the early years are illustrated by his refusal to lie on his back as a very young baby while, on the other hand, being markedly passive about eating; he would eat, without protest, anything his mother fed him. He never objected to being dressed or to having his clothes selected for him. He was always a quiet child, and the parents soon became aware that he did not play with other children. Rather, he would provoke them and then be unable to defend himself against their retaliatory anger; in turn, he would become angry with them. He developed an amazing vocabulary at an early age, and the other children responded to him as someone who did not speak their language. He played happily by himself, talked to himself a great deal, and never responded well when other children wanted to be friends.

Bill had for the most part acted in a loving way toward his brother, and only in the past three or four years has he begun to show anger toward him. Whereas Bill used to enjoy the role of big brother, he now often joins other children in attacking his younger brother.

Bill has always had learning difficulties; these were attributed primarily to his lack of attention and to his unwillingness to work in class. This year, he has been excluded from two classes and is failing a third. He has made attempts to participate in school sports but has failed in them consistently. He has not expressed interest in dating and has never initiated any contact with girls. He is certain they would not accept him. He is a voracious reader, but he will not read material his parents want him to read. He has rebelled against going to church, though earlier he was much interested in attending Sunday school and seemed quite devout. His interests have gradually become increasingly constricted. He was able to handle a paper route until recently, when his customers complained he was not delivering papers properly.

Bill entered a brief course of therapy a while ago. Although his therapist reported much improvement, therapy was interrupted because the parents did not feel sufficiently included in the treatment process. Lately, the school counselor has been seeing Bill regularly. Since the incident in which Bill locked his brother out of the house, the parents have been afraid to leave the two boys alone together.

Physical, Neurological and Laboratory Data: These examinations were all within normal limits.

THE PSYCHOLOGIST'S DESCRIPTION

Bill is a good-looking, articulate boy of almost seventeen, whose mesomorphic build does not dispel an aura of effeminacy. His excellent, although at times somewhat stilted, use of language, his well-developed store of information and his general air of thoughtfulness are impressive. His speech reflects an occasional tendency to think obsessively, and he obviously enjoys intellectualizing about a variety of topics.

THE WECHSLER-BELLEVUE SCALE

Name: __Bill__   Age: __16-11__

	RS	WTS	0 1 2 3 4 5 6 7 8 9 10 11 12 13 14 15 16 17 18 19 20
COMPR.	14-15	12-13	
INFOR.	19	13	
DIG.	13	11	
ARITH.	8-9	10-12	
SIMIL.	16	13	
VOCAB.	31	13	
P. A.	14	12	
P. C.	12-13	12-13	
B. D.	33	15	
O. A.	21	12	
D. S.	43	10	

TOT. VERB.	61-64
TOT. PERF.	61-62
TOT. SCALE	122-126

VERBAL I.Q.: __119-123__   LEVEL: __Bright Normal→Superior__

PERFORMANCE I.Q.: __115-116__   LEVEL: __Bright Normal__

TOTAL I.Q.: __121-124__   LEVEL: __Superior__

[Bill's Scattergram reflects the superiority of his intellectual functioning. The degree of his scatter (from 10 to 15) is considerable, but not really disquieting for his age. In seven out of eleven subtests, he obtains a score of 12 or 13, and this seems to be the level at which he is able to function comfortably. The excellent Block Design weighted score of 15 reflects the efficiency of his (noninterpersonal) perceptual-motor functioning; it suggests that Bill's general intellectual level may be higher than what is reflected by his present total scores.]

INFORMATION

No.	Question	Response and Comments	Score
1.	Who is the President of the United States?	Dwight D. Eisenhower. (Who was President before him?") Harry S. Truman. ("And before him?") . . . . Gosh, uh . . somebody between Roosevelt and him. Just say Roosevelt. [Bill's first response is an indicator of much that is to follow: he gives the middle initial of the previous two	+

No.	Question	Response and Comments	Score

presidents because he takes pride in his exactness. His vague feeling that "somebody" came between Roosevelt and Truman shows how the exactness has rents in it. It is a little as if someone were able to attribute the correct Latin botanical name to many trees without being able to call a birch tree by its common English name. Still, Bill is able to recover—one of his important and abiding characteristics.

[It is understandable that a person tends to reveal so much about himself in his first response; this is a time of major stress, when anxiety is high, so that defenses are alerted. Bill's tendency to be just a bit off the mark, and then to recover, is typical of his performance on structured tests.]

2. *What is a thermometer?* — An instrument to measure temperature. [Such a "clean," well-organized response is also typical of Bill.] +

3. *What does rubber come from?* — Uh .. uh .. it comes from a tree. I don't remember the tree's name. Maybe you should just call it a rubber tree. [This is the type of answer, just a bit unusual, referred to previously.] +

4. *Where is London?* — Capital of England. +

5. *How many pints make a quart?* — Two. +

6. *How many weeks are there in a year?* — Fifty-two. +

7. *What is the capital of Italy?* — Uh .. Rome. +

8. *What is the capital of Japan?* — Tokyo. +

9. *How tall is the average American woman?* — Five feet three inches to five feet four inches. No. I don't know. +

10. *Who invented the airplane?* — Well, it would be the Dwight brothers. ("Are you sure?") No. The Wright brothers, excuse me. [Just another hair off the mark; a hint of contamination, and then recovery.] +

11. *Where is Brazil?* — In .. uh .. it's in South America. On the east side —sort of a bulge. +

No.	Question	Response and Comments	Score
12.	*How far is it from Paris to New York?*	Hm . . Four thousand miles.	—
13.	*What does the heart do?*	It pumps the blood through the circulatory system of the body.	+
14.	*Who wrote Hamlet?*	Shakespeare.	+
15.	*What is the population of the United States?*	One hundred seventy-two thousand . . I mean million. [Again.]	+
16.	*When is Washington's birthday?*	February . . . . . uh . . 12, I guess. ("When is Lincoln's birthday?") February 23. That's just a guess. [Again.]	—
17.	*Who discovered the North Pole?*	You mean who went there first? ("That's right.") Richard Byrd, I guess. I'm not sure.	—
18.	*Where is Egypt?*	In . . North Africa . . Northeast Africa. [Over and over, Bill needs to show precision.]	+
19.	*Who write Huckleberry Finn?*	Mark Twain, or . . . . . Gosh . . Joel Chandler Harris. His pen name was Mark Twain. ("Are you sure?") No . . no . . that's Uncle Remus. [Again precise and a bit off the mark.]	+
20.	*What is the Vatican?*	It's the . . the uh . . city of the Roman Catholic Church. It's a separate country or region where the Pope lives. He never leaves there.	+
21.	*What is the Koran?*	It's the . . equivalent of the Christian Bible for Mohammedans.	+
22.	*Who wrote Faust?*	Goethe (he spells it). I might as well tell you . . the only reason I know that is because someone told me it's on almost every test you take. [Does a too strongly developed superego lead to this admission? Is it a disguised way of showing how he has outwitted me? Do both reasons operate?]	+
23.	*What is a Habeas Corpus?*	It's the . . It's the remains of a murder victim. It's necessary for the proof of murder. [Bill is probably thinking of *corpus delicti*. A fuzziness of the boundaries which should keep areas distinct from each other, with material that brings Bill into less familiar intellectual territory, is typical of his thinking. Were such fluidity to occur with more everyday material, it would represent a more serious indication of pathological thinking.]	—

No.	Question	Response and Comments	Score
24.	What is ethnology?	Uh . . ethnology . . It's . . It's . . Gosh, I don't know. ("Do you have any idea?") Something scientific, I think. It may be the study of earth tremors, possibly.	—
25.	What is the Apocrypha?	The Apocrypha . . uh . . I don't know . . It sounds like something religious.	—

RAW SCORE: 19

WEIGHTED SCORE: 13

(He seems tense, and I ask if he feels nervous.) Not as much as with Dr. E_____ (a female psychiatrist). I can talk with a man better. I'm more comfortable with men. There doesn't seem to be any deep-seated reason for that. [The "deep-seated reason" comment is meant both seriously and sarcastically. Because of his experience with psychotherapy, Bill is primed to see "deep-seated reasons," but he is also using the opportunity to express annoyance about being asked to look beyond the immediate.]

COMPREHENSION

No.	Question	Response and Comments	Score
1.	What is the thing to do if you find an envelope in the street, that is sealed, and addressed and has a new stamp?	I'd drop it in the mailbox. [A clear, direct, non-obsessive response.]	2
2.	What should you do if while sitting in the movies you were the first person to discover a fire (or see smoke and fire)?	Tell . . uh . . to the . . to an usher or somebody . . somebody that worked there . . and tell them there was a fire . . and they take the necessary steps. Quickly, too, but not conspicuously quickly. [Obsessiveness becomes more marked, possibly because Bill guards himself against a tempting impulsive action—e.g., to cry out a warning.]	2
3.	Why should we keep away from bad company?	Because of the impression that others get. Because others seem to think . . have a tendency to think . . . I guess you could just say that a man is known by the company he keeps. [Bill impatiently cuts through his obsessiveness but with some loss of saliency.]	1
4.	Why should people pay taxes?	Because . . uh . . to pay for the services they get from the government . . and necessary defense.	2
5.	Why are shoes made of leather?	Because it's pliable and durable and long-wearing. [He thinks efficiently and to the point again.]	2
6.	Why does land in the city cost more than land in the country?	Uh . . . . Because it . . uh . . I don't know how to put it exactly. There are more people in the city. People want to live closer to where they work, and it's not so far in the city for them to	1-2

No.	Question	Response and Comments	Score
		travel. ("Why is the land more expensive?") Because any business would want to be closer to people so that . . so that would get more business and people could live closer and buy things. ("Why does the land cost more?") Because the land is coveted by both business and living places. [It takes a while and some of the examiner's help before Bill can center in properly. When he is not helped back on the track, he becomes involved in paths which carry him from his goal. The word "coveted" has a somewhat odd ring in the context.]	
7.	If you were lost in a forest (woods) in the daytime, how would you go about finding your way out?	Uh . . well . . I'd decide which way is more likely to . . where people would most likely be closest, and try to keep a straight line by lining up three trees in front of me in a straight line. Sometimes that doesn't work, I guess. [This solution is somewhat out of the ordinary. The answer is scored 1 because Bill makes use of some sort of natural fact.]	1
8.	Why are laws necessary?	Uh . . people . . . . . have to live in . . uh . . in an efficient manner with other people without anyone causing anyone else harm, and they don't do it naturally.	1
9.	Why does the state require people to get a license in order to be married?	Because their . . . . their . . . laws require certain things to . . people to get married . . They must be the proper. age, and so forth.	1
10.	Why are people who are born deaf usually unable to talk?	Because they have no idea what speech sounds like and cannot listen to themselves in order to correct themselves, in order to sound like others.	1

RAW SCORE: 14-15

WEIGHTED SCORE: 12-13

[Although mild fuzziness is apparent in Bill's thinking, his protocol so far does not raise any significant questions about the solidity of his mental organization.]

DIGIT SPAN

(Bill repeats eight Digits Forward and five Digits Backward.)

RAW SCORE: 13

WEIGHTED SCORE: 11

ARITHMETIC

(Bill earns full credit on the first eight problems, none of which requires more than $1\frac{1}{2}''$ for him to solve. On the last two problems, however, he does the following:)

No. Problem	Response and Comments	Score
9. If a train goes 150 yards in ten seconds, how many feet can it go in one-fifth of a second?	Oh shoot . . let's see . . . . . gosh . . . . I can't think anymore. (Twenty-six seconds have passed.) Twenty-two seconds . . I mean feet. Wait . . yeah, twenty-two feet. ("How did you do that?") I divided 150 by twenty . . oh my gosh! I thought one-fifth second goes into ten twenty times, and then I multiplied that by three. (With some help, he is finally able to reach the correct solution.)	
10. Eight men can finish a job in six days. How many men will be needed to finish it in a half day?	It comes out a fraction! ("Take your time.") . . . Oh . . oh it would be . . uh . . I can't think very well. It comes out eight-twelfths and that's two-thirds. ("Would it take more or less men?") Oh, more men. Oh, no wonder. It would take twelve times as many men. ("How many would that be?") Ninety . . no . . yeah . . ninety . . . . . ninety-six.	

[These last two problems show a sudden drop in Bill's ability to think effectively. In both cases he complains of a thought interference, and the change in efficiency is certainly notable. Significant, too, is an increase in obsessiveness as the problems become more complex.]

RAW SCORE:	8-9
WEIGHTED SCORE:	10-12

SIMILARITIES

No. Items	Response and Comments	Score
1. Orange-banana	They're edible, and fruits, and the color's almost alike . . similar. You want all the ways? ("Which way is the one you want to give?") They're both edible. [Bill has a problem in choosing the "best" from the three possibilities which occur to him.]	1
2. Coat-dress	To wear. [Again, surprisingly, he gives a less adequate, functional definition.]	1
3. Dog-lion	Animals. Should I be more specific and say mammals? [Bill's wish to offer a refined abstraction is in surprising contrast to his preceding, much less adequate, Coat-dress formulation.]	2
4. Wagon-bicycle	Vehicles.	2
5. Daily paper-radio	They . . you get news from them.	1

No.	Items	Response and Comments	Score
6.	*Air-water*	They have no definite shape. [This is a rather odd way of expressing this similarity. While the response merits a score of 1, it merits a lifted eyebrow as well. The definition would fit two gases, something which Bill possibly has in mind.]	1
7.	*Wood-alcohol*	Fuels.	1
8.	*Eye-ear*	Organs of se . . sensory organs.	2
9.	*Egg-seed*	Uh . . beginnings of life . . beginnings of kinds of life. [Once again, Bill manifests his need to formulate with precision; he tries to offer an answer which at the same time takes into account various likelihoods. But in spite of his efforts to be super-precise, Bill's answer is not adequate for a full score.]	1
10.	*Poem-statue*	They're . . . . have an appreciation to them . . an appeal to the inner person. [Although Bill puts things poetically, his tendency to bypass the essence is again apparent. While he achieves a more than adequate weighted score on this subtest, he might do even better were his ideas gathered more tightly.]	1
11.	*Praise-punishment*	They are . . the results . . of actions.	1
12.	*Fly-tree*	They're living.	2

RAW SCORE: 16

WEIGHTED SCORE: 13

PICTURE COMPLETION

(Bill correctly finds twelve of the fifteen "missing" items. On Items 4 and 5, however, his thinking reflects two lapses:)

Card. Hm . . the . . uh . . hm . . I don't know . . . . . . The diamonds are in different patterns. (20″) No . . One more big diamond in the center is missing. (28″)

Crab. Two of the legs and back, and I'd say the tail. (19″) ("Are you sure?") One of the legs on the left side. (23″)

[These responses suggest an impairment of reality testing, followed by recovery. Bill's sporadic and mild confusion prevents a correct response from becoming available; in mild desperation, he substitutes an inferior answer.]

RAW SCORE: 12-13

WEIGHTED SCORE: 12-13

(Testing is discontinued for the day. On the following day, Bill complains of his lack of feeling or curiosity regarding the entire examination.)

PICTURE ARRANGEMENT

No.	Item	Correct Order	Time	Arranged Order	Story and Comments	Score
1.	House	PAT	3″	PAT	It's of a carpenter building a house. He puts the foundation down first, and then the skeletal structure, and then the finishing touches.	2
2.	Holdup	ABCD	6″	ABCD	This is a crook who robbed a man and is caught by a cop, and brought to court and sentenced, and is serving his time.	2
3.	Elevator	LMNO	5″	LMNO	The bell ringing means the rising elevator. And the bell's ringing, so the elevator must be rising. And . . . . first you can see two men and then you can see a king. [So far, very good.]	2
4.	Flirt	JANET	24″	JANET	These always seem to have a psychological significance, like a dream. Shall I tell you my impression? ("Go ahead.") The King is riding in his car, and he sees a woman with a big hat. Then he has the chauffeur stop the car and gets out of the car and walks down the street with the woman, wearing the hat. ("What do you think is the psychological significance?") The two men seem to be like parents that he naturally has, and the woman is a . . . . woman. And the hat . . represents his attraction to her and the way of life she offers, and he accepts the hat and wears it himself. He . . that . . uh . . he drops his riches that he has already, and in exchange takes . . uh . . takes what he . . hm . . what he likes about being a woman. ("And what about the parents?") They were waiting for him to	3

No. Item	Correct Order	Time	Arranged Order	Story and Comments	Score
				come back. ("And?") And he doesn't come back. [The unusualness of Bill's "interpretation" is attenuated by his having been asked to make similar interpretations of his own dreams. Nevertheless, Bill seems too much at ease in attributing "symbolic" significances, and an observer would be happier to see him adopt a more down-to-earth view. The facility with which he ascribes "symbolism" leaves one a little ill at ease. A significant, perhaps not fully intended, aspect of the "interpretation" has to do with Bill's conception of needing to leave his parents in order to achieve heterosexuality.]	
5. Taxi	SAMUEL	50″	ASMUEL	He was with a statue, uh . . . obviously the representation of a woman. And he called the taxi to go where he wanted to go. And . . . . hm . . . . discovered that it appeared as if he was with a woman. This embarrassed him greatly, and he tried to make it obvious that he was not. [Bill often tries to attain his goal of appearing intelligent through a stilted use of language. A slipshod and small error results in his obtaining a score of "0" on this item, even though he obviously understands it well.]	0
6. Fish	EFGHIJ	26″	EFGHIJ	The King fishing . . . . and he caught two fish quickly. But it became apparent soon that he was just trying to get a feeling of accomplishment . . and fooling himself by having the diver hook	5

No. Item	Correct Order	Time	Arranged Order	Story and Comments	Score
				fish on the hook. Actually, it accomplished nothing. [Bill is harsh with those who present appearances not based on actual accomplishment. Probably this stern attitude is a projection—he is actually harsh with what he feels to be his own tendency to fool himself and others into believing he is more able than he really is.]	

RAW SCORE: ___14___

WEIGHTED SCORE: ___12___

BLOCK DESIGN

(Bill seems to have no trouble whatever with the perceptual-motor analysis and integration of the block designs. The blocks almost fly together in his hands, and he shows no hesitations and no other behaviors which suggest the slightest bafflement. With a single minor exception, he is exceedingly systematic.) [Bill shows by his excellent performance on this subtest, usually so sensitive to cognitive impairment, how well organized his ego functioning can be and ordinarily is in situations that are well structured and otherwise externally controlled.]

RAW SCORE: ___33___

WEIGHTED SCORE: ___15___

OBJECT ASSEMBLY

(Again, Bill organizes efficiently. He obtains some time credit wherever possible.)

RAW SCORE: ___21___

WEIGHTED SCORE: ___12___

DIGIT SYMBOL

(Bill's functioning here is not as smooth as one would expect from his Block Design and Object Assembly performances. A few symbols are somewhat awkwardly drawn—e.g., lines which should be straight are mildly curved or jagged.) [Bill's difficulties here are so minor that, with the present degree of knowledge, they cannot validly be attributed to anything other than a slightly lowered ability on this type of task. The "difficulty" is such by contrast only, since the final score is average for Bill's age.]

RAW SCORE: ___43___

WEIGHTED SCORE: ___10___

VOCABULARY

No.	Word	Response and Comments	Score
1.	*Apple*	A red, delicious fruit . . . . hanging on a tree . . I mean, it comes from a tree. [Bill's compulsive effort to be precise is once more apparent.]	1
2.	*Donkey*	A stubborn, kicking, small animal with a slightly pretty body. [Another somewhat peculiar formulation. One does not usually think of a donkey as having a "slightly pretty body."]	1
3.	*Join*	Bring together . . to fit.	1
4.	*Diamond*	Uh . . a tremendously valuable, transparent piece of . . of . . hard but . . it's transparent, that's my main . . . material.	1
5.	*Nuisance*	Tommy, my little brother (he smiles). A small brother or small boy. ("What do you mean?") That's my first thought. Anything that bothers you continually. ("How about Tommy?") He pesters me and asks questions all the time, and I just don't like him. [An interesting shift occurs here. Bill suddenly reacts as though this were a word-association rather than a vocabulary task. What does such an arbitrary (even though humorous) shift in the midst of a task signify? Does it reflect (an occasional) inability to maintain a set? Once again, Bill eventually gets back on the track.]	1
6.	*Fur*	Uh . . well . . uh . . it's used in coats usually to keep warm and . . . warm. It's usually greatly valued. ("Can you tell me any more about it?") It comes from animals. It's soft. It's the skin of animals . . with the hair.	1
7.	*Cushion*	Uh . . uh . . it's a protection against a hard . . covered with cloth. It's made of something resilient to protect against a hard surface. Protect a person. [Had Bill said, "a pillow," it would have done as well.]	1
8.	*Shilling*	A piece of money in England . . and England's satellites. I mean, the Commonwealth. [It is becoming increasingly clear that Bill finds it at least as important to make an "intelligent" impression (both to himself and to others) as to give an accurate response.]	1
9.	*Gamble*	Uh . . take a chance . . in order . . Chance of losing what you have, in order to gain what you don't have. Usually the chances are against you. [This response reflects Bill's too decorous, somewhat prudish orientation.]	1

No.	Word	Response and Comments	Score
10.	*Bacon*	It comes from a pig . . a strip of meat . . crisp meat.	1
11.	*Nail*	Uh . . something hammered into wood, to hold two pieces of wood together. It's hammered first into one and then the other. [Bill's compulsivity frequently merges into the pedantic.]	1
12.	*Cedar*	A tree with . . . . . . just a thin tree with small brownish fruit, I guess. I don't really know what a cedar is. It's not edible. I mean, the fruit.	1
13.	*Tint*	Slight coloring.	1
14.	*Armory*	Building for storage of munitions.	1
15.	*Fable*	A myth that is known not to be true.	1
16.	*Brim*	The top and outside rim . . inside . . well, the top rim. [Another sample of Bill's obsessive thinking.]	1
17.	*Guillotine*	An executing device which drops a heavy blade on a chopping block on which is . . uh . . the condemned man's head . . the condemned man's head is on, and it chops his head off. [A striking manifestation of intellectualizing pedantry.]	1
18.	*Plural*	A word denoting more than one of a noun or pronoun.	1
19.	*Seclude*	Isolate.	1
20.	*Nitroglycerine*	A liquid made to explode with agitation . . slight agitation, from which dynamite is made. ["With agitation"?]	1
21.	*Stanza*	Part of a song . . A verse of a song, I guess you'd say.	1
22.	*Microscope*	An optical instrument for the seeing of very small objects. [Intellectualization frequently works well.]	1
23.	*Vesper*	Vesper? Hm . . a wasp is all I can think of. Of course, that's not English. Vespa in Italian. There's a word in Spanish like it. [Bill's intellectualization occasionally carries the stamp of virtuosity but also the hint of a clang association.]	0
24.	*Belfry*	Uh . . an enclosure for a bell on top of a building.	1
25.	*Recede*	Move back.	1

No.	Word	Response and Comments	Score
26.	*Affliction*	Illness.	½
27.	*Pewter*	Powder for something. ("How do you mean?") I think it's white powder, but I don't remember what it's for. [This seems to be a clang association, the seriousness of which is ameliorated by Bill's making clear that he is guessing.]	0
28.	*Ballast*	Weight carried on a ship to . . raise the water level . . or reduce, lower the ship in the water, so that it'll sail more stably.	1
29.	*Catacomb*	. . . . I'm trying to think . . . . A cave or place . . a complicated place, hard to get out of, easy to get lost in. [Such as the dilemmas in which Bill often finds himself.]	½
30.	*Spangle*	A decorative, shiny piece of clothing or paint . . maybe not. Probably only clothing.	½
31.	*Espionage*	Work on . . spying on another country, I guess.	1
32.	*Imminent*	Pending, I guess. Apparent that it's going to happen.	1
33.	*Mantis*	An insect . . that eats other insects . . of a certain kind. [Apparently he needs to ignore that the female eats its mate.]	1
34.	*Hara-kiri*	Suicide. ("Can you tell me anything more?") Japanese.	1
35.	*Chattel*	I don't know.	0
36.	*Dilatory*	I don't know.	0
37.	*Amanuensis*	I don't know.	0
38.	*Proselyte*	I don't know.	0
39.	*Moiety*	I don't know.	0
40.	*Aseptic*	Good . . well . . not good . . promoting growth of bacteria.	0
41.	*Flout*	Uh . . ridicule . . break down of a person. ("How do you mean?") I mean . . uh . . tear down a person.	½
42.	*Traduce*	I guess it'd be . . That's tra*verse* . . I don't know.	0

RAW SCORE: 31

WEIGHTED SCORE: 13

THE DRAW A PERSON TEST

PART I (PLATE 26)

(Bill's immediate response, after being asked to draw a person, is:) I can't draw. (Nevertheless, he begins to draw right away. He wonders whether he should use the entire sheet of paper. As he draws, he says:) It looks terrible. (As he continues to draw, he self-depreciatively laughs several times and says:) It looks like a drawing I saw, that an imbecile drew. (After he finishes the drawing and signs his name, he says:) Boy! That's awful! (He does relatively little erasing on Part I.)

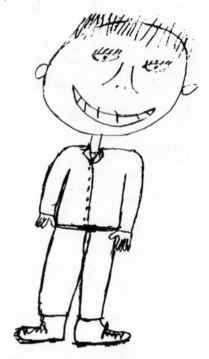

PLATE 26

PART II (PLATE 27)

(In various ways, he indicates his reluctance to begin. As he draws, he frequently erases and otherwise modifies what he has drawn. While doing this, he makes such comments as:) I've never drawn much before, so I'm having a hard time . . . . Oh gosh! (He laughs.) It doesn't look right at all. This writing . . I mean . .

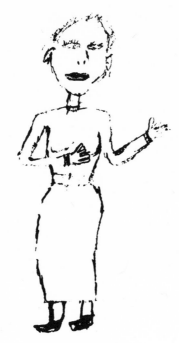

PLATE 27

this drawing doesn't exactly look like the way a person looks to me
. . it's just a crude attempt. ("Does my writing down what you say
bother you?") No, I don't think so. It's just, I have an awfully hard
time putting down the way a thing looks to me in my mind. (As he
works on the hand:) I can't draw a hand. (He attempts to use his own
hand for a model. He does a great deal of erasing, particularly around
the hand, and takes much longer with this drawing than with the
first. He erases the huge, grim mouth he has drawn and puts a slightly
smaller one in its place. He continues to modify obsessively, to add
on, to take away and to change. After he appears to be all done, he
again erases the legs, saying they point the wrong way. After this, he
redraws the eyes. After he completes the drawing, he says:) I could
improve that one of the man. He looks like a basketball. He looks
monstrous.

[A comparison of Bill's two drawings points dramatically to the
difference in his conceptions of male and female. His male is a little
boy who presents a smiling, somewhat hydrocephalic countenance
to the world and who seems to say, "Look how simple I am! I
wouldn't hurt anything or anyone. There is certainly no reason for

you to want to hurt *me!"* His drawing of the woman, with which he
has considerably more difficulty, is of a much older person, who can
best be characterized as a forbidding vamp. Although Bill has already
said that he is much more at ease with men than with women, his
drawings fill in more of the particulars. His representations suggest
he sees women as calculating, stern persons who take advantage of
somewhat simple-minded and rather helpless, if superficially well-
meaning, little-boy males.]

RORSCHACH TEST

RORSCHACH SCORING SHEET

Number of Responses: 24

Manner of Approach (Location)

W	4	Ws	2
D	13		
Dd	1		
Do	(1)		
Dr	3		
De	0		
S	1		
Total	24		

Location Percentages

W%	25
D%	54
DR%	21
De%	0

Form, Movement, Color and Shading Determinants

F+	6
F−	1
F±	1
F∓	3
M+	3
FC±	2
FC−	1
FC(C)∓	1
CF	4
C(C)F	1
CFC'	1
Total	24

Groups of Contents

A	7
Ad	2
H	4
Hd	(1)
Obj.	3
At.	0
Ats.	0
Pl.	2
Blood	3
Gooey stuff	1
Geol.	1
Reflect.	1
Total	24

Determinant and Content Percentages

F%	46/75	Obj.%	13
F+%	64/67	At.%	0
A%	38	P%	21
H%	17		

Qualitative Material

Popular	I III V VIII X
Combination	VI VIII IX X
Fabulation	11
Confabulation	1
Peculiar	6
Queer	1
Confused	3
Deteriorated	1
Symbolic	1
Aggressive	1

EXPERIENCE BALANCE: 3.0/8.0

[Bill's Rorschach performance confirms the initial impression that his psychological situation is worrisome. A look at his psychogram reveals that he is psychologically too "open" and, therefore, too undefended. Eleven of his responses—almost half the total—are Fabulized; five are designated Peculiar, one Queer, one Symbolic, one Deteriorated and three Confused. Only 46 percent of his responses are determined exclusively by formal characteristics, and in only 75 percent of his responses do formal characteristics play the predominant role. The percentage of responses with good formal quality, although within "normal limits," is nevertheless low for someone so intellectually, obsessively and compulsively organized as Bill. Most opposed to expectation is the Experience Balance, which is much more unconstrained than one would wish to see in a "healthy" obsessive-compulsive character organization. A closer look at Bill's Color responses reveals that the majority are poorly organized. Such suggestions of limited intellectual control (in someone who prizes it so highly) strongly point to an active disorganizing process at work. While a major adolescent reorganization with some necessary disorganization is desirable to permit optimal growth into adulthood, Bill seems far to exceed the limits of the ideal loosening of boundaries which one expects and wants to occur at that time. One is again face-to-face with the problem of how much "abnormality" is "normal" in adolescence or, stated more accurately, how much behavior usually and correctly designated as "abnormal" (at a later or slightly earlier age) falls within the boundaries of appropriate adolescent behavior.]

RORSCHACH PROTOCOL

Card #	React. Time	Score	Protocol	Inquiry and Observations
I	12″	WsF+AP Fab.	1. It looks like a bat, or something. It looks like a bat, flying over and looking down. ("Do you see anything else?")	1. ("Tell me about the bat.") It looks as if it's against the sky, flying over, looking down. ("Why does it look that way?") Because . . it just looks like it . . It just reminds me of flying low over me and like the sky was behind . . up above it. ("What makes it look like the sky?") Through the wings kind of. It looks like the wings had holes in 'em. And around the outsides. [Bill articulates his

React.			
Card #	Time	Score	Protocol	Inquiry and Observations

Inquiry and Observations column continued:

thoughts easily, but this ease of expression lulls one into thinking he offers more than he actually does. It is apparent, for example, that his second and third responses are not really new ones, but only very mild variations of the first.]

Pec. Fab. Agg. Confus.

2. It kinda looks like a caterpillar . . not a caterpillar, but a butterfly. Not the outside of it, but the inside of it, like rather seinister (sic) . . sinister. Hm. What should I say now? Describe the butterfly? Oh, the different things, all the *different* things . . . .

2. First when I looked, it seemed like the wings of a butterfly . . sort of big. When I looked closer at it, it looked more like a butterfly wings . . smoother and more solid, but bat wings have those little claws on them and sort of more webbed. ("What made it seem sinister?") The ominous way it seemed to fly over, looking down.

Do Tend. Fab. Pec.

3. Well, these holes in here . . the eye spaces . . makes it look like something flying, that spreads over a wide area, with their wings, that's wide . . . .

3. The wings seemed to spread out, like thin wings, as far as they could. It seemed like cloth or paper spread out over fingers. [One response has artificially been made into three because of the examiner's wish to create discrete order out of what is so poorly ordered in the first place. What starts out to be a simple flying bat becomes more complex, but not actually very different. Bill's imagination goes beyond the easily shared as he is carried away by his descriptions. He becomes arbitrary and his logic becomes difficult to follow. Why, for example, should the eye spaces make the animal look like "something flying, that spreads over a wide area, with their wings, that's wide"? Bill's response *may* not be badly organized, but it is difficult to determine whether

React. Card # Time Score			Protocol	Inquiry and Observations

it is or not. One has difficulty both in ascertaining what Bill's determinants are and in clarifying how they determine what Bill says they do. Even more serious, it never becomes altogether clear, not only *how,* but *what* Bill sees.]

DrF—Ad 4. It looks like . . this part here looks like the head of an insect . . sort of like a fly . . the head of a fly, I mean . . . . (He looks at the card some more.) I guess I'm through.

4. ("How about the fly?") The eyes were bulbous and seemed to take up the whole head, as flies' eyes do. (The four small upper central promontories.)

II   3″   DCFC′   Blood

1. I don't know. It looks like something on the ground. Something splattered on the ground. This part on the bottom looks like blood splattered.

1. The black part (of the bottom red D) looks sort of like it was dropped on the ground . . splattered. That blot didn't mean as much to me as the first ink blot. ("Tell me about the blood.") Some people get actually sick when they think of blood, and they don't like the thought of it. Blood doesn't always suggest a wound or something bad to me, so much. [Such a preoccupation with blood is almost invariably an ominous sign.]

SF+Obj. 2. I don't know if this means anything, but this part in the center looks like a delta-wing jet.

DCF   Blood   Fab.

3. This part looks like cloth that's been pushed against a wound, and the blood's on it . . . . One thing, my connotation for blood isn't as bad as most people. I don't think of it as horrifying.

3. (Top red D's.) [More blood.]

| React.
Card # Time Score	Protocol	Inquiry and Observations
DdF+ Obj.	4. The part up here looks like the point of a pen . . a fountain pen. I don't know, I guess I'm through.	4. (Top central Dd.)
III 24″	Hm . . (He smiles.) Here the red doesn't mean much.	[Nevertheless, he is apparently first drawn to the color, which he cannot organize.]
WM+ HP Fab. Confus.	1. It reminds me of two funny-looking people talking. Hm . . (He shakes his head and smiles.) . . . . Just two women talking, like at a bridge party . . or . . or . . with a glass of ice water or ice tea. I guess that's about all.	1. ("Where was the ice water?") Oh, I didn't see that . . but two women talking. You know, like they do at bridge parties. ("What made them funny looking?") They look like . . in a comic book, for instance. They have characters with beaks, animated birds, for people, I imagine. ("What made them seem like women?") I don't know . . I . . . . they're talking I guess, and below their heads and in front of their bodies there were sort of bumps that look like female breasts. [Several things are striking about this response. The first involves the nonexistent ice water. Bill does not say, "just two women talking looking as though they had a glass of ice water"; rather, he says they have a glass of ice water which, it turns out, cannot be seen. As he talks about this almost confabulized response, the basic identity confusion (already hinted at in the obsession about the bat-butterfly on Card I), emerges more clearly. The "women" he sees are less than human: they are "comic-book" characters with "bird heads." Such a putting together of the real and the comic-book reflects not only Bill's need satirically to derogate women, but also the identity confusion he experiences. One might reasonably

React.			
Card #	*Time*	*Score*	*Protocol*

Inquiry and Observations

ask, "How much greater is this identity diffusion than what one should normally expect of any sixteen- to-seventeen-year-old?" The answer to this question becomes increasingly clear as we follow Bill through his Rorschach, as again and again he testifies to his confusion, not only about who *he* is but about who and what the people and things around him are. Although some adolescent diffusion is, as has been said, a good and necessary state, Bill's is too intense and too ubiquitous to be anything but worrisome.]

IV   16″   WM+H

1. This is kind of far-fetched, but it looks like a great big, kinda old man—one of these ape-kind of men, with this very small head, kind of, and suggestive of low intelligence. And he's sitting on a stump . . . . I guess that's about all.

1. ("Tell me about the man.") Just a . . like, kinda like a guy with . . huge, fat legs and body. And two little lines that came out of the sides of the trunk of the man were mere suggestions of his arms . . . . and he was sitting on the stump with his huge legs and feet sticking out in front of him, with his feet on the ground. ("What made him look apelike?") Because he was so heavy for his height, and his huge fat legs and the trunk. [Once again Bill sees a distorted human figure, this time of a man. So far, he has seen an animal and a female figure about whose identity he was uncertain; now he sees a great, big, kind of old man who looks like an ape and whose very small head suggests low intelligence. Bill's tendency to be either uncertain about the consistent nature of living things, or to degrade them and make them unattractive and ridiculous, comes forth clearly. One should assume, of course, that when Bill talks about

React. Card #	Time	Score	Protocol	Inquiry and Observations
				other living things, he is frequently telling about the way he perceives himself.]
V	9″	WF+AP Fab. Confus.	1. It looks sorta like a butterfly with these light . . tendrils, I guess. Little projections from the rear of his body, the tail sort of like part of the wings. But the head looks like the head of a snail, and the wings look like a hawk's wings, or falcon's. And it looks as if I'm looking down at him while he's flying—as if I'm above him. I guess that's about all for now.	1. ("Tell me about the snail-like head.") It's sort of fat but has two projections out the front of the head, that look like snail's eyes . . eye stocks. (Bottom center Dr.) ("And what about the hawk wings?") They were too thin and sort of swept back for butterfly wings . . and they were pointed. [Once again we see Bill's effort to make consistent sense out of a living thing, by attributing a composite of identities to it. Over and again, he says that nothing is true to type—the identity of all living things is mixed up.]
VI	20″	DrF∓ gooey stuff Fab.	1. It looks like uh . . some . . The bottom part looks like something splattered on the ground . . some gooey something (said with disgust).	1. ("Tell me about the gooey something.") Sort of a yellowish gooey stuff [the card is achromatic] that sometimes caterpillars . . Sap . . I guess, tree sap, that's what it is . . Sticky, yellow sap that comes out of a tree. It looks like its trail line through the middle of the picture. It looks like its trail.
		Comb.		
		DF∓A Pec. Deter.	2. And this top part looks like a caterpillar that's just almost through crawling through it. It has . . . fuzzy sort of antenna sticking out of its neck . . to the side . . and wings too small to lift it off the ground. I think that's all.	2. ("Tell me about the caterpillar.") It was long and looked sort of like it had the head of a caterpillar. A fat sort of body. And it had those four antennae sticking out of its neck. Sometimes caterpillars have just spines and things sticking out of their body all the way up and down. ("Would a caterpillar have wings?") No, a caterpillar wouldn't naturally have wings. ("What was gooey?") The caterpillar looked as if it was, and the stuff was sort of sticking to the caterpillar and all

React.			
Card #	*Time*	*Score*	*Protocol*

Inquiry and Observations

over him. It's hard to know where his body ends. [It would be difficult to find a more graphically portrayed metaphor—the caterpillar whose wings are too small to lift him off the ground, stuck in a gooey mess, without definite boundaries. In this way, Bill tells how hard he finds it to change from the caterpillar child into the butterfly adult. The caterpillar may have some characteristics of a butterfly (i.e., the wings) but, of course, caterpillars do not actually have wings—i.e., Bill is not grown up in any real sense. The "gooey mess" may be Bill's representation of his present dilemma, of the realization he has of his inability to tear himself from childhood. Just as one cannot see where the caterpillar ends, so Bill is unsure about his own boundaries. It is becoming increasingly apparent how serious Bill's identity disturbance is, how, under his façade of intellectual competence, he suffers from a major inability to know either who he is or where he is headed.]

VII	17″	WM+(H)		

1. This looks like two dwarfs or elves . . looking at each other, with this topknot sort of hair . . Like a tribe of African women; a tribe of women of Africa tying their hair in a tight knot. And they're just looking at each other, as if something is funny about the other one. I guess that's about all.

1. ("What made them seem like dwarfs?") Their small bodies, compared to their big heads. They look more like elves, but sort of deformed, somehow. [Once more Bill's "people" turn out to be deformed, slightly ridiculous; in fact, not people at all. They even find each other "funny."]

Card #	*React.* *Time*	*Score*	*Protocol*	*Inquiry and Observations*
VIII	12″	DF+AP Fab.	1. These red things on the side . . look like two tadpoles, almost frogs . . . . . climbing up a side of an island, out of the water.	1. ("How about the tadpoles?") They still have tails that are shrinking, and feet, too, and they're just dragging themselves up on the shore. [Here is another metaphoric description of the way Bill perceives his growing up. He is still mostly a tadpole—not yet a frog. Growing up is a "dragging" process.]
		DCF Reflect	2. And this bottom part looks like the reflection of the island in the water.	2. The reflection in the water was a different color. Instead of green, it was red and yellow. Reflections look better than the actual thing. ("How do you mean?") The colors are brighter, so that there is a mere suggestion. The proportions are wrong. (Bottom D.) [Bill once more shows his tendency to see things that are out of proportion. The phrase "reflections look better than the actual thing" harks back to Bill's indignation at the Little King's fooling himself into thinking he had caught many fish. Although Bill said he disapproved of the Little King's distortion of reality, he now says unreality sometimes "looks better."]
Comb.		DFC± geol.	3. It looks like it's got a green mountain like a volcano, coming out of the island.	3. ("Tell me about the volcano.") It had a . . the top of the picture looked like the cone of a volcano curving up to a point. And there's a lot of volcanoes in the middle of islands. (Top D.) [It is significant that Bill sees a volcano in the midst of the landscape where this major metamorphosis is trying to take place.]
		DCFpl	4. The green part at the foot of the mountain, and the blue part in the middle,	4. (Middle D.)

React. Card #	Time Score	Protocol	Inquiry and Observations
		are trees and stuff down to the shore. I guess that's all.	
IX	25″ WSFC(C) ∓pl	1. It looks sorta like a flower . . a big old flower. And it's growing out of one of those gunnysacks that they used to keep dirt in . . or planting the plants. And this right here is the stem, and I guess the pistil of the flower. The whole thing seems to be the flower. I can see where this green part could be part of the plant that wouldn't be the flower, but nevertheless, the whole thing seems to be the flower. And down here in the base of it, it looks like it's cut away. It looks like one of those cutaway biology diagrams. And the base is the place where the pollen is caught . . and it looks like stamens. I guess that's all.	1. ("What kind of flower did it seem to be?") Sort of a long . . I mean, tall, thin flower that opens at the top. I don't know what kind it would be. ("What made it look like a flower?") Because of its color and the way it opened at the top, and the thing that stuck up at the center looked like the pistil. (He suddenly remembers facts about pistils and stamens which are contrary to the way he saw the flower, but "it may not be important to write it down.") [Although, on the surface, this seems to be a well-differentiated response, it is neither well perceived nor adequately described.]
X	20″ DF∓Ad (Hd) Pec. DrFC−H Queer Confab. Symb. Comb. (See elaboration following Response No. 5)	1. This looks like a . . the top part . . in an insectlike way, like a head. It looks like the head of a . . of one of the real snob queens. (Top center gray D.) . . . This sort of a . . this red part (central side long reddish D's) . . here looks like the . . . . dress of the queen. And this	1. ("Tell me about the queen.") The first part I looked at . . like the head, and a very snobbish expression . . a tall, thin head. It reminded me of the queen in *Alice in Wonderland.* ("What made it look like a snob?") It looked like a thin head . . and features that are small, and stretched and elongated vertically. It gave the impression of a very snobbishlike expression. ("What made it look like a

React. Card # Time Score	Protocol	Inquiry and Observations
	green part (bottom green D's) looks like legs of the queen.	queen?") There was a queen in every movie I saw about Alice. And partly because it was very colorful. [Again, one comes across Bill's apparently defensive need to derogate. And once more, Bill's ways of communicating his perceptions are filled with gaps, which make it difficult to follow his thinking.]
DF+AP	2. And these blue parts to the side look like spiders or crabs.	
DCF± Obj.	3. And these two yellow things on the side look like . . uh . . kinda sea shells . . hm.	3. Everything away from the dress is not the queen. (Outside yellow D.)
DF±A Pec.	4. And these black things to the side look sort of like shrimp, somehow.	4. ("What made them look like shrimp?") I don't know. Just sort of short feet . . and the body projections, and the way he curved out. (Green-gray outer D.)
DC(C)FA	5. And the things at the bottom look like coral. I guess the reason why these things on the outside look like sea creatures is because they're so brightly colored.	5. ("Why coral?") Its . . its color . . the same all over the blot . . that part of the blot. But it had sort of variations that looked like gentle roughness. It wasn't smooth and shiny. (Outer orange-brown D.) [Bill sometimes has an almost poetic way with words— e.g., "gentle roughness."]
	6. (1. cont.) The queen has a thin head but a sort of snobby expression so it looks that her mentality is probably low. And these parts of her body somehow, and they're detached, and very	6. ("And the parts of the queen's body?") Inside her dress, there were a whole lot of colorful . . they didn't look like specific parts of her body. They were . . they looked like parts of her. Maybe her personality ("How do you mean?") I mean, maybe . . parts of her. The way she was . . in her . .

React.				
Card #	*Time*	*Score*	*Protocol*	*Inquiry and Observations*

Protocol

small. I think that's about all. I mean ..... yeah, about all.

Inquiry and Observations

inner parts, yeah, like organs. ("Would you explain more about that?") By being detached, they were separate, sort of, and they were very small. ("What did you mean about her personality?") Actually, her mind . . her way of thinking and acting. ("What made you think of that?") The first thing it reminded me of were organs of the body . . and they might also be. But they didn't seem to be specifically of her body. It was very abstract. The queen's dress was reddish but dilapidated. It was old and . . it reminds me of dry blood . . the color of dry blood . . that's died and lost its usefulness. ("How do you mean?") I think of blood like life. When the blood drains out of a person, he dies. [Bill's response to this last card is extraordinary. Although he has given hints of unusual thinking previously, this response is far beyond the realm of the "somewhat" odd. Were Bill more playful, the pathological implications of the response would be ameliorated. But he is altogether serious about what he sees; for the moment, at least, fantasy has taken over, and reality has little significance. Bill's arbitrary, symbolic thinking, his peculiar ways of expressing himself, and the difficulty one experiences in trying to empathize with his perceptions and interpretations all combine to suggest that Bill has the beginnings of a severe thinking disorder, that he is experiencing the advent of a major disorganization.]

Thematic Apperception Test

Card 1 (A young boy is contemplating a violin which rests on a table in front of him.)

What is this? A riding mask or something? This kid . . This is a dark room, except for his reading light . . . . . He . . . . is . . isn't concentrating. And is . . doesn't want at all to do what he wants to . . I mean, what he's supposed to do. Violin, I just now noticed. I couldn't figure it out. I thought he was reading for a second . . . . His parents have locked him in his room . . I probably told you that, and taken away other objects of interest out of the room, away from him . . . . so that he can do nothing but practice on the violin without getting awfully bored . . . . . He isn't going to practice, as long as there is anything he can do to avoid it . . . . This is his parents' method . . . . . of making him practice . . . . . He's . . . . . he's thinking about everything he can think of and tries to find everything he can do . . . . oh to occupy his mind and to avoid doing practicing the violin. He's even memorizing the serial numbers on the violin (he smiles) . . . . His parents have found that . . . . that even through any kind of punishment they cannot get results out of him with the violin, unless they make it so he can't do anything else. He has no choice . . I don't know . . . Now I'm getting a little vague. (He takes time out from telling the story to tell about his tendency to "get vague" in his thinking every once in a while.) ("What does the boy do?") I don't know. He's just building up a personal hate for his parents and building them up in his mind as very mean. [This story reflects the warfare going on between Bill and his parents. He sees his parents as trying to trick or force him into doing things he will not do, even when he would basically like to do them (see his slip). He feels that the only recourse left to him is to resist them with all his power, not even giving them the satisfaction of watching him go through the motions of doing what they want. The resentful hatred Bill feels toward his parents comes up frequently in future stories. He cannot account for the hatred, can think of no reason for it, but the intensity of feeling results in acts on both sides which increase the resentments between parents and child. Although this type of intrafamily warfare and lack of understanding is a common enough adolescent phenomenon (perhaps even a hallmark of adolescence), most adolescents have all sorts of "good" reasons at their fingertips for hating parents—e.g., the parents are "mean," "heartless," "old-fashioned," "nongiving," "unfair" and so on. What is particularly disturbing about Bill's hatred is his inability to rationalize it. The hatred simply, unaccountably, exists.

[Bill complains of experiencing "vagueness," both here and on other portions of the tests. He says such feelings occur every once in a while, and occasionally he finds it difficult to think clearly. This vagueness is represented in Bill's mistaking the violin, first for a riding mask, then for a book. Such distortions further substantiate one's increasing conviction that Bill's confusion goes well beyond the bounds of the "normal" turmoil of adolescence.]

Card 2 (Country scene: in the foreground is a young woman with books in her hand; in the background a man is working in the fields, and an older woman is looking on.)

Well, this is the daughter of these two people . . . and she wants an education . . . . uh . . but . . his parents . . her parents, I mean . . want her to live her life the way they do . . the way they live their lives . . . . . . and . . . . disapprove of her trying to get an education . . . . uh . . She feels guilty going ahead, getting an education, when her parents don't want her to . . . . but she has ideas of her own and feels it an insult to her parents to want a definite way of life . . . . Her parents just feel as if she doesn't like them at all and is deliberately trying to do what they don't want her to do . . . . . . but . . . uh . . (he shrugs) I guess that's all. ("How does it all come out?") . . . . Well, she's probably gonna . . . go ahead with her education and . . but feel bad about it. ("What do her parents feel or do?") . . . . They will try to talk her out of it. ("Why don't they want her to go ahead?") They're not educated themselves at all . . . and feel she's leaving the good life, as they call it. And they think she should leave well enough alone. [The exchanging of sexual pronouns (e.g., "his" for "her") occurs frequently among children and adolescents. In part the mix-up probably reflects a developmentally not yet established sexual identity. In Bill's case, however, an added reason probably operates: he finds it difficult to maintain the test fiction that he is talking about someone other than himself.

[It makes no sense when Bill says, "She feels guilty going ahead,

292   THE TROUBLED ADOLESCENT

getting an education when her parents don't want her to, but she has ideas of her own *and* feels it an insult to her parents to want a different way of life." A listener expects the "and" to be followed by an idea consistent with the first part of the phrase. Bill is apparently so caught up in guilts about opposing his parents that he is unable to present his cause logically and reasonably. The awkward sentence represents still another example of Bill's disturbance of thinking and demonstrates the degree to which his logic can become the victim of one of his predominant affects—intense guilt which he feels about opposing and degrading his parents. The story he tells to Card 2 follows by a day the story he tells to Card 1. It seems likely that the first story aroused guilts which Bill now tries to expiate or, at least, ventilate. A major aspect of Bill's guilt toward his parents appears to involve his being ashamed of them.]

Card 3 BM (On the floor against a couch is the huddled form of a boy with his head bowed on his right arm. Beside him on the floor is a revolver.)

This looks like a gun on the floor . . I'm not sure . . . . . He's probably . . or she, I guess . . has probably killed somebody accidentally. I guess it's "he," with those high English-style pants, I guess . . . . . Probably a good friend or . . someone . . . . . and he's overwhelmed with guilt . . . . I guess all sorts of thoughts are raising . . are racing through his mind. About how he'll never allow himself to come near a gun again . . and all the things that should happen to him. His thoughts are exaggerated by . . . . what he's done . . and . . . . and eventually his thoughts will fade . . and he'll . . . . . fade in the background and . . . . . he'll either believe they're gone . . although they shouldn't be . . or he believes they shouldn't be . . . . and live an unhappy life, haunted by his guilt . . . . He believes inside that . . . that he should not try to eliminate this guilt or . . be happy, though he tries to suppress it . . . . I guess . . hm . . I guess that's all. ("Why does he believe he shouldn't be happy?") Because he feels indebted to . . . . he feels he should feel guilty. His conscience should bother him. ("What should happen?") All the things that should be done to him. ("Such as what?") Very severe punishments. [Bill demonstrates an obsessive preoccupation with determining the sex of the pictured person. While this particular figure frequently raises questions about its sexual identity, Bill's concern, together with such things as his calling "women" the Popular "men" on Card III of the Rorschach, his calling the girl in the previous card "he," and his much greater comfort when he talks with men are probably some indices of confusion regarding his sexual identity. His generally somewhat effeminate manner further substantiates the impression that he finds it extremely difficult to make an age-appropriate heterosexual adjustment. This state of affairs is not in the least surprising to find within the context of Bill's more generalized confusion regarding what and who he is, who he has been and who he will become.

[The guilt theme in this card is again striking. The impression that Bill is heavily self-accusing, seeks punishment and thinks he neither merits nor can ever achieve happiness is becoming increasingly confirmed. Making his hero's crime an "accident" helps very little to ameliorate and disguise self-destructive, self-punitive needs.]

Card 4 (A woman is clutching the shoulders of a man whose face and body are averted as if he were trying to pull away from her.)
This man . . uh . . is mad at somebody . . . . He hates another man . . . . . . and is obsessed by the idea of revenge . . . . . He's been kept from this man and his . . . . and his hate has mounted considerably . . . . and . . . . he wants only to . . uh . . get back at this man for whatever he's done to him . . . . And this is his girl holding him back . . . . . She doesn't like the other man either, but she's trying to keep him away from him, to keep him from being hurt . . . . . or . . . . doing something to him that . . . . would get him arrested— murder, for instance . . or assault . . . . . She will be successful in keeping him from the other man . . . . but through his life . . this man's life . . . . he will hate the other man . . . . and be snappish and mean . . . . . . to everyone he knows . . . . and grow old before his time . . . . That's all, I guess. ("Why does he hate this other man?") He doesn't really know why, but he just . . . . but his hate has grown over the years. [Bill tells another story involving unreasoning hatred, hatred which will make his hero grow prematurely old. Echoes of oedipal themes are apparent: the girl friend (mother) sides with her boy friend (son) against "somebody"; she wishes to protect her son "from being hurt," possibly by a retaliating father. In a later story, Bill successfully eliminates the father, and his hero has his mother all to himself; this arrangement, however, turns out not to work either.]

Card 5 (A middle-aged woman is standing on the threshold of a half-opened door looking into a room.)

This woman has come back home after a long time . . . . . and
. . . . . . finds it apparently the same as when she left . . . . But she
finds that . . . . . it isn't as happy a place as she thought it would be
. . and it brings back more unpleasant memories than good ones
. . . . . . She's rather old, and the place is along the styles of . . oh
. . old style, I guess . . and she realizes the good old days aren't . .
aren't really so good after all . . . . And I don't know . . that's
all. ("What had she hoped to find?") She's been in a dismal mood
and frustrated, the way things are going . . have been going . . and
she hoped to return to find her old lost happiness . . which never
really existed. [One of the meanings which can be inferred from
this story has to do with Bill's once more dealing with the problem
of whether to grow up. Although he yearns to be young again, he
wonders if he has too greatly romanticized the past.]

Card 6 BM (A short elderly woman stands with her back turned to a tall young man. The latter is looking downward with a perplexed expression.)

This is this man's mother . . . . . He's come back from . . to his
home, after a long absence, and she finds him changed for the
worse . . . . She's disappointed in his . . . . his job, his personality and his future . . . . She had such high hopes for him when
he was younger . . . . . . She didn't . . I mean, *he* didn't realize she'd
react this way . . . . . He thought she'd be glad to see him back and
. . . and they'd have one of her old-fashioned dinners . . . . . He's
found his father has passed away . . . . And things have generally deteriorated . . . hm . . I don't know . . I guess that's all. These
are rather melancholy stories, and I don't seem to fit along the same
pattern I was telling yesterday. [This story suggests that Bill thinks
he has turned out to be a disappointment to his mother. Once he
has left home (i.e., once he is no longer a child), he cannot recapture
the "good old times," including the "old-fashioned dinners." Even
though an unreasoning hatred may exist between Bill and his
father, things "generally deteriorate" once the father is no longer in
the picture. This story continues the theme of the last with some
modifications: "You can't go home again," even when things are the
way you think you want them.]

Card 7 BM (A gray-haired man is looking at a younger man who is sullenly staring into space.)

This . . . . older man . . . . . . looks like a judge, I guess . . . . This younger man has done something . . . . and the judge has asked him why . . . . Then he says "Just punish me" . . and whatever happens to him as punishment . . . . . he believes . . . . . that what he did was worth it . . I mean, he'd suspected this punishment beforehand and knew that it'd happen . . and done it anyway . . . . . . I think he knew he'd have to take the punishment . . in order to get back at somebody. This man, instead of being vindictive . . the older man . . is more . . . . understanding . . he tries to be . . . . than this boy had expected . . I mean, this man . . . . He wants to be punished so that he will feel justified in his hatred for people . . . . I guess that's kind of all. My mind kind of fogs. ("Why does the young man hate like that?") Differences of opinion, I guess. He's always thought that he's right . . and . . he felt as if all his life he's been condemned. ("Condemned how?") Just been treated unfairly. [Although he does not say so, the young man's (i.e., Bill's) hatred is probably again directed toward his father. While Bill says that whatever the hero does is worth the punishment, one wonders whether the main point of the angry act is not to *be* punished (i.e., obtaining punishment may well be the primary motive for the hero's behavior). The older man whom Bill creates is not nearly so vindictive as the hero expects; he is quite understanding, in fact. This particular theme appears to reflect Bill's ambivalence toward his father, the ambivalence which generates such intense guilt and perhaps makes his "mind fog."]

Card 12 M (A young man is lying on a couch with his eyes closed. Leaning over him is a gaunt form of an elderly man, his hand stretched out above the face of the reclining figure.)

This is a . . hypnotizing another boy . . . . The hypnotist . . . . . . is a . . . . He dislikes the first boy . . . . He's only hypnotizing him because he likes hypnotism . . . . . though he may . . . . not be as careful to remove harmful suggestions before waking the patient . . I mean, his subject . . . . and without knowing, he may . . harm the subject . . . . The subject is an innocent sort of boy . . . . but the hypnotist is . . unbalanced and knows it . . . . . but he may not let himself realize . . . . . . that it can be dangerous to hypnotize a person without . . . . being able to concentrate on it and doing it properly . . . . . . The subject is . . . . . aware of the boy's dislike for him and if he is hypnotized at all . . . . and will awaken . . . . What'll I say? ("Anything you wish.") He will awaken . . if the hypnotist does anything he doesn't like. And he won't allow himself to be hypnotized deeply, into a deep sleep. I guess that's all. [Bill's identifications seem to change as he tells this story. At first he identifies himself with the malevolent hypnotist, but he becomes more and more the hapless victim who tries to resist the hypnotist's influence. Bill also seems intent on creating an image of himself as an "evil person." But as he reveals himself more, his fearfulness and helplessness emerge and make clear how "victimized" he feels by his surroundings.]

SENTENCE COMPLETION TEST II

(Only a small portion of this test was administered; time was running out, and the examiner felt he had obtained enough pertinent information to present a fairly complete diagnostic picture.)

He hoped that when he grew up he would be better. ("Better how?") Better at doing something . . having more skill.

When he saw what the other kids were doing he wanted to join them.

When he compared himself to his friends (he smiles) I don't know. He found a great deal of difference. ("How was that?") It seemed that others thought he was different. ("Different how?") I can't think very well. [Not thinking "well" has an obviously avoidant meaning here. Bill finds it hard to speak about his isolation.]

He was sad whenever he thought of . . oh . . his chances of leading a useful life.

When he was asked about his aches and pains he . . uh . . tried to cover them up.

The person he admired most . . . . hm . . I don't know . . (He returns to this item after completing the next.) He is probably afraid to admire somebody. ("Why is that?") Gosh, I don't know. I have a fear of having my mind controlled. [See the apparent connection with the TAT "Hypnosis" card.]

His brother was . . always seeking . . trying to get the best of him. ("Trying to get the best of him how?") In everything. [No wonder Bill wants to lock his brother out.]

When his father came into the room he . . turned and . . and tried to look as if he was paying attention to something else. ("Why was that?") It would be hard for his father to understand the workings of his mind. [Once again the theme of the intellectually inferior father.]

When he was with his sister I don't have a sister, and I don't know about that. ("Make up something.") It embarrassed him to be watched . . not by her, but by other people. [Shame about family again.]

At school he . . . . . hm . . . . . was . . uh . . not able to concentrate.

When he looked at the work the others were doing he . . tried not to want to do it himself. ("Why was that?") I don't know if I'd have answered these questions the same before.

THE PSYCHOLOGIST'S REPORT

Bill's fine use of language, his well-differentiated store of information and his general air of enjoying reflection and abstraction suggest that his Wechsler-Bellevue Intelligence Quotient of 121-124 is lower than his optimal ability. His Verbal Quotient of 119-123 and his Performance Quotient of 115-116 place his abilities in the Bright Normal to Superior range.

Bill's intelligence test performance is fairly homogeneously distributed, and he never does less well than the average for his age. Nevertheless, he occasionally seems satisfied with less than his best performance; at times he loses full credit because his answer is not clearly stated, or because it is slightly odd, at times even inappropriate. An example of an unusual, although not actually incorrect, response is his explanation of how air and water are alike: "They have no definite shape."

Frequently it seems that Bill has difficulty "centering in"; he appears to hover around the periphery of an answer, not getting to its crux. His record is filled with temporary inefficiencies—unexpected errors of fact, which he quickly and spontaneously corrects. He says, for example, the airplane was invented by the "Dwight brothers," an apparent mild contamination from a previous correct response involving "Dwight Eisenhower." Before he corrects himself, he says the population of the United States is 172,000 and Mark Twain's real name was Joel Chandler Harris. Together with failing to hit dead center on occasion, and temporarily giving mildly incorrect answers, he complains of periods of vagueness and confusion during which he is empty of idea and feeling. He is most troubled by an inability to "care" and says feelings of uninvolvement have plagued him for years.

Bill depends a great deal on intellectualization, a process which causes him both to search for knowledge and to become involved in pseudopsychological matters that lead to an overpreoccupation with such matters as dreams, hypnosis and similar psychic phenomena. He often focuses this interest on himself, treating himself as an interesting psychological specimen. But once introspection involves something more serious than playing a psychological game, he shies away from it. Bill's "psychological mindedness" at times takes rather startling forms. For example, he tells the following story to the *Flirt* sequence on Picture Arrangement:

> These always seem to have a psychological significance, like a dream . . . . . . ("What would the significance here be?") The two men seem to be like parents that he naturally has, and the woman is uh . . a woman. And the hat represents his attraction to her, and the way of life she offers, and he accepts the hat and wears it himself . . . . He . . that . . uh . . drops his riches that he has already and in exchange takes . . uh . . takes what he . . hm . . what he likes about being with a woman . . . . [His parents] were waiting for him to come back. ("And?") And he doesn't come back.

Although Bill explains that some years ago his therapist taught him how to "analyze dreams," his readiness to interpret material in this "symbolic" fashion is nevertheless disquieting.

A Rorschach response indicates how "wild" and arbitrarily determined Bill's interpretations of reality can become. The following is so capricious and erratic that, together with the signs of unusual thinking already mentioned, one cannot avoid the conclusion that Bill's thought disorganization is already quite advanced. He interprets Rorschach Card X as follows:

> This [top gray D] looks like uh . . in an insectlike way . . It looks like the head . . . . It looks like the head of a . . of one of the real snob queens . . . . She has a thin head with a sort of snobbish expression, like her mentality is sort of low . . . . It reminds me of the queen in *Alice in Wonderland* . . . . . . [Later, he adds:] Inside her dress there were a whole lot of colorful . . it didn't look

like specific parts of her body. They were . . they looked like
parts of her. Maybe her personality. ("How do you mean?") I
mean, maybe parts of her. The way she was . . in her inner parts
. . yeah, like organs. By being detached, they were separate, sort
of, and they were very small. ("How do you mean, her personality?") Actually, her mind . . her ways of thinking and acting.
("Could you explain that more?") The first thing they reminded
me of was organs of the body . . and they might also . . but they
didn't seem to be specifically her body. They were very abstract
. . . . The queen's dress was reddish, but dilapidated. ("What
made it look that way?") It was old and . . it reminds me of dried
blood . . the color of dried blood . . that's died and lost its usefulness. ("What made it look like that?") I think of blood like life.
When the blood drains out of a person, he dies.

Other Rorschach responses are also (if rather less) strange. Bill
sees such things as "splattered blood" and "cloth pressed upon a
bloody wound"; he sees "something splattered on the ground . .
some gooey something." Although this particular blot is achromatic,
Bill speaks of it as "yellowish."

Bill's disturbance probably has its core in the problem he experiences in crystallizing an identity. It is apparent he cannot accept
any of the alternatives—growing into adulthood, returning to childhood, or remaining where he is. He metaphorically captures his
unsettled situation when, on the Rorschach, he perceives a caterpillar turning into a butterfly; it is stuck in some "gooey stuff," part
of which adheres in such a way that it is hard to know where the
metamorphizing animal ends. Even as Bill cannot accept or solve
growing up, so the caterpillar's wings are "much too small" to lift
him off the ground. Elsewhere, Bill perceives tadpoles turning into
frogs: "They still have tails that are shrinking, and feet, too, and
they're just dragging themselves on to the shore." The island on
which they are "dragging themselves" has a volcano on it. But difficult as growing up is, childhood is no better. Bill tells the TAT
story of a woman who has returned home after a long absence. She
finds things are not nearly so good as she remembers them, and she
cannot find her lost happiness because, she discovers, it never really
existed.

Bill's identity diffusion is further apparent in his tendency, on
the Rorschach, to see combination animals that are a patchwork of

different species. A bat, for example, has the head of a snail and the wings of a falcon. Evident, too, is a rather marked fear of and dislike for women, along with considerable evidence which suggests an uncertain sexual identification. It cannot be ascertained with the present material to what extent Bill's sexual confusion represents one part of the more general identity diffusion, and to what extent the whole identity diffusion is more apparent than real and serves primarily as a defense against heterosexuality.

Bill is intensely isolated. He experiences an impossible-to-transcend distance from his family and peers, all of whom he defensively considers his intellectual inferiors. He feels immense, often unrationalizable anger toward his parents, an anger which results in crippling guilt feelings. Because he views his parents so ambivalently, he feels an extraordinary need to be punished for his derogating, hateful, feelings toward them. While he claims that the pleasures he would gain from any parent-directed destructive act would be well worth any subsequent punishment-pain he might receive, it seems that the goal of the aggressive action is not only the wish to hurt, but also the wish to *be* hurt (punished).

While Bill longs for help, he distrusts the "helpers" and fears the passivity that he thinks receiving help would necessarily impose. In telling a story to the TAT "Hypnosis" card, Bill seems to identify himself both with the evil, unbalanced hypnotist and with the naïve, hapless subject (to whom he once refers as "patient"):

> This is a boy hypnotizing another boy . . . . the hypnotizer . . . is uh . . . . he dislikes the first boy . . . is only hypnotizing him because he likes hypnotism, though he may . . . . not be as careful to remove harmful suggestions before waking the patient . . I mean, his subject . . . and, without knowing, he may . . harm the subject . . . The subject is an innocent sort of boy . . . . but the hypnotist is . . unbalanced and knows it . . . . But he may not let himself realize . . . . that it can be dangerous to hypnotize a person without . . . . being able to concentrate on it and doing it properly . . . . The subject . . . . is aware of the boy's dislike for him, and if he is hypnotized at all . . . . and will awaken . . . what'll I say? ("Say whatever comes to mind.") He will awaken . . if the hypnotist does anything he doesn't like . . . and will not allow himself to be hypnotized deeply, into a deep sleep. I guess that's all.

In summary, Bill's quite severe disorganization is rather poorly hidden by a relatively well-functioning ego façade which contains intellectualizing defenses that are often not adequate to prevent the occasional emergence of arbitrary, illogical thinking. Bill's pronounced need to expiate guilt raises the dangerous possibility that he may act destructively in order to receive punishment. Although he tends to derogate the people close to him, he has by no means closed off communication between himself and them. While he is fearful to reveal himself, he also expresses his need to reach and be reached by others, to discuss his problems and to obtain help. He does not feel ready to enter adulthood; neither does he wish to stay where he is or to go back to an earlier time.

DISCUSSION

Bill presents a striking example of the young person who is trapped in adolescence, who can move neither toward childhood nor toward adulthood. He sees no great point in growing up, since the future holds so little promise—all he can see there is that he will (should) suffer and do penance indefinitely for his "badness." Although he has the physical and ego equipment to enter adulthood, he is otherwise not at all prepared for the transformation. He is so intensely, so ambivalently bound up with his parents that he cannot free himself sufficiently even to begin to enter into any sort of relation with peers of either sex. He cannot give up childhood in order to achieve true autonomy. His defensive but highly superficial rejection of his parents, and his equally defensive rejection of his peers, leave him with only himself. Since he does not know who or what he is, what the quality of his "humanness" is, what his boundaries are, the busy world passes him by. He keeps whirling around in a small eddy, while the main body of life forges ahead. Quite possibly there is still time to reverse Bill's isolation and disorganization. Perhaps it is not too late to give him a helpful boost into a maturing process which will facilitate the desirable life-steps.

CONCLUSION

Al and Bill were both diagnosed as "schizophrenic." But what do these two adolescents actually have in common? Is the difference between them only one of degree, or do major qualitative distinctions separate them? By giving both boys a diagnosis which suggests such severe pathology, does one intend primarily to convey the disorganization of the two? While both are certainly disorganized, Bill's disorganization seems to bear little relationship to Al's. Al operates on a level where biological needs are paramount, where they almost constantly and totally take over awareness and drown out subtler agencies (e.g., shame, pleasure, aesthetic involvement). Bill, on the other hand, has been able to achieve considerable differentiation, a fairly high degree of sophistication and rather effective sublimation. Another major difference between the two involves Al's never having been able to achieve much beyond his present very limited level. He has been more or less the way he is at present ever since an early age, if not since birth. Bill, however, was able gradually to develop a rather high (if narrow) level of functioning, from which he is now regressing.

Whatever the final decision on the matter, it is obvious that the category "schizophrenia" includes an extremely wide range of personality organizations and behaviors (a statement which can be made about most diagnostic categories). While it undoubtedly helps to create at least some order out of the varieties of personological organizations and disorganizations that one meets, it is a temptation to categorize arbitrarily, so that significant differences are glossed over and not given their full importance. Three types of adolescents have been presented in this book so far: the "retarded," the "organically damaged" and the "schizophrenic." Major differences have been at least as prominent as similarities, both within and between the categories.

How are Al and Bill handling their adolescence? Because Al has only the most rudimentary defensive structures, he gives in easily to what his body demands, just as he has apparently given in all his life. The major change at this time is the *content* of what Al gives in to —the sexual feelings which have been developing as he has been physically maturing. But his handling of what might be considered an "adolescent" sexual need actually has little to do with adolescence. Psychologically, Al is a very young child with a growing body, with physical desires which he can not adequately control and which often take over.

Bill, on the other hand, is trying to deal with *all* psychological aspects of adolescence, of which overt sexuality is only one. Although we learn from his history that some problems (e.g., peer relations) have been lifelong, others (e.g., the deteriorating relationship with his younger brother) seem to stem from about the onset of adolescence. Although Bill seems to have been disturbed all his life, the demands of adolescence require better solutions than he can offer. Because he experiences adolescent demands so intensely and finds himself so unable to handle them effectively, he becomes increasingly disorganized.

5

The Doubt-Ridden Adolescent

This chapter continues the progression toward disorders which, as far as one can feel relatively certain at this time, are increasingly "functional." Again, we arbitrarily categorize the adolescents whose test protocols follow on the basis of one major characteristic, i.e., the role of thought in their psychological organization. The present continuity includes, at one extreme, those adolescents who defend themselves by flooding their consciousness with thoughts which are only distantly and disguisedly related to the relevant impulse, and at the other extreme, those who defend themselves by allowing themselves as little reflective thought as possible. That is, in a sense the former group is made up of persons who think at the expense of appropriate action, while the latter is made up of those whose actions are insufficiently based on reflective thought.

The types of reaction to which we refer, which are also called "neurotic," "obsessive," "mixed," "hysterical," "inhibited," etc., can certainly be found as much among older and younger persons as among adolescents. But while, for example, obsessive defenses are in no way the exclusive domain of the adolescent, they are often brought forth or strengthened by the impact of the adolescent developmental period. A young person, previously not particularly obsessive or doubt-ridden, may develop these characteristics as he is required to deal with the new quality and quantity of his impulses. This obsessive (or hysterical, or narcissistic, or other) organization may be temporary and acute, to be discarded once adult equilibrium is achieved, or it may be retained as a part of a permanent character organization. It is possible, too, that adolescence may enhance and sharpen a pre-existing part-organization, so as to give it added prominence. In one way or another, adolescence is almost certain to affect the growing individual's thought organization.

In this chapter, the protocols of two adolescents who can be described as overideational are presented. The first, Paul, at times becomes almost immobilized as a result of his doubts and obsessions. The second, Wes, presents a so-called "mixed" organization and demonstrates both obsessive (i.e., overideational) and hysterical (i.e., underideational, repressive) features.

CLINICAL SUMMARY: Paul

Paul is almost thirteen, the older of two sons. His difficulties are lifelong and have gradually engulfed every aspect of his functioning, crippling him in his social, emotional and intellectual adjustment. He has failed in school, has been alienated from all friends, and lives a solitary and withdrawn existence, punctuated by battles and rebellion at home.

Paul's mother was severely nauseated during her pregnancy with him, and she gained much weight during this time. Paul was born three weeks prematurely and weighed five pounds, five ounces at birth. His mother describes him as having been a very ugly baby who looked "like a baboon." His arms and legs were in constant motion, partly because he apparently suffered from a calcium deficiency. The mother became so tense that she was unable to enjoy her baby. This tension increased when her infant also showed irritability and feeding problems. In order to keep his food down, he required phenobarbital fifteen minutes before each feeding. Considering this feeding problem to be a rejection of her, the mother in turn became rejecting of the child. Paul was fed according to a strict schedule and not picked up but left "to cry it out." Toilet training was begun early, but neither parent recalls when Paul established toilet control. He started to walk before he was one year old, but his coordination was not good. The mother thinks that Paul's speech was late, but he was able to talk fairly well by the age of two.

When Paul was two, the entire family moved to be near the mother's parents. Both grandparents felt that Paul was "mean." When his younger brother was born, the mother and grandparents apparently abandoned Paul psychologically and gave him no emotional warmth. Paul's father attempted to make up for the rest of the family's neglect of Paul, and as a result serious conflict arose between the parents.

Six years ago, Paul's three-year-younger brother, who had been a close playmate, died of nephritis after a ten-month illness. Paul, having at times mistreated the brother, felt responsible for the death and subsequently became more hostile and withdrawn. Paul's mother could only think, "Why wasn't it Paul who died?"

Almost as soon as he entered public school, Paul became a disturbing element; as a result, the school had him tested by a psychologist. Subsequently, he attended and was withdrawn from several private schools. He saw a psychiatrist until two years ago, when his parents terminated his psychotherapy. Paul's mother, who first suffered a miscarriage (and said that Paul caused it through his misbehavior), gave birth to another boy about four years ago. A short time later, Paul was sent to camp, but he had so many difficulties with his fellow campers and counselors that he was sent home. Following the camp experience, he was sent to a private, out-of-town school because his mother felt she could not bear to have him around home. He was withdrawn from this school within two weeks because he apparently received severe physical abuse from the other boys. He was then sent to another private school, was again withdrawn, and began therapy with another psychiatrist. This psychiatrist felt that it was not possible to treat Paul while he stayed at home and that Paul had to be admitted to a residential treatment center.

Physical and Laboratory Findings: The physical examination and laboratory blood studies are within normal limits. The EEG is mildly abnormal, suggesting a disturbance in the left temporal region where minor irregularities occur consistently and increase during hyperventilation. The neurological examination reveals an imbalance to the external ocular movement but is otherwise within normal limits.

THE PSYCHOLOGIST'S DESCRIPTION

What strikes one immediately about Paul is his doubt-ridden, hesitant, ruminative approach. Trying to explain his need to overclarify, overamplify and overcorrect, he says, "Sometimes I just *have* to say things. I can't seem to help it, even if it hurts me." He frequently checks to make certain I know precisely what he means and that I write down his exact words. Often he returns to comments he has made the previous day, correcting them, explaining them further or merely conveying his preoccupation with them. He constantly attempts to explain himself "fully," so that no area of vagueness can remain. Frequently he makes comments that are superficially irrelevant, and it is apparent that he must first rid himself of extraneous thoughts before he can continue with the present, pertinent topic. Occasionally he interrupts himself to write a memo about something he needs to tell the psychiatrist the next hour or the next day. He explains that he must write himself these memoranda because his memory, which had already been poor, has been getting much worse during the past two months.

Because of his delaying activities, it took Paul an unusually long time to complete the tests. He required three hours to finish the Wechsler-Bellevue, two and a half hours for the Rorschach, one-half hour for the Draw A Person and one and a half hours to tell seven brief Thematic Apperception Test stories.[1] When I encouraged him to go a little faster, he became angry and sarcastic. He was aware, however, of the irritation his symptomatic behavior could arouse. One time, for example, he asked, "Do you get aggravated when I ask you so many details?"

THE WECHSLER-BELLEVUE SCALE

Name: Paul   Age: 12-10

	RS	WTS	0 1 2 3 4 5 6 7 8 9 10 11 12 13 14 15 16 17 18 19 20
COMPR.	14	12	
INFOR.	15-17	11-12	
DIG.	10-11	7-9	
ARITH.	6	7	
SIMIL.	14-15	11-12	
VOCAB.	23½	10	
P. A.	15	13	
P. C.	10	9	
B. D.	22	10	
O. A.	21	12	
D. S.	35	8	

TOT. VERB.	51-53	
TOT. PERF.	52	
TOT. SCALE	103-105	

VERBAL I.Q.:   114-117   LEVEL: High Average

PERFORMANCE I.Q.:   112   LEVEL: High Average

TOTAL I.Q.:   115-117   LEVEL: High Average

[1] Although it is a temptation to try to cut through such delaying tactics and to hurry the subject along, it becomes apparent how persons of this sort, who have such an overwhelming incapacity to cut through their cerebral flotsam, can simply not be hurried in the usual way. At most, the examiner is wise to avoid responding to any delaying byways.

[Paul's Wechsler Scattergram shows a rather marked instability, ranging as it does between weighted scores of 7 and 13. His two lowest scores (Digit Span and Arithmetic) are on tests which are particularly vulnerable to the effects of tension. His next lowest performance is on Digit Symbol, a test also highly susceptible to apprehensiveness. A good Picture Arrangement performance such as Paul's is frequently found in the so-called "character disorder," and it is alleged to reflect a refined capacity to understand others' motives for purposes of exploitative manipulation. Persons interpersonally alert to this degree are ordinarily highly sensitive to environmental detail, but Paul's lowered Picture Completion performance shows that this alertness does not apply across the board. Apparently Paul's interpersonal sensitivity is isolated from other sensitivities; i.e., it is not part of a more general, outwardly directed, reality appreciation. Because Paul's skills wander over such a wide range, he may well be subject to some sort of acute, rather than chronic, psychological encroachment.]

(When I try to put Paul at ease by asking him about his trip here and about his reaction to the town, he replies that the psychiatrist had already asked very similar questions.) [He tries to convey, in this way, both his "seeing through" my "small talk" and his doubting my genuineness. Suspiciousness regarding the sincerity of others is typical of Paul, but it soon becomes obvious that his distrust relates primarily to himself. His speech reflects the degree to which he doubts both his impulses and the observations of other events that go on inside and outside himself. It reflects the uncertainty he feels about all that surrounds him—even matters about which a less disturbed person would have developed an easy assuredness and an unquestioning conviction.]

INFORMATION

No.	Question	Response and Comments	Score
1.	Who is the President of the United States?	President Eisenhower . . (He is biting his nails.) ("Who was president before that?") President Truman. ("And before that?") Roosevelt.	+
2.	What is a thermometer?	Uh . . It measures . . It measures temperature. It has mercury in it, and the mercury expands when temperature gets hotter, and . . I don't know how you'd say that. (He makes contracting motions.) ("Contracts?") Yeah, it contracts when it gets colder. It ranges usually from zero up to over one hundred. [Here is the first test example of Paul's	+

No.	*Question*	*Response and Comments*	*Score*
		tendency to present all the data so as to leave out as little as possible and so as not to be found wanting. This need to fill in potential informational gaps is, of course, typical of an obsessive-compulsive orientation.]	
3.	*What does rubber come from?*	It comes from the sap of a tree. I believe it's grown in Malaya. I know it's grown in parts of South America, and I think in Africa.	+
4.	*Where is London?*	It is in England. [For the moment he is able to give up the compulsive presentation of all sorts of data. He does not for example, need to say that London is the capital of England, or that it is the home of Parliament, or that it is located on the Thames.]	+
5.	*How many pints makes a quart?*	Four. ("Are you sure?") Wait a minute. Yes (Several responses later, he spontaneously corrects this answer.) [Paul's push to display accuracy does not prevent his making a fairly obvious error on a rather easy item.]	−+
6.	*How many weeks are there in a year?*	. . . . . I'm afraid I don't know that. ("What would you guess?") Well, let's see . . . . . . forty-eight. ("How did you figure that?") I know there's four in a month and twelve months in a year. [Once more it is apparent that the urge for precision does not prevent a rather astonishing gap in knowledge. While Paul can later tell who discovered the North Pole, he is unable to furnish the present, basic sort of information which is ordinarily assimilated without conscious effort at an early age. One can see how the obsessive-compulsive defenses, which, one assumes, let Paul function with less felt anxiety, do not necessarily result in greater intellectual efficiency.]	−
7.	*What is the capital of Italy?*	Rome.	+
8.	*What is the capital of Japan?*	. . . . . I don't know that. ("What do you think it might be?") Tokyo. ["I don't know that" might mean, "I'm not positive."]	+
9.	*How tall is the average American woman?*	. . . . . . I would say about six feet. ("How tall are you?") I don't know. I grow so fast. Let's see, I think I'm about . . . . I don't think I know. About five feet seven inches. ("Would you be taller or shorter than the average American woman?") I know I'm taller. ("So how would that affect your answer?") Make it about six feet two inches. ("But I thought you were taller than the average American woman.") Oh, woman! I thought you said the	+

No.	*Question*	*Response and Comments*	*Score*

average man. ("So how tall do you think the average American woman is?") About five feet four inches? What I said sounded awfully silly for a woman. I think I made a mistake on that. I'm kind of nervous . . . On that pints question—it's two. I should have known that. Are you timing me? [Paul's response reflects his momentary confusion, the modification of his conceptions by intruding thoughts and preconceptions (in the past, on the WISC, he was asked to estimate the height of the average American *man*). Just as is true later, on the Rorschach, Paul here does not permit himself to respond spontaneously. He relies on what he has already performed, on what he has put together before, and in that way tries to avoid showing others and himself how disorganized he can become when he cannot depend on his memory. His returning to the "pints" question shows how he continues to ruminate about ideas that others can finish with and dismiss from their minds. Paul finds it hard to forget about even a minute problem—unresolvable tension states are forever being triggered off in him.]

10. *Who invented the airplane?*

Well . . . the Wright brothers made the first successful flight. [This sort of hairsplitting is what one expects from Paul.]   +

11. *Where is Brazil?*

It is in South America . . uh . . the upper part . . and . . uh . . . it's a very large country . . larger than the United States, which covers *most* of the upper part. [Again, one expects Paul to elaborate in this way. Although elaboration was lacking in his answer to the "London" question, it appears that, as Paul becomes increasingly uncomfortable, his need to refine his response increases.]   +

12. *How far is it from Paris to New York?*

. . . . (He sighs.) I don't know that. ("Make a guess.") I seem to remember something. I don't think it could be true. As a matter of fact, it sounds awfully . . but about 2,800. [Again, Paul feels great uncertainty, even about facts he "knows" accurately.]   +

13. *What does the heart do?*

The heart . . uh . . pumps blood and keeps the blood circulating through the body. I think it filters it too. ("Which answer would you choose?") Well . . uh . . maybe it doesn't . . but . . uh . . it filters the blood and makes it pure. At least I hope it does.   −+

14. *Who wrote Hamlet?*

Shakespeare.   +

No.	Question	Response and Comments	Score
15.	What is the population of the United States?	. . . . Uh . . this might not be right, but . . uh . . four billion. [He is apparently thinking of the earth's population.]	—
16.	When is Washington's birthday?	. . Uh . . it's in January. I believe it's in the latter part. I'm not sure. I get it mixed up with Lincoln's. Well . . uh . . I think it's in the first part. [So far, all answers which involve numbers have caused extra uncertainty.]	—
17.	Who discovered the North Pole?	Uh . . Peary. I don't know his first name, but it was Peary, I believe. [Paul demands that he know, that he have every detail accounted for.]	+
18.	Where is Egypt?	It's in North Africa. [Not simply "Africa," but "North."]	+
19.	Who wrote Huckleberry Finn?	Mark Twain. That was a pen name. His real name was Samuel Clemens. [One must be aware, of course, of another aspect of Paul's tendency to marshal facts—his pride in his knowledge.]	+
20.	What is the Vatican?	It's the . . uh . . it's the capital of the Catholics. It's where the Pope lives, who's the head of the religion. [Note the excellence of this response in comparison to No. 6, the "weeks in a year" question, an objectively much easier one.]	+
21.	What is the Koran?	. . . . . . I don't know.	—
22.	Who wrote Faust?	. . . . I don't know. I haven't even heard of these.	—
23.	What is a Habeas Corpus?	Uh . . I've heard of it, but I don't know what it means.	—
24.	What is ethnology?	I don't know.	—
25.	What is the Apocrypha?	I don't know.	—

RAW SCORE: 15-17

WEIGHTED SCORE: 11-12

COMPREHENSION

No.	Question	Response and Comments	Score
1.	What is the thing to do if you find an envelope in the street, that is sealed, and addressed and has a new stamp?	. . . . I'd throw it in the nearest mailbox. [Following the preceding equivocation, this response is surprisingly straightforwardly presented.]	2

No.	Question	Response and Comments	Score
2.	What should you do if while sitting in the movies you were the first person to discover a fire (or see smoke and fire)?	Well . . I've never tried to think of that. I don't know what I'd do. I'd try to keep calm. I wouldn't scream "fire!" At least I hope I wouldn't. I'd tell the usher. ("How would you sum up your answer?") The usher . . was . . uh . . I'd keep calm and tell the usher. [Paul's problems with commitment emerge again. So do his difficulties with controlling impulsivity. The Comprehension questions, which cannot be answered with a simple fact, are particularly stimulating to obsessive processes.]	2
3.	Why should we keep away from bad company?	Because it has a bad influence on us. Or it *may* have a bad influence on us. [The need to be precise once again.]	2
4.	Why should people pay taxes?	Well, the government needs money to keep going . . to run the country. So people pay taxes to the government.	2
5.	Why are shoes made of leather?	Uh . . Leather is the best material for that purpose. It can stand a lot of hard wear. ("Can you think of any other reasons?") Well (he shrugs), it's attractive. On that other answer I gave, "I guess it can stand a lot of wear"—I *know* it can. [Because he needs to express himself precisely and to avoid showing himself lacking intellectually, Paul overvalues the importance of meaning nuances. As far as he is concerned, words have immense power.]	1
6.	Why does land in the city cost more than land in the country?	Well, I would say it's more valuable in the city because cities are growing and need more land . . and more resources. I'm not sure about that. End. Tell me, I've been thinking some time . . like that little thing I said at the end about resources. Would it be better not to tell you at all? ("Tell me whatever seems right to you.") . . . . . . On those shoes, leather is probably also more comfortable. [Paul's inability to let an old response be is further underlined. His saying "End" apparently represents one of his efforts to control his poorly contained outpouring of words.]	1
7.	If you were lost in a forest (woods) in the daytime, how would you go about finding your way out?	Well . . uh . . These are little details, but have I been lost a long time? (He tells a rather long story about a friend who became lost in the Badlands.) Well, I would try to backtrack myself. If it came night, I'd try to take shelter, probably. Probably what I'd really do would be to climb a nice high tree and see if I could see civilization, and maybe try to find out where I was and how	1

No.	Question	Response and Comments	Score

to get out. [Paul is simply unable to approach a problem directly.]

8. Why are laws necessary? Well, laws are necessary to keep order. And . . uh . . well, that's the best definition I can give. Keeping law and order, that's just the best definition I can give. That makes good sense. [Again, the inability to let go.]   **1**

9. Why does the state require people to get a license in order to be married? I don't know. Probably if I thought hard enough, I could figure it out. I'll have to ask my father that. But I don't know offhand. ("Could you make a guess?") To know *when* they got married or *where* they got married and who *got* married. [Even though he gives a perfectly acceptable response, Paul implies he is too young to know facts that deal with such adult matters as marriage; he will obtain this type of information from his father.]   **2**

10. Why are people who are born deaf usually unable to talk? Well . . uh . . their vocal cords. I thought you said death . . I didn't get it. Their vocal cords are undeveloped or damaged in some way, and their vocal cords are where the voice comes from. ("So why would people who are born deaf usually be unable to speak?") Well, their vocal cords were not developed with the rest of them. And, as I said, the vocal cords are where the person's voice comes from. Of course, there might be some damage at birth. [Paul offers his answer with certainty, as though it were based on scientifically established fact. He presents his unusual information without apology, as though it were well known and a part of generally accepted knowledge. Paul's uncritical judgment suggests a fairly severe "fault" in his thought functioning. The (grammatically meaningless) misperception—"death" for "deaf"—points further to the vulnerability of his psychic organization.]   **0**

RAW SCORE: 14

WEIGHTED SCORE: 12

DIGIT SPAN

(Paul accurately repeats six Digits Forward and receives alternate credit because he correctly repeats seven digits on the third trial. He cannot correctly repeat more than four Digits Backward, even though he is given three opportunities.) [As mentioned earlier, Paul obtains his lowest weighted scores on Digit Span, and on Arithmetic, which follows below. His major difficulty on Digit Span involves repeating the numbers in reverse order, a task which is probably more affected by generalized tension than the simple "forward" repetition of numbers. Ordinarily a person repeats about one less digit backward than forward, so that Paul's discrepancy of three digits is greater than usual.]

RAW SCORE: 10-11

WEIGHTED SCORE: 7-9

ARITHMETIC

(After he is given the instructions:) That's the worst thing. ("How do you mean?") It's the one I dislike the most.

(Paul solves the first seven problems correctly within the time limits, except for Problem 4 to which he gives the incorrect answer "twelve." On Problem 8 he answers "seven hundred" in one second. When I ask how he came to this answer, he says:) Well . . oh . . two-thirds . . uh . . oh! Did I get it wrong? Do you want me to do it again? . . . . 600!

(On the ninth problem, Paul's tension level is still greater. After he reads the problem silently to himself, he says:) I'm just so darn nervous. ("Just do the best you can.") I shouldn't be nervous. I've had it so many times. But I just can't think. (He has to reread the problem several times to himself but complains:) It seems like looking at a blank wall. Nothing comes through. (Because he seems so uncomfortable and because his tension level is increasing so greatly, I do not present the last problem.) [The anxiety so often mobilized by the Arithmetic problems is probably brought about by the demand that the person who tries to solve them directs himself intensively to his inner (thought) processes. Although persons with certain types of (repressive; action-oriented) character organizations are typically unable to turn their attention inward in this way, such a disinclination tends not to be found among the obsessive-compulsively organized. When, as in Paul's case, a clinician nevertheless comes up against a problem of mental immobilization on Arithmetic in someone who is not primarily organized along repressive action-oriented lines, he suspects the effects of a process that makes looking inward particularly anxiety arousing because it seems so dangerous. This "process" is frequently one that involves a decompensation of defenses.]

RAW SCORE: 6

WEIGHTED SCORE: 7

SIMILARITIES

No.	Items	Response and Comments	Score
1.	Orange-banana	They are both fruit. Do you want me to say more? ("Like what?") I was going to say they both have skins you can peel off. Also, I might say, both have to be peeled off to be eaten. ("Which answer would you choose?") Both fruit. [Paul's questioning reflects his need for an outsider's help to cut through his uncertainty, so he can achieve more effective organization.]	2
2.	Coat-dress	Both clothing.	2
3.	Dog-lion	Both animals.	2

No.	Items	Response and Comments	Score

4. *Wagon-bicycle* — Both vehicles. [Apparently Paul has received enough external support to help him determine what types of test responses are acceptable. Up to this point in the subtest he is able to give short, adequately formulated, abstract responses.] — 2

5. *Daily paper-radio* — They . . they both give the news . . and we . . Yeah . . they give you the news. ("Were you going to say something else?") Well, they give you every-thing . . advertising . . variety. So they give you the news on everything. — 1

6. *Air-water* — Both are . . gases. ("Is water a gas?") Well, I think it is. It sounds like it. Uh . . you could say it's atmosphere. Both are atmospheres, then. Maybe it is, I don't know. Of course, an atmosphere is something that covers something, isn't it? An at-mosphere . . . creatures live in it. [This response is certainly not a usual one.] — 0

7. *Wood-alcohol* — Well, you got . . I know there's some resemblance because they have wood alcohol . . and alcohol comes from wood. ("Can you think of any way they might be alike?") I don't even know if that's true. (He is biting his nails.) I'm afraid I can't get that one. I just know about that . . Oh, well, they both have liquid content. Here's the answer, but it's not the one you're looking for . . I know that. [As the items get harder, Paul's responses become increasingly "peculiar."] — 0

8. *Eye-ear* — Both senses. — 2

9. *Egg-seed* — They're . . both products . . or . . that . . are . . to reproduce. Or . . well . . (he shrugs) they're both things that reproduce whatever they came from. — 2

10. *Poem-statue* — Uh . . well . . they're both . . uh . . . . I don't know . . I've heard that before. I've heard it asked lots of places . . Well, they both tell you things. ("How do you mean?") Well, they both tell you about a certain thing. [This is a vague answer for someone who values precision as much as Paul.] — 1

11. *Praise-punishment* — Oh . . am I supposed to relate these? ("Tell me how they're alike, the way you did with the others.") They're opposites! ("Can you think of any way they might be alike?") Well, I know there's something . . but . . . . . I know there's a word for it, but I can't explain it. It's not because of nervousness. What made me nervous was what you first asked me, like about arithmetic and about — 0

No. Items	Response and Comments	Score
	Japan . . I think I was wrong . . Okinawa maybe. Well, I'll stick to what I have and hope for the best. [This response is interesting for a number of reasons. As Paul finds items more difficult, he loses his set and asks to have the Similarities redefined. Also, as his tension continues to increase, he underscores his very evident anxiety through denial. Rumination increases, and he concerns himself with old responses once again.]	
12. *Fly-tree*	They're both things that stand . . You know, they can go into the air. They can go high above things. Also, both grow. ("Which answer would you choose?") The second one wasn't very good, but now that I think of it I'll take the first one. Or maybe I won't. I don't know. Which shall I take? Do I have to take a definite one? ("Yes. Choose one of them.") They're both possible. (He finds it so difficult to commit himself to a decision that I finally tell him he doesn't need to choose.) [Here we witness the obsessive person's ultimate problem—his inability to decide.]	0-1

RAW SCORE: 14-15

WEIGHTED SCORE: 11-12

PICTURE COMPLETION

(This test is administered the following day. Paul begins the hour by reviewing aloud a number of Similarities items about which he was unsure the previous day.

(As far as Picture Completion is concerned, he remembers one of the items—the missing shadow—from the previous time he took it. He misses two early items, but his errors are not particularly significant. He correctly solves Nos. 5 through 11, and then he continues as follows:)

No. Item	Time	Missing	Response and Comments	Score
12. *Man*	25″	tie	All I could see here . . his hair might be over a little too much on this side. There's not as much hair on this side.	0
13. *Bulb*		thread (or prong)	(He looks at the room's flourescent ceiling light and checks it against the drawing.) Oh, it's phosphorescent (*sic*). I can't use it as a model. Well, I don't know much about a light bulb. I don't know that at all . . . Oh, I see! The wire should come down to here. See what I mean? (He shows me.)	0
14. *Girl*	13″	eyebrow	The ear is missing. [The face is drawn so as not to show the ear.]	0

No.	Item	Time	Missing	Response and Comments	Score
15.	*Sun*	5″	shadow of man	The man's shadow is missing. I expected the shadow of the tree to be pointing toward the sun. (He is apparently aware of my stop watch for the first time.) Were you timing me on the whole for that? (He asks many questions about how "phosphorescent" lights work.) [Paul's response to Nos. 12 through 15 are not exceedingly odd, but are peculiar enough to give pause.]	1

RAW SCORE: 10

WEIGHTED SCORE: 9

PICTURE ARRANGEMENT

No.	Item	Correct Order	Time	Arranged Order	Story and Comments	Score
1.	*House*	PAT	3″	PAT	The man is building a foundation for his house. In the second picture, he's started the structure. And in the third, he's finished the house and is painting it.	2
2.	*Holdup*	ABCD	8″	ABCD	In the first picture, the man is being held up by a robber. In the second, the policeman was taking him away. In the third, he was standing trial. In the fourth, he was in jail. [Paul's emphasis on isolated detail, at the expense of inclusive meaning, is illustrated by his tendency to tell the story by telling about the individual pictures, even though they have been taken away.]	2
3.	*Elevator*	LMNO	8″	LMNO	On the first it showed the . . uh . . what do you call those things? ("Elevator?") Yeah, elevator, not open but closed, and the sound of the motor coming from underneath. In the second, the elevator just is starting to open. In the third, it was halfway up. In the fourth, the Little King was walking	2

No. Item	Correct Order	Time	Arranged Order	Story and Comments	Score
				off. The two workmen were on it still.	
4. *Flirt*	JANET	19″	JNAET	You sure have enough of these Little King ones! In the first picture, the King was being driven along by his chauffeur in a car. I think I arranged those wrong. I think I should show the woman before he pointed. Should I give it in that order? ("Give it in the order that you think makes the right story.") Then it showed a picture of a woman. Then it showed the King getting out. Then it showed him walking away with the woman. [Paul's tendency to fragmentize, to emphasize detail at the expense of totality is again striking. Although his elements are correctly placed and interpreted, one has the feeling that he misses the point (certainly the humor) of the situation. It may well be that Paul approaches his entire life in this same kind of compartmentalized, detailed fashion, which causes him to lose sight of the main points of situations.]	3
5. *Taxi*	SAMUEL	48″	SAMUEL	("Try telling the story, without saying what's on each card.") A man was walking along with a statue of a woman. And he signaled a cab. It's a lot easier this way (referring to my suggestion). He got in the car. The woman was leaning against him. Then he looked around. And then he got kind of embarrassed—frightfully embarrassed. And he moved the statue to the	3

No.	Item	Correct Order	Time	Arranged Order	Story and Comments	Score
					other side of the car. ("Why did he get embarrassed?") The way he was leaning against her, it looked like they were loving it up between each other. [It is apparent that, even after he is encouraged to loosen up, Paul still needs to give a painfully detailed exposition. Two of his phrasings do not ring altogether true: the first is his description of the man as "frightfully embarrassed"; the second is his speaking of the man and the dummy as "loving it up between each other." Particularly the second phrase sounds as though Paul were much more easygoing about such matters than one would expect. Undoubtedly he is unaware of the connotations of the phrase. Both unexpected word usages occur in conjunction with a sexually toned situation, and one may infer, from these and other examples, the degree to which Paul needs to assume an artificial, nongenuine attitude in the face of a situation which arouses his sexual impulse life.]	
6.	*Fish*	EFGHIJ	41″	EFGHIJ	Well, the Little King is fishing off a pier. At first he had no fish at all. Then it seemed . . it seemed to have a bite. He got a little interested, and then he pulled one fish up. Then he was fishing again. He already had one fish in his basket. And . . uh . . then he was catching another fish. He had two fish in the basket. Then I think he caught one more. Then he whistled out over the	3

No.	Item	Correct Order	Time	Arranged Order	Story and Comments	Score

water, and out of the water popped a diver. The diver had ap . . ap . . . appa . . . (He has difficulty saying the word "apparently.") How do you say that word? I've always been able to say it. ("Apparently?") That's it! The diver had been putting the fish on the line. [Not only does Paul again organize by stressing isolated detail; he also uses the detail accurately and in an alert fashion. Because of this evident alertness, it is all the more significant (and puzzling) that he is unable to find several easier missing details on Picture Completion, where this same talent is required. Perhaps he is simply more alert whenever *interpersonal* situations are involved.

[The unavailability of a word he has "always been able to say" is noteworthy and suggests the presence of a process which impairs smooth functioning.]

RAW SCORE: ___15___

WEIGHTED SCORE: ___13___

BLOCK DESIGN

No.	Time	Accur.	Description of Behavior and Comments	Score
A.	9″	Yes	Should I make it exactly like that? (He constructs the copy easily.) [It is difficult to know what function this type of unnecessary question may have. Paul asks such apparently superfluous questions frequently. In part, they may serve to put off for a little while his involving himself in activities that he finds difficult. They also seem to permit Paul to put himself in a dependent position, where he can demonstrate helplessness vis-à-vis the adult whom he (ambivalently) endows with great knowledge and power.]	—
B.	12″	Yes	(He places the blocks quickly and correctly.)	—

No.	Time	Accur.	Description of Behavior and Comments	Score
1.	10″	Yes	(He fumbles somewhat with the blocks, his hands tremble, and he is otherwise tense. But again he seems to know what he needs to do and proceeds without major difficulty.)	5
2.	10″	Yes	(He deals with the blocks in the same way as above.) This isn't on the subject right now, but what is your full name? [This tendency to "leave the field" suggests that Paul is beginning to experience more difficulty than he can easily handle. It is likely, too, that he wants to know more about the person with whom he will spend considerable time. In order to be more at ease, he tries to "peg" and categorize him.]	5
3.	18″	Yes	(Initially he erroneously rotates a few blocks, and seems mildly confused.) They don't have to be perfect, do they? They can be a little off. ("Try to make it exactly the same as on the picture.") I don't mind doing this stuff, it's pretty interesting. The only thing I don't like is arithmetic. And I don't care for the ink-blots. ("Why is that?") I'm tired of them. [He experiences the Block Designs as increasingly hard to solve and handles difficulties by using denial, and by trying to manipulate the explicit and implicit instructions. His questions reflect the demandingness of a harshly developed, but bribable, superego.]	3
4.	58″	Yes	(He shows considerable trial-and-error behavior and occasionally does not know how to proceed. He frequently checks his construction against the model and catches several errors he has made.)	3
5.	63″	Yes	Brother! (He has difficulty in reproducing corners and is uncertain whether they face correctly or not.)	3
6.	1′ 46″	Yes	(After some initial fumbling, he recognizes how to make stripes. He reverts to occasional wrong moves but eventually always finds the correct way again. At 1′ 30″, he first says he is finished but then exclaims, "Oh, oh! I see what I've done wrong here." After encouragement, he corrects his wrong version.) Do you get tired of giving these, or do you enjoy it? [Paul's reliance on various defensive maneuvers (in this instance, projection) in the face of difficulty is becoming increasingly conspicuous. Perhaps he is also responding to an examiner attitude which the examiner may be hiding ineffectively.]	3
7.	3′ 23″	Yes	What a challenge! (He says this sarcastically. He proceeds slowly and makes a number of errors. At 2′ 4″ he declares himself finished, but he has two blocks rotated. When I wonder whether his copy is exactly	0

No.   Time   Accur.   Description of Behavior and Comments   Score

the same as the model, he says, "Oh brother!," sees his errors and corrects them. He achieves no alternate credit because he finishes overtime, even with help.)

RAW SCORE: 22

WEIGHTED SCORE: 10

OBJECT ASSEMBLY

(He proceeds at a fairly rapid pace, with some mild confusion on the *Profile* item. After he has finished putting the *Hand* together, he says, "It looks like a deformed hand." He compares what he has made to his own hand and explains that it seems "stretched.") [The need to compare bodily parts and the tendency to see them as "deformed" suggests significant identity problems. The "bad" hand may also signify a rejection of a part of the self which is considered to do unacceptable things.]

RAW SCORE: 21

WEIGHTED SCORE: 12

DIGIT SYMBOL

(His symbols are neatly, accurately, but slowly drawn.)

RAW SCORE: 35

WEIGHTED SCORE: 8

VOCABULARY

No. Word	Response and Comments	Score
1. *Apple*	You mean, I tell you what it is? ("That's right.") A fruit which is eaten by people. It has a red skin. The inside is sort of light. ("That's fine.") It's juicy. You can make juice for drinks, like cider. [Once again, he asks the apparently superfluous but anxiety-reducing question. Paul's compulsion to list detailed information is obvious. It is a compulsion which is clearly stronger than the examiner's implicit encouragement that Paul stop going on and on.]	1
2. *Donkey*	A donkey is a . . in the horse family and is related to the burro . . jackass. And it has the reputation for being a stubborn animal. And big ears, and it's smaller than a horse. And . . uh . . you could say it's used by miners, but that's a burro.	1
3. *Join*	. . . . Joining? (He seems not to comprehend the word, and I show it to him.) Oh, join! Come together; make contact. "He joined the club." "The two rivers joined."	1
4. *Diamond*	A diamond is a . . very valuable rock. It comes from coal, which has turned to diamonds over years and years and years because of pressure. It is very valuable. A lot is found in South Africa.	1

No.	Word	Response and Comments	Score
5.	Nuisance	A bother.	1
6.	Fur	The hair of animals.	1
7.	Cushion	A soft thing to lay on, or sit on, or rest on. Uh . . it's made of cloth . . cotton, or whatever.	1
8.	Shilling	A piece of money used by the British.	1
9.	Gamble	To . . uh . . to bet. [On the last five responses Paul has been able to be quite direct.]	1
10.	Bacon	Uh . . it comes from . . uh . . a pig . . and . . . . . . It's laid in strips. ("How do you mean?") You buy bacon in strips. Can I ask you a question? Is it related to ham, or pork, or both? ("I think to both.") Where does the bacon come from? (I explain as best as I can.) Boy, a pig can sure be used for a lot. [Again, as he experiences difficulty, he turns passivity into activity and asks questions.]	1
11.	Nail	It's . . uh . . a long piece of metal which is used to attach things by means of driving in or hammering in.	1
12.	Cedar	You mean a cedar tree? A cedar tree is an evergreen tree which is in the pine family. It has needles . . and . . uh . . is . . uh . . and is . . has the same physique as a pine or fir tree. Where I come from, it grows in the mountains. ["The same physique" is a rather unusual formulation.]	1
13.	Tint	Tent? (I spell the word.) Like you tint hair? ("What would that mean?") I don't know exactly what it means, but . . add color to the hair? Add color to the hair. Do you have any aspirin? ("Do you have a headache?") Yeah, over my eye. (He tells about his headache and how his mother won't take him to a doctor because she says that this would be nonsense. He tells me that he wants to ask the psychiatrist a question, but he's forgotten what it is. He says again that he's become very forgetful during the last three months. He says his forgetfulness is "horrible.") [Paul's tension is obviously rising again, not only because the subtest items are becoming more difficult, but also because the entire examination forces Paul to become increasingly aware of himself. Days filled with examinations have an additive effect, and Paul's capacity to bind tension and to remain organized is being progressively undermined. [Using his headache, Paul is trying to encourage his examiners to take sides with him against his "unreasonable" mother. The effort to enlist a sympathetic adult outsider's commiseration to create a division between the adolescent and "unfair" parents is frequently seen. The same need to "divide and rule"	1

No. Word	*Response and Comments*	*Score*

occurs when the adolescent tries (often successfully) to enlist his parents' sympathies against the examiners. This two-pronged campaign, involving parents and examiners, is often carried on at the same time, and the examiner must be alert not to fall into this divisive trap. Once he feels he has successfully seduced his examiner into antagonism toward his parents, the adolescent typically becomes so frightened that he attempts to deny what he has done by developing antagonism toward the entire examination. The examiner's wisest initial reaction is, as always, to remain neutral.]

14. *Armory*

(He looks puzzled.) . . . . . . Wéll . . this probably won't help when you score me down, because it'll show I don't know. I didn't know what it was until yesterday. I might as well be frank. I drove past one. An armory—if it's the same thing—is a place where weapons and ammunition is kept. [This type of honesty may well be another instance of Paul's need to deny an aspect of himself which he considers unacceptable, in this case, dishonesty.]

    1

15. *Fable*

A legend . . something that is not necessarily true. Many times it isn't. It's a story, like Aesop's *Fables*. Do you get aggravated when I give you so many details? Sometimes I just *have* to say things. I can't seem to help it, even if it hurts me. I can't stand to see anybody fooled. (He goes on to tell how he has to tell people information which he has and they don't. He tells how he must cut a loose thread on his trousers, since he would otherwise pull on the thread and tear his trousers apart. He speaks of this as "another temptation.") [It is difficult to know to what extent Paul himself is aware of the aggressions he indirectly expresses this symptomatic way and to what extent he is aware only of the reactions others have to his symptoms. But, in addition to whatever aggression he may recognize, and in addition to the counteraggression he induces and recognizes in others, he is also painfully aware of his helplessness to do things differently, so that he *must* express himself in these particular ways, even when they "hurt" him.]

    1

16. *Brim*

Grim? Rim? (I show him the word.) I don't savvy that one. Grim or rim I have. I think I've heard it, but I don't know what it means. Is this for vocabulary? Or knowledge? Can you tell me the meaning now? (I explain I can't answer specific test questions.) [As Paul is puzzled by a meaning, he once again wishes to have test requirements redefined.]

    0

No. Word	Response and Comments	Score

17. *Guillotine* Guillotine is uh . . it might . . uh . . a thing for executing people by ways of detaching their heads. Shall I tell you how it works and what it looks like? It's hard to explain. ("Would you like to draw it?") (He makes an accurate drawing of a guillotine, showing the place where the person to be executed puts his head and the basket that catches it after it is severed. He draws the knife which cuts the rope and writes "All you need to do is cut it!") I hope this drawing is all right. Are you testing my drawing ability? I can draw a lot better. — 1

18. *Plural* Uh . . plural . . now how would I say that? You wrote that down too? Well, it's . . uh . . more than one, like "ducks" is plural. [He begins to express concern about my writing down what he says, i.e., about his committing himself. If we think of obsessiveness as having as one of its major goals the avoidance of commitment, then my making his statements relatively permanent constitutes a considerable threat.] — 1

19. *Seclude* I believe—I'm not sure, though—it means to be alone by oneself. Away from other things . . of its kind. But that's "seclude." [The examiner should have inquired into the "but." Does the "but" mean that Paul somehow lost track of the fact that *seclude* was the word he was asked to define?] — 1

20. *Nitroglycerin* A very . . a highly explosive chemical. — 1

21. *Stanza* (He sighs.) That's a line . . used . . for . . in the form of a paragraph or sentence, but I don't know exactly what it is. ("Where would you find it?") I know it's in music. Lines of music. — ½

22. *Microscope* Is a thing that highly magnifies small objects. Usually an object that cannot be seen by the human eye. And it studies them closely. Do I have to say what kind of object? ("No. That's fine.") — 1

23. *Vesper* I don't know. — 0

24. *Belfry* (He tells a joke about bats.) You didn't write *that* down! That's supposed to be a joke! Belfry. I believe it's a tower where there's a bell. Like the schoolhouse had a belfry. The bell in a belfry calls people to church. [The rising concern about my writing down what he says is apparently associated with his fear of its being made increasingly difficult for him to change the impression he is creating. He apparently wishes to be known as highly serious.] — 1

25. *Recede* To contract . . that's it. I learned that yesterday. (See Information question No. 2, "What is a thermom- — 1

No.	Word	Response and Comments	Score

eter?") Or was it the day before? Me and my memory. To contract. I'll give you an example: "The flood waters began to recede." ("What would they do then?") Contract. ("How do you mean?") Back up. [Paul again shows his need to be "honest."]

26. Affliction — I don't know. I know confliction. There's no relation, is there? I think of affection when I look at it. (He wants to know about the training I've received and is particularly interested to know whether I've ever worked in an insane asylum.) [The slipperiness involved in the progression affliction→confliction→ affection certainly suggests mild loosening, particularly when there is no such word as "confliction." Paul's asking the examiner whether he has worked in an insane asylum makes one think that Paul wonders whether the examining team considers him "crazy."]   0

27. Pewter — I don't know.   0

28. Ballast — I don't know. Am I expected to know these words or are they pretty high? ("No one's expected to know all the words on this test.")   0

29. Catacomb — I've heard it so many times, but I don't know what it means.   0

30. Spangle — I don't know. When I think of spangle, I think of spaniel. [A single clang association of this type is not usually noteworthy; but when it is accompanied by additional clangs, by loosening and peculiarity in other portions of the protocol, then this type of association has more pathological significance.]   0

31. Espionage — Oh . . uh . . I believe it's a form of sabotage. [A mild clang association.]   0

32. Imminent — I'd like you to write these words down for me, because I like to learn new words. (He means he would like to take the last few Vocabulary words home with him.) I'm curious . . too curious. Someday it's going to kill me. Do other kids comment on your writing things down? ("Sometimes.") How it's awfully silly? [A juxtaposition of a worried, with an aggressive, comment. Doing and undoing.]   0

33. Mantis — I don't know.   0

34. Hara-kiri — Don't write this down, but does it have any relation to what the Japanese did during the war? I always heard them talk about that, but I didn't know until this year. The Japanese did that. They committed   1

No.	Word	Response and Comments	Score

suicide by jabbing a knife into themselves rather than be captured . . and die gloriously for the emperor. To be captured is a disgrace, but to die like that is glorious. [He does not want me to write whenever he is not sure. Perhaps, on an unconscious level, he does not want the verbal evidence of his sadistic preoccupations preserved.]

(Paul is unfamiliar with the remaining words.)

RAW SCORE: 23½

WEIGHTED SCORE: 10

(Paul is becoming more and more tense, so we take a short time out after we finish the Wechsler-Bellevue. He wonders how long I have been working here and says the psychiatrist has been here a long time. He complains that I ask him questions in the same way as the psychiatrist, whereas I should be concerned just with testing him.

(He asks about various hospitals in town and wonders whether "insane persons" go to the Adult Menninger Hospital. He also wonders whether we are able to take care of a person who has an accident on the street. At one point he says, "Maybe you're preparing me for the insane asylum." When I wonder how much he is worried about such a possibility, he denies the concern and says he was only joking. He comments that this is the trouble with psychiatrists and psychologists—they think they can figure out what things go on in a person's mind, but they may have a totally wrong idea.

(He explains that he has been very worried that we would think him a "gruesome" person [i.e., "insane"?] because of his description and drawing of the guillotine.

(He is becoming increasingly disturbed by my verbatim recording.)

THE BENDER GESTALT TEST

PART A (5″ EXPOSURE) (PLATES 28 AND 29)

(Paul's 5″ Bender drawings require him about forty-five minutes to complete. His drawing pressure is so heavy that the pencil impression goes through three to four sheets of paper. As he draws the designs from memory, he makes such comments as the following:)

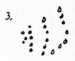

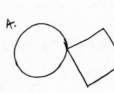

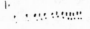

PLATE 28

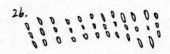

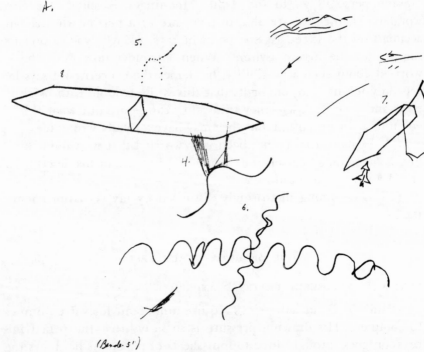

PLATE 29

Design 1. Wait a minute. Don't take it away yet. I thought that was a dud or something. Let me see it again; I wasn't paying any attention.

Design 2. On this, it looks like an exclamation point. I can't help it. It comes out as an exclamation point. It's supposed to be dots. It's supposed to be this. (He makes an accurate circle.) I'm going too fast.

Design 3. I hope this is right. (He makes a circle instead of a dot.) That's not right, but it's something like that.

Design 5. Do you have to know the exact number of dots? I know it has a curve in it.

Design 6. (He draws the design in the air, while looking at it.) It's awfully tricky. Is it normal to make these mistakes? I sure hope it doesn't matter how crude you do it. Things that are crude like this, it isn't going to matter, is it?

(He talks about how hard it is to control his hand to do exactly what he wants. Then he wonders whether it ever rains here during the day. He mentions that he is frightened of lightning and says that when the lightning strikes nearby, the thunder is awfully loud.) Why doesn't the lightning break your eardrum? Of course, you're no doctor, so you wouldn't know.

[Paul's performance is paradoxical in a number of ways. For example, while he expresses his wish to be exceedingly accurate, and while he makes a great to-do about accuracy, his drawings are fairly *in*accurate. Although his final drawing of Design 2 represents a second effort, it is badly put together because he is going so fast. His organization is poor, even sloppy. His drawings thus vividly demonstrate how his obsessive-compulsive symptoms seem to represent a reaction formation to a wish to be messy.

[His comments reflect other inner contradictions. Thus, while he anxiously clings to the examiner and implicitly and explicitly expresses his inability to go it alone, he at the same time attempts to degrade him and expresses much aggression toward him. While he asks the examiner for help in self-understanding (e.g., of his fears), he makes clear that he does not consider the examiner capable of doing the job adequately.]

PART B (COPY) (PLATES 30, 31 AND 32)

(Before beginning the Copy portion of the Bender, Paul asks many questions about the Children's Service. He wonders, for example, how the children are roomed. He asks, "Is it permissible to ask you these questions?") [It is apparent how much of his time Paul spends in doing and undoing. He aggressively *demands* to know, then he wonders whether this way of trying to find out is "permissible."]

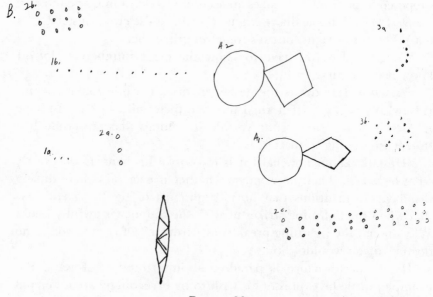

PLATE 30

Design A. Oh, oh, I tried to draw it while I was holding the card this way (rotated at a 90° angle) but it didn't come out right. Can I do it over?

Design 1. Do I have to have them the same farness apart? I did better on this one (Design A) the first time, when I was racing for time.

Design 2. Does it help first to do the outline on paper? I have a big problem trying to make things perfect. I have to fight with myself . . . . Oh, oh, it's not the right size, is it? [Paul sees part of his problems accurately.]

Design 3. Do these have to be perfect dots? (He has rotated the model 90°.) You might not like this, but do you mind not smoking? I hate the smell of tobacco, and besides it gives me a sore throat. (I stop smoking.) There it is. Something like this. Do you mean there's no time limit on these? ("No, there isn't.") [For obvious reasons Paul is not encouraged to take as much time as he needs.

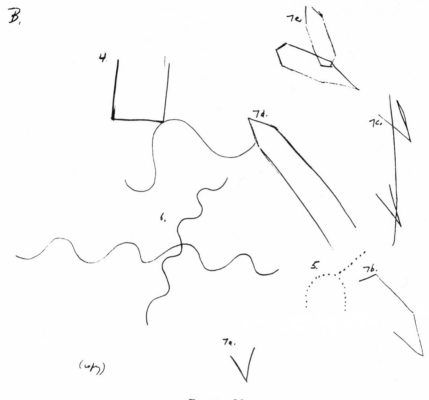

Regarding the examiner's heeding Paul's request not to smoke—
the examiner considered this a reasonable, nonmanipulative wish.]

Design 4. Most of them I draw smaller than they really are. This
one sure isn't. You're not allowed to use a ruler, are you?

Design 5. Are these optical illusions? ("How do you mean?")
I've seen optical illusions before, and they are funny-looking designs.
I didn't mean that you're trying to fool the kids, but I think there
might be some optical illusions lying around. (He slowly and carefully counts the dots, but he immediately has to count them again
because he has forgotten his total. After he erases a portion, he
counts all over again. He counts and recounts several times more.)
Oh! It isn't quite right . . . . . I'm going to see spots before I leave
here. I'll have my fill of spots.

Design 6. Are you trying to hypnotize me? ("How do you
mean?") Oh, I didn't . . . . (He counts the waves and sees that he

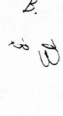

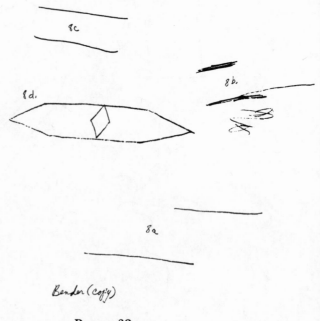

Bender (copy)

PLATE 32

drew them right.) Oh! They're right! (In a surprised tone.) That line was supposed to go up, I see. I made it go down. Do you think that's a bad mistake?

Design 7. Is it all right if I erase some of these others to get this one right? ("Don't erase what you've already finished.") I didn't think you'd want me to. Where were you born? . . . The poor things run off (i.e., the design goes off the paper).

Design 8. These double (parallel) lines I get scare me. (He makes a large line across the paper.) Oh, oh, that's going to run into something. (He takes a new sheet of paper.) I'm going to make this into a rocket ship. (He keeps trying to make straight lines, even though the ones he has drawn are quite adequate.) Is it possible for a human being to make straight lines? (He tells about his family background, saying that he is a distant cousin of President Monroe. He tells how his great-great-grandparents went across the country by wagon train and how one of them was killed by Indians. He mentions that one relative was the captain of a clipper ship and says that he is related to everybody, maybe even to me. He shows me a sore on his finger and says that it tears him apart to have to draw with it. He asks how long I think it will take to heal but right away says he will ask the psychiatrist who, after all, is a medical doctor who will be able to answer this question more satisfactorily.)

[Paul's drawings on Part B are individually more neatly and accurately done than the ones on Part A, the 5″ Exposure. So great is the apparent demand he makes of himself to be accurate (i.e., "perfect") that he rarely produces a design for which he has not first made at least a few trial attempts. What is again striking is Paul's haphazard organization of the designs on the page. One would certainly not suspect Paul's final results to have come about only after considerable preliminary practice. The component elements of his designs reflect a lack of consistent graphic control, for which Paul sometimes corrects but just as frequently does not. Inconsistent control is particularly reflected in the sudden size enlargement of Design 4. Design 5, unaccountably, is small again.

[Paul shows how often he needs to go in opposing directions. Thus, while he appears to strive for neatness and accuracy, his product is actually sloppy and inaccurate. A conflictual problem is similarly apparent in the interpersonal area. He wishes to draw near but, at the same time, to keep away. Such multidirectional impulses result in his being torn, and in his wanting to do things now one way and now the opposite. As soon as he tries to commit himself to one direction, another offers inviting possibilities.

[Paul's expectation that others will try to fool him (e.g., through optical illusions, hypnosis) is very evident. Such a chronic expectation of being poorly treated is well conceptualized as "basic mistrust." While he obviously mistrusts the examiner, he also (possibly for this very reason) continues to want to know more about him.]

THE DRAW A PERSON TEST

PART I (PLATES 33 AND 34)

(Only Part I is administered to Paul because it takes him such a very long time—one-half hour—to complete it. Time is running short, and Part II has to be sacrificed. Part Ib is included to illustrate the quality of Paul's false starts and rehearsals, as well as other try-outs which Paul requires of himself.)

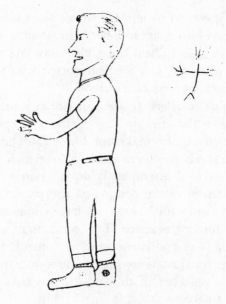

PLATE 33

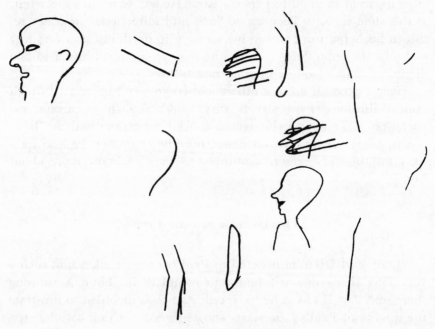

PLATE 34

(Before he begins the drawing, Paul wonders if one person might be able to write just like another. He says:) Somebody might arrest me because sometimes I write differently than other times. [An age-appropriate identity instability.] They might accuse me of trying to forge my own name. But you keep the same style all the time. (Paul is expectedly self-critical of his drawing. He makes five false starts and eventually says:) Let's face it; I can't draw a body.

(As he draws the face, he says:) The eye came out bad, and he's got a bad expression. Does that matter? He looks mean and cunning. What if I take a great deal of time on this. Does it matter? I'm rusty. I haven't drawn for a long time . . . . . Ah! There go the lips. (He is having trouble making the lips look light enough. He finally finishes the head.) This is just about the time when I should stop. I can't draw bodies any better than when I was in kindergarten. I might as well draw like this! (He illustrates with a stick figure.)

(As he continues to draw, he says:) I don't mind telling you—this upsets me, to draw the body, but I can't tell you why. (He works carefully and meticulously.) The head's too big for the body. It's better than I've done in a long time, though. I gave him tennis shoes. Is that all right? Oh, oh! Tennis shoes don't have a heel. (He erases and corrects some more.) He's an awfully short person.

(After he completes the DAP, he says:) Tell me, why are you having me draw this? (As I begin to explain, he interrupts:) You sound like you're trying to explain it to a little boy. You know, when I talk with people like you who know so much, I feel so small and insik—is—inig— (He can't get out the word "insignificant" until I help him. He explains different parts of the person he has drawn, to make sure I understand what he has intended. He wonders whether at the end of the hour he can quiz me about his drawing, to see if I know what everything is supposed to represent and so that his drawing won't look so "funny." As he draws, he continues to ask whether something or other is all right to do.)

(As he looks over his completed drawing, he says:) I didn't give him a good elbow. I didn't give him any elbow. (He practices draw-ing an elbow on the second sheet of paper.) I'll say the other hand is at his side. Okay? Can you remember that? . . . . Should I put a design on his shirt?"

[Paul's reaction is almost exactly as one would expect. Since he cannot copy, he must depend on internal models. As difficult as the Bender drawings were for Paul, they were much easier to do than the present drawing, which offers (demands) much more freedom. The freedom makes his work immensely harder; each impulse is met and negated by an immobilizing counterimpulse and by a negative self-comparison. Paul needs constantly to check whether something is right for him to do. He has so little internalized on which he can depend that he is constantly on the lookout for an external standard. But he resents having to depend on someone other than himself, so his compliments and pleas for direction are forever interlaced with demeaning and belittling comments. In this way he strives to bolster his self-regard. He cannot say why it upsets him to draw the body. It is probable that the activity triggers thoughts and impulses which, with more effective intellectual control, would never appear in awareness. That the thoughts nevertheless do appear to Paul reflects the ineffectiveness of his inner organization.]

[While in many aspects Paul's Rorschach Scoring Sheet looks exactly as one would expect, in some others it differs a good deal. He gives an unusually high number of responses, but perhaps not as compulsively many as one would look for. Similarly, it is surprising to see his relatively few Dr responses and the absence of any De responses. The high percentage of Paul's Animal responses suggests a lack of originality and a reliance on what he is given, rather than on what he himself creates. Yet he sees only seven Popular or near-Popular responses, so he apparently also avoids the obvious. Paul's Experience Balance is not nearly so constricted as one might expect and reflects a healthy intellectual and emotional evenness. The ratio of "acceptable" to "not acceptable" form responses is well within "normal" limits.

[Only the many qualitative notations make it apparent that all is not so well organized after all. Particularly noteworthy is the marked "aggressive" pressure and the "peculiar" and "castrative" aspects. Although Paul's tendency to fabulize might reflect a well-developed imagination, one nevertheless tends to look at the very high number of Fabulized responses with suspicion. Is Paul's view of things determined too much by internal, at the expense of external, reality? Then one notes the Confabulized response, the two Fabulized Combinations, the two Contaminatory Tendencies and the Arbitrary response.

[When one looks at Paul's Rorschach Scoring Sheet one is left, in other words, with the initial impression that, from a formal standpoint, he seems better organized than one expects. Yet, as one notes some of the more pathological qualitative indicators, the initially optimistic picture begins to fade, and one feels impelled to look more closely at actual responses before coming to a definite conclusion about the solidity of Paul's present mental organization.]

RORSCHACH TEST

RORSCHACH SCORING SHEET

Number of Responses: 40

Manner of Approach (Location)

W	8
D	27
Dd	0
Dr	4
DrS	1
De	0
Total	40

Groups of Contents

A	21
Ad	8
H	2
Giant	1
Hd	1
Mask	2
Obj.	1
Pl.	3
Geog.	1
Total	40

Location Percentages

W%	20
D%	68
DR%	13
De%	0

Determinant and Content Percentages

F%	80/97	Obj.%	2
F+%	75/78	At%	0
A%	73	P%	17
H%	10		

Form, Movement, Color and Shading Determinants

F+	13
F−	4
F±	11
F∓	4
M+	3
FC+	1
FC±	1
CF	1
F(C)+	1
FCh+	1
Total	40

Qualitative Material

Popular	II III V (VI) (VII) VIII X
Combination	III VIII X
Fabulation	9
Fabulized Combination	IX X
Confabulation	1
Contamination Tendency	2
Castration	3
Aggression	9
Peculiar	3
Confusion	1
Arbitrary	1

EXPERIENCE BALANCE: 3.0/2.0

RORSCHACH PROTOCOL

Card #	*React. Time*	*Score*	*Protocol*	*Inquiry and Observations*
I	3″	WF±Ad	1. It looks like a goat . . a billy goat. ("Anything else?") Can you analyze it from the other side? < . . ∧	1. ("What made it look like a goat?") It had two ears and horns . . and uh . . it had the beard, or whatever you call it. What *do* you call it? ("That's right—beard.") And the head seemed pretty much shaped like one. A billy goat . . You get that, Don't you? I wonder why they call them that? [Again, Paul's asking whether he can turn the card does not represent a "real" request for information. As will become increasingly clear later on, he has taken this test many times before. He must know he can turn the card any way he wants. The question, therefore, once again seems to mean that Paul wants to put himself in a helpless, submissive position—from which he can then attack.]
		DM+H Fab. Cast.	2. Part of it looks like a woman without a head, trying to direct an orchestra. ∧ < > ∨ There is something else, but I can't remember just what it is ("Just tell me whatever you see now.")	2. ("Tell me about the woman.") I saw one in the center. ("What made it look like a woman?") She had on the dress. (Center D.) [Paul sees "the woman" as inadequate in two ways: (a) she has no head, and (b) she is "trying" to direct an orchestra. [Apparently Paul is making an effort to give the same responses he has given previously; in this way he can avoid spontaneity.]
		WF+Obj.	3. I think the middle looks like a jack-o-lantern. ∨ > ∧ (He looks at me.) I could see a million of 'em if I kept going. Is it kind of cheating when you know 'em so well?	3. ("Tell me about the jack-o-lantern.") Oh, that's a very . . . . I shouldn't have said jack-o-lantern. Because it's shaped that way. Boy! (In response to a firecracker explosion outside.) There are enough firecrackers in this city. Bang! Bang! Bang! They don't allow

Card #	React. Time	Score	Protocol	*Inquiry and Observations*
				firecrackers in Wisconsin, but they do it anyway. ("Tell me a little more about the jack-o-lantern.") The trianglish . . not very good language, that . . eyes. And the mouth. [Apparently Paul is trying to discipline himself not to list all the percepts he sees. This capacity to withstand somewhat the demands of his obsessiveness reflects strength.]
II			(As I am putting out the card:) I bet a lot of kids say that's (last card) a jack-o-lantern.	
	8″	DF+AdP	1. It's two dogs. Wait, I've got to ask a question. It's two dogs, nose to nose, but . . . . I got to ask you. What kind of dogs do you call these? ("It depends on how you see them.") (He becomes very upset as I write down his question about how you call the dogs.)	1. ("Tell me about the dogs you saw.") Well . . I . . uh . their head was shaped . . not like Scotties . . like dogs. The nearest thing to them was a Scotty. Their head was shaped like it. I saw two ears. They had a nice long nose. They had the neck drawn to their body . . and all four legs. ("Could you see all four legs?") Their feet were in the background. (He wants me to write as quickly as he speaks.) Write down about the perfect head. (Black side D's.) [Paul's efforts to control are becoming increasingly open as his anxiety continues to mount—about the examination in general and more specifically about the verbatim recordings—and as he feels increasingly at ease with the examiner.]
		DFC±Ad Fab. Agg.	2. In the red I see two kinds of birds. I don't know what kind they are. Kind of like a cardinal, but not quite. They are birds from another dimension,	2. ("What about the birds?") (He is still angry from the previous inquiry.) They had a real long straight-up topnotch. And they had their beaks wide open . . as wide as it would go. You could see the teeth in there. And they seemed to be chatter-

	React.			
Card #	Time	Score	Protocol	Inquiry and Observations

screeching and chattering at each other. They look like they're real mad at each other. On the first one, two small dogs. They look like two Scotties (he names them after he draws them for me and after I say his drawing looks as though it is of Scotties). It looks closest to me like two small Scotties. (He explains that he does not mean that the birds are different kinds of birds but, rather, that they are two different strains of birds.)

ing . . or screeching at each other very loudly. Most of the dots in the last two paragraphs and in the last paragraph . . all of them, I think . . I'm pretty sure . . at least the last few . . but not in this sentence, dots have been there . . I've slowed down so that you could catch up. ("Could you tell me some more about the birds?") They're really not a very good resemblance but . . uh . . they had the topnotch. It was nothing like the cardinals. And they were red. P.S. I saw my first cardinal yesterday. (As he is outlining the cardinals on the card:) Oh, oh! Birds don't have teeth. Write down what I just said. So solly! It's a long-necked bird.

[Is Paul object or subject of the chattering and screeching, or is he both object and subject? The much increased obsessiveness that takes place at this time in part probably represents Paul's effort both to control and indirectly to express aggression. Even though he corrects himself, it is still strange to hear him speak of a "bird's teeth." Paul's comments regarding the examiner's dots, intended to show Paul's speaking pauses, reflect his conviction that he is being treated unfairly—a conviction which may eventually well serve as a paradigm for treatment.]

DrF(C)+
Ad
Agg.

3. Shall I say something about this one or isn't there time? (He becomes angry because I take down what he is saying. He waits a long time be-

3. It seemed like a dead ringer for the horn of the unicorn. ("How was that?") It looked like one. Its indentations. (He is referring to the markings. He looks at the card again.) It looks like a barber pole.

React.		
Card # Time Score	Protocol	Inquiry and Observations

Card # Time Score	Protocol	Inquiry and Observations
	fore he gives his next response, and in the interim he makes intensely angry comments about my taking verbatim notes.) Horns, like on a unicorn. What do you call them? They're the kind of horns you see on a mythical unicorn or on a narwhal (he pronounces it "narwhale"). (When I don't understand this word, Paul very sarcastically draws a narwhal for me. He looks it up in the dictionary to show me.) See, a psychologist doesn't know everything.	The lines are actually slanted on the true horn, but it doesn't matter that much. (Projections on red bottom D.) [His anger is by now almost chronic; at least, it takes very little to trigger it, and this is almost invariably linked to his feeling that the examiner is trying to make him appear ludicrous. He spends much time and energy trying to demonstrate that the superiority with which he has endowed the examiner is not really so great after all (e.g., "See, a psychologist doesn't know everything").]
DrF—Hed Pec.	4. I see two eyes and a mustache. Those birds are really going! They're good drawings.	4. ("Tell me about the eyes and mustache.") The reason I saw that . . It reminds me of seeing a comic book, with a cat in it. A little kid's book. This is one of the reasons. (Tiny Dr areas at the top, between two red D's.) [This is a poorly differentiated and rather capriciously interpreted percept. It reflects the type of obsessive and compulsive preoccupation with minutiae which one expects (much more of) from Paul.]
III 12″ Comb. ⎰WM+H ⎱Fab. ⎰DF+Mask	1. This looks like two . . uh . . two natives with a mask . . each holding a mask . . a war mask or something like that. > ∧ Do you want me to see what else there is?	1. ("Tell me about the natives.") I don't know. I called them that a long time ago . . because they're holding that primitive-looking mask. There's another reason, but I don't have the decency to say it. I saw that now. I didn't see that before. It wouldn't be decent to say. I always thought

React. Card #	Time	Score	Protocol	*Inquiry and Observations*

that that was natives because it seemed to be a very primitive kind of mask. And it looked to me like they were jumping around . . in motion. ("Were they men or women?") Well (he laughs), now you're getting it, aren't you? They always looked like men, but they look like women this time. But what would they be doing around a council fire? That's what spoils it. Why would they be doing a war dance?

[This response epitomizes Paul's confusion about others and about himself. First, he somewhat dehumanizes the Popular "people" and makes them into "natives"; then he gives them masks behind which to hide; then he wonders if they are men or women; then he speculates about their functions as men and women (i.e., "What would women be doing around a council fire? Why would they be doing a war dance?"). The seductiveness concerning his awareness of the figures' sex is noteworthy. Even though the examiner makes it a point not to ask him to explain his "mysterious" comments, he volunteers again that he will not tell him whatever it is that he does not have "the decency" to say. The "decency" slip suggests that Paul is aware that his "decency" is not as uncomplicated as he likes to make it seem.]

DFC+AP   2. I see a butterfly coming down the middle . . a pretty, pretty red one.

DF±A   3. Hey, that's something I never noticed . . kind of a . . some

3. ("How about the hyena?") It had the head of one. (Upper side red D's.)

React.				
Card #	Time	Score	Protocol	Inquiry and Observations

kind of a cat . . the cat family. > The large cat family. Oh, now I know. Like kinda like a hyena. That's what I was trying to say. The kind that go (makes a "fierce" face).

IV 10″ WM+
Giant
Agg.
Fab.

1. That's the one with so many things in it. I see a giant squashed all over. A flattened-out giant. He looks flat to me . . his face is all flat. He's sitting on a stool. He's got a big body and no brains.

1. ("What makes the giant look flat?") Well . . uh . . it seemed that way. The head just seemed to be flat. The head gave it a good portion of the flatness. [There is apparently nothing in the blot which makes the giant look flat; the flatness seems rather to result from Paul's need to degrade the giant (father?) who, after all, has no brains.]

DF±A
Cast.
Agg.
Pec.

2. I'll tell you one thing. (He complains again about my writing this comment down. As before, I try to interpret his anxiety about his feeling trapped by what he says.) It looks like something . . two eyes . . it looks like a squid minus four tentacles. And what there are, are cut off. Wait. It looks like a squid with his tentacles cut off, but four aren't completely cut off. (He draws a squid with all tentacles intact.) What he does have are just as good as nothing at all. Let's see now. Can I turn it around, or are you in a rush? (This is a sarcastic

2. (Bottom center D.) [Partly at least, one interprets this response as reflecting the (castrated) powerlessness Paul feels. A squid uses his tentacles both to attack-defend and to gather food. Paul is expressing the helplessness he feels about protecting and fending for himself.]

React. Card # Time Score	Protocol	Inquiry and Observations
	comment in response to my perhaps too-obvious wish to finish Paul's testing within the next three hours.)	
	Do the kids seem to have a trend to say the same things about these? Like this one? I knew this thing looked like something, but I had to figure out just *what* it looked like. It had the eyes, shape and mouth of *some* creature, but I had to figure out a creature that would look like that. V What's this?	[Paul is concerned to know how deviant he is.]
WF±A Contam. Tend. Fab.	3. Some kind of a bat . . a prehistoric one. Upside down it doesn't look like one. Some kind of a bat. With the head of a squid.	3. On that last one, the uh . . What are these? (He motions.) ("Projections?") The side projections don't make much sense. I don't mean the wings, which do make sense, and the . . a little, that is . . the head, too . . taken off would make a more sensible-looking bat, but that's a matter of degrees because it doesn't look much like a bat anyway. But the next card, that looks like a bat. [Paul's giving the bat a squid's head is not a full-fledged contamination, as it would be if he called it a "squid bat." Nevertheless, the response contains qualities of a mild contamination. [Again, he conveys that the Rorschach is old stuff as far as he is concerned, by telling what the next card will contain. Although he superficially complains about having had the Rorschach many times before, it is likely that he is grate-

React. Card #	Time Score		Protocol	Inquiry and Observations

ful to have the control which comes with knowing what to expect. Probably Paul was much more anxious when he took the Rorschach the first time, when he had no idea what would come up next. He is able to permit himself only rare excursions into the previously unexplored, as when he says, "Here's something I didn't see before."]

React. Card #	Time Score		Protocol	Inquiry and Observations
V	Imme-diate	WF+AP	1. It looks like a bat. V .... ∧ V ∧ And it's a darn good-looking bat, too . . . Wait! It looks just like a bat. Just about in all details: head, ears. Certain bats have longer ears than others; this one is like one of those. The legs seem pretty good. And so much for the wings, too.	
VI	5″	WFCh+ A(P) Contam. Tend. Agg. Cast. Confab.	1. That is a dead ringer for a thoroughly squashed, run-over cat. Second thought: . . it looks like . . uh . . like a . . uh . . solid steel cube . . about . . it would take about two yards in diameter . . fell on this cat. Bang! That's a good-looking cat (he laughs). That wasn't a joke, either. The fact that the head was so detailed. But I wouldn't exactly say the cat was good-looking in any way . . if it was squashed. I'm a gory creature, aren't I?	1. Are you going to keep this record? ("Yes I will. What made the cat look squashed?") Well, its body for one, looked like a rug . . a bear rug. The body really doesn't make too much sense, but it looked good enough. P.S., no tail, either. ("What made it look like a cat?") The ears, the snout, the cat whiskers. The head is shaped like a cat . . or it *was* like a cat. ("What made it look like a rug?") Well, it was gray. It seemed fuzzy, I guess. [Paul has combined two percepts usually seen separately: a cat's head and a bear rug. He combines the two by making it a "squashed, run-over cat." Once again, the response does not reflect a true contaminatory process. One has the feeling

Card #	React. Time	Score	Protocol	Inquiry and Observations

that Paul is usually able to keep separate what should be kept discrete. Nevertheless, one senses what things don't always remain as distinct as they should.

[When Paul says he is a "gory creature," it shows that he is aware of and concerned about the extent of his aggressive and destructive impulses.

[The reason the examiner gives Paul a short, factual answer to the question about "keeping the record" is that, although Paul's question obviously expresses his anxiety, the examiner believes the anxiety will be best relieved by a brief, factual approach rather than by an approach involving a long discussion of "feelings" which would only further stimulate Paul's obsessive processes. The examiner's point of view may, of course, represent little more than a rationalization whose purpose is to disguise the wish to complete testing quickly and "successfully."]

VII 1″ WF±A(P)

1. I see two rabbits. (He says this before he even looks at the card, wishing to convey that this is all very old as far as he is concerned.) ∨ > I just see those rabbits.

1. ("Tell me about the rabbits.") They seem to be turning around and looking at each other.

VIII 2″ Comb. { DF+AP / DF±pl

1. I see two wildcats . . mountain lions . . or something of that sort . . climbing up a tree. It's a fir tree of some sort.

1. ("What makes it look like a fir tree?") The shape. The top was shaped remotely like one. It would be the only tree where these things live, I think. But it's odd that they would be climbing on the outer branches. And I wish I could have seen it as a rock,

React.			
Card #	Time	Score	Protocol	Inquiry and Observations

React.
Card # *Time Score*   *Protocol*   *Inquiry and Observations*

but I didn't. [Paul takes himself very, very seriously. His comment, "I wish I could have seen it as a rock, but I didn't," reflects his inflexibility and the "yes/no" quality of his outlook. With more or less directness he needs to criticize whatever he is exposed to. The fact that the fir tree looks only "remotely" like one is Paul's way of saying it is an inferior likeness.]

DrSF∓Ad   2. The top looks kinda like a skeleton or something. I see ribs, and a snout . . and I see the eyes. I know what they look like . because I've seen cows' skulls and I have a horse skull at home, that's the gray part.

The back leg (of the mountain lion) is really perfect. You can see the foot. The foot and the thigh . . you never write what I want you to write.

2. ("How about the skeleton?") The gray part I said looks like a skull. ("Do the outer edges of that [top D] belong to it?") They have to be part of it, but it doesn't make any sense. [Paul organizes this otherwise not unusual response in such an idiosyncratic way that it is scored ∓. It is not clear why the outer edges of the top detail "must" be part of the skull. Is he stimulus bound to such a degree? But although there are quite acceptable elements in his "skeleton" percept, Paul makes it so difficult to empathize with it that the end result is arbitrary.]

DF+A   3. A little like a sting ray. Yeah, it does look like a sting ray. Do you know what a sting ray is?
Agg.

3. (Top D.) [Paul's sarcastic question is intended to remind the examiner of his ignorance concerning the narwhal.]

IX   8″   Fab.   1. I see two elks or . . mooses . . sitting on a . . yeah . . sitting on the top foliage of a tree.
         DF∓A
         Comb.
         DCFpl

1. (Orange and green D's.) ("What made it look like a moose?") Well, its body is shaped a little like it. Its head isn't too good. And its horns. ("What about the foliage?") Well, the greenery there . . big globs of green . . it looked like the top of a tree; or in a bush. In a bush! In a bush! [He succeeds in making his

React. Card # Time Score	*Protocol*	*Inquiry and Observations*
		response much less arbitrary than it seemed at first: mooses in a bush make a good deal more sense than mooses sitting on the top foliage of a tree.]
DF∓Ad	2. If you look at the tree closer, it looks like something, but I cannot comprehend what. I see the possible mouth, the snout and the eye.	2. ("What did that 'something' seem like?") It looked like something dumb. ("How do you mean?") A Warner Brothers' moose. The kind you see in Porky Pig. The droopy snout. The kind in the Bugs Bunny comics. [Paul's perceptual and associative processes are not well synchronized. Although he sees "something," he does not know right away what it might be. Such lack of perceptual-conceptual meshing suggests impaired intellectual organization, an observation about Paul's functioning which is no surprise by now. He is able to recover, however, to the point of calling his percept "something dumb." He is thrown back, in other words, on his hypercritical, derogating view of the world, its people and its things—a giant Warner Brothers' cartoon.]
DrF+Ad	3. Yi! ∧ Oh boy! An elephant, an elephant. I see an elephant (speaking in a little boy's voice). I never saw that before. It's an African elephant. The ones with the big ears. You ought to record all this, you know. It would be a lot easier. The trunk is awfully skinny!	3. (Bottom pink D, including Dr section which merges into Space area.) [Once again, Paul finds enough freedom to allow himself to see a "new" response. The elephant's skinny trunk undoubtedly represents another self-perception of the same sort as the squid's cut-off tentacles and the squashed cat's missing tail. [The degree to which he is bothered by the examiner's writing is remarkable. He has modified his attack somewhat, and his reproach now emerges as a "helpful suggestion."]

React.			
Card #	Time	Score	Protocol	Inquiry and Observations

			The next card has a lot of crabs.	
			∨	

X   3″   DF+pl   1. You know, those crabs don't look so much like crabs. They look more like kelp . . off La Jolla. (He becomes upset again when I write the last phrase.) Not La Jolla. You misunderstood me. It comes any place . . any place in the ocean. I was just commenting. I went to fish there with my mother and father. That's kelp.

1. ("What made it look like kelp?") It just looked like it. The way it was all spread out. (Side blue.) [Evident again is Paul's fear of being misunderstood and his consequent anger.]

DF+AP   2. There's a crab and there's a crab. (Same blue D on other side.)

2. (Popular side "crab" D's.)

DF+A   3. There's two sea horses. Ocean aquarians.

3. (Bottom green D's.) ["Ocean aquarians"!]

DF±A   4. There's a duck-billed platypus. It's the closest thing I can come to it. It looks familiar. What is it?

4. (Bottom brown side D.) ("What made it look like a platypus?") It has a bill like one. [Although Paul can call the sea horses "ocean aquarians," he acts as though he does not understand the true nature of the blots (i.e., "What is it?"—as though it must be a "real" picture of something). Is this pseudo or actual naïveté?]

DF—geog.   5. I know that's Arb.   something. This reminds me of Idaho. I don't know why.

5. (Large central pink D.) ("What made it look like Idaho?") That isn't Idaho. I don't know what it is. A piece of land somewhere. Yes, it is Idaho. It reminds me of Idaho. ("In what way?") I don't know. It just does. [An arbitrary interpretation.]

React. Card # Time Score	Protocol	Inquiry and Observations
DrF−A Fab. Agg.	6. It reminds me of some funny creature . . big eyes sticking out. A comical creature, screeching . . Moo! ∨	6. (Bottom portion of "Idaho," upside down.) ("What kind of a funny creature did it seem to be?") A comical cow. A snout is here. It looks like a big horn.
DF±creature-mask Fab. Agg.	7. And I . . uh . . I see two more . . uh . . oh-oh! I see a mask. I see something from another planet! It's a perfect thing. Those eyes are perfect. It's some creature, I don't know what. Some of these don't look like they did last time.	7. (Top central gray D.) ("What does the creature seem like?") It's going to dive down at you. ("How much of that was the creature?") The whole thing. [This reaction reflects both Paul's rigidity and his flexibility.]
DF+A Fab. Pec.	8. I see uh . . I see two kinds of birds climbing down a mountain side . . the heads together. I don't know what made me think of that. I guess it was like Idaho. There better no one ever have thought of that before. Okay, okay. You'll write it down later anyway. I don't know why I come to see a psychologist anyway. They're just a bunch of tricksters.	8. (Central blue D's.) [Paul's anxiety about being trapped resists the examiner's helpfully intended, mildly interpretative comments. It almost seems that the only action which by now could effectively decrease Paul's deeply disturbed state would be to terminate the examination. Such an extreme act would, of course, create problems of its own. Although the examiner has enough information by now to be able to contribute helpfully to a discussion of Paul's case, a premature end of testing would affect Paul very negatively. He would be frightened to find that he had the power to cow the adults whose ostensible purpose is to help him. He would feel guilty about using his behavior in such a self-destructive fashion. Finally, he would feel hopeless at realizing that he effectively prevented those who could help from understanding him as well as possible. [The tests themselves, and

	React.		
Card #	*Time Score*	*Protocol*	*Inquiry and Observations*

<table>
<tr><td></td><td></td><td></td><td>testing as such, do not create Paul's anxiety; rather, his fear of being discovered, of being found wanting, of revealing himself unintentionally, build his anxiety to the present intense pitch. Paul's major conscious anxiety is that he will appear stupid or lacking in intellectual and other ways. He is angry because he feels forced to say things which may be "misinterpreted."]</td></tr>
<tr><td></td><td>DF±A</td><td>9. Right smack in the middle . . not quite in the middle . . I see . . What does it look like to you? Put "hee-hee," so that they won't think I really asked you. Make it a joke. It *was* a joke! (He insists I write this down.) ("What does it look like to you?") I don't know. It's *something.* It looks like some bug. Here's the eye, and there's the nose. If you took those balls off the ends of the wings it would be a butterfly.

I'm not through. Why did you say "Fine?" I refuse to talk on the basis of the Fifth Amendment. It will incriminate me. And it does! Is this a courtroom? Am I on trial for murder? ∨ Every insignificant thing I say has to be written down.

What does it say there? Dictate what you've written!</td><td>9. (Upper central "maple seed.") [Paul's anxiety, anger, suspiciousness and tyranny emerge in full flower. Although he attempts to dilute the intensity of his reaction with some humor, e.g., "the Fifth Amendment," the intensity of his discomfort is apparent.]</td></tr>
</table>

	React.		
Card #	*Time Score*	*Protocol*	*Inquiry and Observations*

Fab. { DF—A / Confus. / Comb. { DF+A

10. Now this is a perfect chicken, with a great big long neck. Whose head is sticking into the eyes of a perfect donkey, burro, jackass, mule. Take your pick. It looks more like a donkey to me. But maybe it looks more like a burro. Ah, forget it.

10. (Bottom central "rabbit's head" and green "caterpillars.") ("Would you tell me about the chicken and the burro?") It was a fairly perfect body of the chicken. A chicken with the neck and head of an eel. It's fifty-fifty. [This response gains extra strangeness when Paul declares the chicken to be "perfect"—even though it has the neck and head of an eel, even though the rest of it is impossible to recognize as a chicken—but mainly because he presents this Fabulized Combination deadpan, as though there were nothing at all odd about a chicken that sticks its head into the eyes of a "perfect jackass." This response alone would suggest that Paul is undergoing a fairly active process of decompensation.]

Now I see a . . Say something. Say something! Say a poem.

[Paul requires an outside reaction to help him keep going. When the external response is lacking—in this case because the examiner is so busy writing that he seems removed—Paul feels lost.]

DF+A

11. Oh! There they are! If you really want to write, I can say so darn many things that you'll be at my knees. When you want to write, you write. When I want you to write, you don't. Come on now! Let's get to business. Here's two *perfect* looking ah! Cocker spaniels. They're just *perfect!*

11. (Central bottom yellow D's.)

	React.			
Card #	Time Score		Protocol	Inquiry and Observations

DF±Ad

12. Next . . there are a lot of things in this . . I see a . . a swan. It looks a little like a swan.

12. (Side central yellow D.) ("Tell me about the swan.") I see the head and bill. Certain features make it look like a swan, rather than a duck. And its bill is longer.

DF∓A
Comb.

13. I see . . uh . . two just about perfect . . goats. Just plain goats. Two goats climbing on something . . climbing up.

13. (Top side green D's.) ("What made them seem like goats?") Well, they're shaped like an animal, and they're down on their haunches, and they have a horn.

DF±A
Agg.
Fab.

14. And I see two creatures that . . I don't know what they are. They seem to be like around a pole or something. They're very mad and fierce-looking. They seem to be looking at each other in the eye.

14. (Topmost gray D). [Although Paul is able to restrain the volume of his output on previous cards, Card X, with its many isolated details, offers the temptation to respond to each separate area, sometimes more than once. Card X does not require Paul to exert the sort of perceptual and cognitive control which preceding cards have required and which, apparently, Paul is no longer capable of exerting.]

(As we complete the test, he asks many questions about the final conference. He says, "You'll all probably talk about five minutes or so, like in court. Then you'll say, 'Next case!' " He continues to mimic a ridiculous court procedure. I tell him about the final conference and explain that it lasts about two hours. Apparently somewhat mollified, he says, "Well, that's better.")

[It becomes entirely obvious again to what degree Paul's aggression is associated with his fear of being given too short shrift. He is convinced that nobody wishes really to understand, to help or to spend a decent amount of time on him and his situation. People are interested only in "convicting" him and in dealing with him in an offhand, superficial way.]

THEMATIC APPERCEPTION TEST

(It takes Paul one and one-half hours to tell seven brief, unrevealing stories.

(He needs to prepare his stories and to know ahead of time exactly what he will say. Before he commits a story to the dictaphone, he rehearses it aloud. He stares at each new card a long time, apparently trying to remember what stories he told before. Occasionally he gets up from his chair, in order to think more effectively; some-times he interrupts his storytelling to write himself memos.

(He continues his diatribe against psychiatrists and psychologists and says they are "bluffers."

(He plays his voice back on the dictaphone and reacts disgustedly to it. He says he wanted to make a good impression and to sound very intelligent, but he complains that, as he listens to his voice, he sounds "like a moron.")

[Although he rather successfully avoids self-revelation in his stories, he is occasionally impelled to tell the examiner things he did not include in the original story. For example, he tells a brief story about a boy who is crying because he accidentally shot his friend to whom he was showing a new pistol. After he finishes dic-tating the story, he says that he does not want to dictate that the wounded boy's arm had to be amputated, because this would make us all think he was "gruesome." Similarly, on Card 6 BM, he says the woman's son was taken to a prisoner-of-war camp; after he has finished his story, he explains that he does not want to say that the son was killed in action.

[In spite of his efforts to avoid telling about himself on this test, Paul reveals a little about the probable relationship between himself and his parents. He tells that, although his father may mean well, when something really needs to be done it is best done by Paul him-self, with his mother's help. Although the father puts on the appear-ance of being the strong male, he is really not strong at all.]

The Psychologist's Report

Paul interprets his examination as a trial, and he sees me as prosecutor, judge and jury. During one of his frequent exasperated outbursts, he says, "I refuse to talk on the basis of the Fifth Amend-ment. It will incriminate me. And it does! Is this a courtroom? Am I on trial for murder? Every insignificant thing I say has to be written down!" He requires himself to be without flaw and needs to avoid showing the slightest weakness, uncertainty, or lack of knowledge. His frequent outbursts of derogating anger seem caused primarily by fear that he will be trapped into exposing inadequacies so that the clinic staff will think disparagingly of him. When he hears his voice on the dictaphone playback, he is keenly disappointed and says, "I wanted so much to sound intelligent and to make a good impression, and here I sound like a moron." On the Thematic Apperception Test, to avoid seeming unpolished because of hesitations and because of corrections he might have to make, he inwardly prepares and rehearses bland, brief, nonrevealing stories before he allows a single word to emerge out loud. Once, I coughed as he was dictating; he became extremely disturbed because he feared the secretary might believe he was the one who had "spoiled" his story in this way. Although he is usually extremely defensive about the excellence of his intellectual capacities, he apparently has at least preconscious awareness that his underlying disorganization may be quite extensive. He is concerned, for example, that certain of his preoccupations may seem "gruesome" to others. Partly in order to avoid exposing these "gruesome" (i.e., blatantly aggressive) aspects, Paul avoids spontaneity and tends to respond in ways which have worked, and which have helped him to avoid trouble, in the past.

Paul's chronic and ever-mounting anxiety makes him into both an extremely angry and an extremely controlling person. He insists, for example, that I write or not write whatever he wants me to, and he invariably becomes irritated whenever I "disobey" him and write down what he feels might show him up to poor advantage. At times his anxiety causes him to erupt in accusations that I am dishonest, untrustworthy and undependable.

Paul is plagued by easily aroused guilt feelings which he tries to evade by applying hyperscrupulous, compulsive "honesty." For example, when I ask him to define "armory," he says he might as well be frank and tell me he had not known this word until the previous day. For this reason he should receive no credit for his correct definition. He makes a number of other comments of this sort. On the Rorschach, for example, he says, "Isn't it like cheating on these blots, when I've seen them so many times before?" It seems that, unconsciously, Paul feels he is basically dishonest and a fraud; on a conscious level, he does everything he can to demonstrate that he is thoroughly truth-loving, and for that reason has no need to feel guilty.

One of the major ways Paul uses to reduce his feelings of inadequacy, which create both anxiety and guilt, is to focus on what he determines is the inadequacy of others. He explains that he feels compelled to tell others about their "ignorance" and "errors." On the Rorschach, he interprets an area as a "narwhal," and when I admit to never having heard of the animal, he shows me its picture in the dictionary and triumphantly says, "Even a psychologist doesn't know everything." Later on, as he sees a much more familiar animal, he pointedly asks whether I have ever heard of it. Expressions of inferiority can usually be found nearby whenever Paul launches one of his externally directed personal attacks.

How feelings of belittling anger and personal impotence are juxtaposed is illustrated by Paul's partial reaction to Rorschach Card IV:

> *Response 1.* I see a giant squashed all over. A flattened-out giant. A big body, no brains.
> *Response 2.* It looks like a squid without enough tentacles. It looks like a squid minus four tentacles. And what there are, are cut off . . . . . What he does have are just as good as nothing at all.

One wonders to what extent Paul's second response, expressing such a degree of helplessness, represents a placating effort to undo the belittling attack which precedes it. Such doing and undoing is characteristic of Paul; he often alternates an attack with an expression of passivity and inferiority. (Such a formulation does not, of course, exclude the probability that the first response also embodies significant self-reference, while the second embodies significant projective reference.) Be that as it may, Paul is forever turning passivity into activity (via accusing attack) and activity into passivity (via assertions of helpless inferiority).

Although Paul attempts to hide, or at least to disguise, the extent of his psychological disorganization, he is aware that he functions ineffectively. He expresses concern about his disorganization indirectly by asking about the Menninger Children's and Adult Hospitals in great detail, e.g., wanting to know whether "they" keep "insane" people here. He laughs and says he guesses we are preparing him for the "insane asylum." When I wonder about other thoughts he has about such things, he angrily says that his question was meant only as a joke, and he complains about psychologists and psychiatrists always reading incorrect things into people's statements. Paul frequently employs denial in this way.

Paul fears the unexpected. He needs to control the present to avoid surprise in the future. Although he "complains," on the Rorschach, that he knows what cards will follow, one senses that this familiarity is reassuring and is the major factor which permits Paul to deal with the test at all. Only rarely does he gain enough freedom to see "something I never saw before." He also reacts fearfully to loud, persistent or unexpected noise. He complains about the hum of what he calls the "phosphorescent" light fixtures; about the explosion of prematurely set-off Fourth of July firecrackers; about nocturnal thunderstorms. He deals with his fear partly through counterphobic mechanisms. For example, although he thinks he might receive an electric shock from the dictaphone, he touches it and then quickly withdraws his hand, laughing tensely.

While Paul places very high value on intellectual competence, he actually functions on no more than the High Average level. He obtains a Total Intelligence Quotient of 115-117 on the Wechsler-Bellevue (Verbal Quotient 114-117; Performance Quotient 112). His immediate Memory and Concentration are significantly impaired. On the Arithmetic subtest, for example, he has to reread one of the more difficult problems several times to himself because, he complains, his mind is like a blank wall on which "nothing registers." He complains that his memory has been becoming particularly bad the past several months, and that he writes himself numerous memos in order to remind himself of various things. This activity probably has primarily obsessive-compulsive (ordering), rather than merely memory-strengthening, meanings. He is well informed in certain areas, particularly those related to nature and natural phenomena, but occasional surprising gaps exist. For example, he does not know how many weeks there are in a year.

Even on the more structured Wechsler tasks, Paul's thinking is occasionally marred by confusion. When he is asked, for example, to estimate the height of the average American woman, he says it is six feet. Only after a while is it clear that he means the average man. Sometimes Paul's mishearing makes no grammatical or logical sense. For example, when I ask the Comprehension question which deals with why people who are born *deaf* are usually unable to speak, Paul has difficulty answering because he hears *deaf* as "death." Some difficulty is also suggested by Paul's occasional inability to pronounce a relatively simple word; he may make five or six false starts before he either succeeds in saying the word or gives up on it altogether. Occasionally his explanations become so involved and confused that he waves his arms in a hopeless, angry, embarrassed way and says, "Oh, never mind. Skip it!" A thinking peculiarity is suggested by

Paul's tendency to shift suddenly, without warning, from one topic to an entirely different one.

Disordered thinking patterns become much more evident on the Rorschach. While Paul is able to see a fairly adequate number of Popular responses, and while other formal aspects (i.e., the F+%, the Experience Balance) are within "normal limits," a number of individual responses suggest the workings of a rather severe pathological process. Paul shows a tendency toward contamination and toward peculiarity, both of perception and of expression. Many responses contain strong fabulized elements which reflect the degree to which Paul embroiders reality, making it into what he wants or needs it to be. On occasion, his thinking becomes highly arbitrary, as when he describes chickens with heads and necks of eels, who are sticking their head "into the eyes of a donkey, jackass or burro." Nine of Paul's forty Rorschach responses contain angry, aggressive, destructive elements, and several give further testimony to his self-image of being an impotent, incomplete little boy.

The turbulence and bewilderment which accompany Paul's efforts to grope toward a mature, stable identity are epitomized by his interpretation of the Popular figures often seen on Rorschach Card III. Paul first sees these figures as two natives who are holding a primitive-looking mask. When I wonder what makes them seem to be natives, he says, "They are holding that primitive-looking mask. There is another reason, but I don't have the decency to say it. I saw that now; I didn't see it before. It wouldn't be decent to say . . . ("Is it a man or a woman?") Well, now you're getting it, aren't you? They always looked like men, but they look like women this time. But what would they do around a council fire? That's what spoils it. Why would they be doing a war dance?" Paul is not only taken aback, by the physical, sexual aspects of these "natives," he is preoccupied and made uneasy by the appearance of women behaving like men. Paul finds the tableau so disturbing that he says the opposite of what he consciously intends (i.e., he apparently means to say, "I have too much decency to say it."). His need to clarify the distinct functions different people perform is apparent, too, in his first wondering exactly how my professional activities differ from the psychiatrist's and then becoming upset when he believes that our activities overlap, merge, or lose their separate character in other ways.

Paul's disrespect of his parents stands as an obstacle in the way of his feeling as dependent on them as he would like. One wonders if he is thinking of his mother when he interprets a portion of the Rorschach as "a woman, without a head, trying to conduct an orchestra." Not only a disorganized but also an aggressive mother may be represented by Paul's percept of "birds from another dimension, screeching and chattering at each other. Their beaks are wide open, as wide as they'll go. You can see their teeth in there." In other words, the birds not only chatter, they bite as well. Paul's Thematic Apperception Test themes suggest that he also sees his mother as adamant in her demands, forcing him to do things against his will. Paul evaluates his father as a person who, while he may mean well, is too weak to put his good intentions into effect.

In summary, Paul is strikingly obsessive-compulsively organized. Both the obsessiveness and compulsivity make it difficult for him to function efficiently, and one can see sufficient evidence of peculiar and disorganized thinking to suggest that a process of decompensation is taking place. Paul is extremely afraid of revealing himself, and he makes (not particularly successful) perfectionistic demands on himself to maintain a front of effective organization. Although he wants to be highly intellectual, he functions only in the High Average range on the Wechsler-Bellevue. Depression and feelings of inadequacy are suggested by his frequent expressions of worthlessness and pessimism. He reacts with anger whenever he fears he is losing the upper hand with another person. This anger, which also appears whenever he fears exposing himself to poor advantage, is often interlarded with hypersuspiciousness and frequently followed by expressions of personal helplessness, harmlessness and inadequacy. He seems vitally concerned with questions involving the identities and functions of others and, hence, of himself. He has little respect for either of his parents and does not feel he can safely depend on them.

DISCUSSION

The reasons for Paul's having been designated "overideational" are of course apparent. He is immobilized by the many contradictory thoughts which bombard his awareness, contradictions which make it difficult for him to move into any kind of planful action. Almost every tendency to go in one direction is negated by a counterimpulse, so that the original impulse is transformed into ruminative, unproductive thought. The end result is that Paul stands still; he stands immobilized at the threshold to the threshold of adulthood—i.e., he is unable to enter adolescence.

As we look at the next protocol, we can see a somewhat different characterological solution. Although Wes employs mechanisms which are similar to Paul's, he additionally relies rather heavily on an opposite mode of dealing with disturbing thought and impulse: rather than exerting control efforts by hyperideation alone, Wes also tries to keep himself organized by pushing ideas out of consciousness (i.e., by repression). To use a common diagnostic categorization, Wes may be thought to have a mixed (i.e., obsessive-compulsive and hysterical) personality organization. Wes's protocol serves as a transition between the overideational Paul and the underideational adolescents whose protocols follow in the next chapter.

Clinical Summary: Wes

Wes is sixteen years old and is now an only child.

A month before the present examination the police accused Wes of having exposed himself to three nine-year-old girls. Several months earlier, Wes had been accused of the same behavior, but at that time he had denied it and charges were dropped.

For many years the parents have been concerned about Wes's lack of interest in applying himself to any kind of work. He has characteristically been stubborn and resentful toward authority. His earliest grade cards indicate slowness, lack of interest in work and lack of initiative. Teachers have commented on his physical clumsiness. He has never participated in competitive games but has been active in Boy Scouts, the 4-H Club and the young people's organization of his church. Although he has not been a major troublemaker at school, the principal reports that he usually picks one teacher whom he bothers with resistant behavior. He has always been slow to hand in his school work, generally receives grades of C and D, and shows no leadership qualities. At school he is regarded as a lone wolf, and others consider him rather odd. He was recently dismissed from a job of delivering newspapers because he was not dependable.

Wes's mother was nineteen when he was born. She had a difficult pregnancy and delivery, with nausea, uremia and convulsions. The obstetrician said that there was great doubt that either she or the baby would live. Wes weighed eight pounds, eleven ounces at birth. He cried a great deal and seemed always to be hungry. He walked when he was thirteen months old. Bowel and bladder training were accomplished when he was two years old, but he had a relapse at the age of two-and-a-half, when a brother was born. Enuresis continued until age seven. He has consistently eaten a great deal and has spent all his allowance on candy. He has always been a big person, and all his life others of his age have teased him about his weight, his awkwardness and his slowness. He has always chewed his fingernails. He attended public school until the fourth grade; then his parents sent him to a small country school, where he achieved better grades and played well with other children. Also, he was elected president of the local 4-H Club when he was twelve and has been active in Scouts, where he is about to receive his Eagle badge.

Three years ago, Wes's two-and-a-half year younger brother was accidentally shot at a YMCA camp. This tragedy had an enormous impact on the family, and all family members still feel much guilt concerning the event. Following the brother's death, the parents became the sponsors of a young people's church group. Wes has been active in this group, both as president and vice-president. In high school last year, Wes failed math. His parents do not feel that he will have enough credits to be graduated next year.

By the age of five, Wes had had pneumonia three times; at ten he was hospitalized for one week with virus pneumonia. The family had a serious automobile accident when Wes was twelve; although Wes was not hurt physically, he was very restless at night following this event. He cried in his sleep for several months afterward.

The father has had four massive gastric hemorrhages. He has accused Wes of causing some of them because, he says, Wes has upset him so. The father is thrown into a rage at the least hint of Wes's rebelling or individually expressing himself. The father has frequently punished Wes severely with a stick or strap, and on occasion has become so enraged that he has bruised Wes in beating him. Once he threw a glass of milk at Wes. Although Wes's mother is usually the mediator, she has at times taken part in the argument; at such times, while the mother and father argue, Wes sits quietly watching. Although the father often feels contrite after an argument, he can never say that he was wrong. The father has recently decided to go into training for the ministry.

Physical and Laboratory Findings: Physical examination reveals a scarred right tympanic membrane, and obesity without evidence of endocrinological disease. The neurological examination reveals no definite clinical signs of organic disease of the central nervous system. Routine blood, urine, serological tests, and x-rays of the skull and chest are negative. The EEG was first interpreted as mildly abnormal, suggestive of paroxysmal dysrhythmia, but a repeated EEG, with sleep, appears entirely normal.

THE PSYCHOLOGIST'S DESCRIPTION

Wes is tall and heavy for his age; he makes a phlegmatic appearance, even though his gait is rather mincing. During testing he shows almost no tension. His expression is quite bland, and although he smiles occasionally, the smile seems primarily polite and dutiful. He cooperates easily, although he sometimes says he would "rather not" elaborate an enigmatic comment. He goes out of his way to be helpful, e.g., replacing test items in their boxes after he has finished with them, or showing solicitous concern about speaking too quickly or too much. Occasionally his helpfulness seems somewhat overdone, as when he explains well-known slang expressions or slows his speech as if he were dictating to an intellectually limited secretary. In spite of what he intends as pleasant helpfulness, it is difficult to feel warmth toward or from Wes. He seems too self-sufficient and unconcerned about establishing a significant relationship. He explains how, in football, he always avoids blocking at the last moment because he fears bodily contact. This avoidance is prototypical of the way he fends off psychological contact as well.

THE WECHSLER-BELLEVUE SCALE

[Wes's final score on the Wechsler-Bellevue, although it locates him only at the 27th percentile of the general population, still falls within the Average range. His scatter is fairly marked, ranging from 5 on Similarities to 12 on Vocabulary and Object Assembly. It is not easy to ascribe immediate meaning to the seven-point disparity between Wes's scores on Similarities and Vocabulary, both of which are assumed to make use of similar functions; nevertheless, the discrepancy must eventually be accounted for. Offhand, one wonders if the difference in these two verbal abilities might relate to an impaired ability to discover significant *relationships among elements,* while *isolated elements* can be dealt with effectively. If the alternate score is taken into consideration, the Comprehension-Information relationship is seen to be of the type commonly found among persons with a "hysterical" personality organization (i.e., a sensitivity to the socially condoned and valued, with a concomitant devaluation of factual information).]

Name: _____Wes_____   Age: ___16-3___

	RS	WTS	0 1 2 3 4 5 6 7 8 9 10 11 12 13 14 15 16 17 18 19 20
COMPR.	10-13	9-11	
INFOR.	10	8	
DIG.	12	10	
ARITH.	5	6	
SIMIL.	6-7	5-6	
VOCAB.	28	12	
P. A.	9	8	
P. C.	10	9	
B. D.	19	9	
O. A.	20	12	
D. S.	35	8	

TOT. VERB.	40-43
TOT. PERF.	46
TOT. SCALE	86-89

VERBAL I.Q.: ___92-96___   LEVEL: ___Low Average___

PERFORMANCE I.Q.: ___93___   LEVEL: ___Low Average___

TOTAL I.Q.: ___92-94___   LEVEL: ___Low Average___

INFORMATION

No.	Question	Response and Comments	Score
1.	*Who is the President of the United States?*	Eisenhower. ("And before that?") Truman. ("And before that?") You got me. (He laughs.) ("Does any name come to mind?") (He shakes his head.) This might be silly or something, but might it have been MacArthur? [From this first response one hardly obtains the conviction that Wes is particularly well informed. His suggesting the name "MacArthur" as a former U.S. president indicates a both naïve and careless organization of knowledge. General MacArthur was frequently in the news at the time of testing. Wes uncritically picked the first name he could think of which had a wide reputation. This very first response makes apparent how little Wes seems to value knowledge for its own sake.]	+

No.	Question	Response and Comments	Score
2.	What is a thermometer?	To take the temperature with . . of the human body.	+
3.	What does rubber come from?	Latex tree . . from India. Would you like one of these? (He offers me some candy.) [Under the guise of being extra well informed, Wes offers a naïvely incorrect definition. And what does it say about a sixteen-year-old when he eats candy during the very first moments of an examination and offers some to his examiner? Behavior of this sort is much more appropriate to children of latency age.]	−
4.	Where is London?	England.	+
5.	How many pints make a quart?	Four. ("Are you sure?") Uh-huh. [When their answers are challenged, most people tend to pause momentarily for reconsideration. Giving the correct answer does not, however, seem important enough to Wes to make him question himself.]	−
6.	How many weeks are there in a year?	Fifty-two.	+
7.	What is the capital of Italy?	It . . uh . . Uh-uh (he shrugs). ("Can you think of any Italian city?") Nope. (He laughs.)	−
8.	What is the capital of Japan?	I think of one, but I don't know whether it would be right. Would it be Tokyo?	+
9.	How tall is the average American woman?	Around . . between five feet nine inches and six feet. ("How tall are you?") A little over six feet one inch. ("Is the average American woman just about your size?") No. She'd be a little shorter . . about three inches.	−
10.	Who invented the airplane?	Wright brothers.	+
11.	Where is Brazil?	South America.	+
12.	How far is it from Paris to New York?	It all depends on which way you're going. (He laughs.) Around 4,000 miles. Somewhere in there. [It is apparent that Wes handles intellectual problems altogether differently from Paul. Wes is satisfied with approximations and is not much concerned when these are somewhat wide of the mark. Paul, who requires himself to be superexact, often ends up being just as wrong as Wes, but for very different reasons.]	−

No.	Question	Response and Comments	Score
13.	What does the heart do?	It circulates the blood around .. uh .. to the body .. and oxygen.	+
14.	Who wrote Hamlet?	Hmm .. Shakespeare?	+
15.	What is the population of the United States?	You got me again. (He laughs.) ("Make a guess.") . . . . . Around seven or six million. Somewhere around there. [On the surface Wes seems to accept major gaps in his knowledge rather calmly.]	—
16.	When is Washington's birthday?	I don't know. ("Do you know the approximate time of the year?") Uh-uh.	—
17.	Who discovered the North Pole?	Byrd.	—
18.	Where is Egypt?	By Africa. ("How do you mean?") Either in it or by it. It's right alongside it. I know that. [This response excellently captures Wes's approach to knowledge. He feels no particular need to be exact, precise, or to hit the nail on the head. "In it," or "by it," or "alongside it" is close enough.]	+
19.	Who wrote Huckleberry Finn?	Tom Sawyer. [A fairly frequently made error which, by now, seems typical of Wes.]	—
20.	What is the Vatican?	The what? ("The Vatican.") I think it'd be a city somewhere. I don't know where. ("Could you guess?") No.	—
21.	What is the Koran?	Come again? ("Koran.") Would it be a river? That's just a wild guess.	—
22.	Who wrote Faust?	Never even heard of it. (He smiles.) [Wes's casual attitude toward knowledge is underscored by his easy dismissal of more difficult questions. He does not appear troubled by not knowing answers; instead, he conveys that he believes the questions involve the examiner's somewhat outlandish preoccupations.]	—
23.	What is a Habeas Corpus?	A dead person, I think .. a corpse. [A clang association which probably reflects carelessness much more than pathological loosening.]	—
24.	What is ethnology?	I don't know.	—
25.	What is the Apocrypha?	I don't know.	—

RAW SCORE: 10

WEIGHTED SCORE: 8

COMPREHENSION

No.	Question	Response and Comments	Score

1. *What is the thing to do if you find an envelope in the street, that is sealed, and addressed and has a new stamp?*

I'd do one of two things. Three things, I imagine. One, take it to the police station and locate the owner; two, put it in the mailbox; three, take it there myself. ("Which would you choose?") I believe I'd take it there myself . . locate the place. [It is difficult to determine whether this answer reflects "true" obsessive uncertainty. Although Wes's doubting has this appearance at first glance, the doubting might actually reflect only a pseudo obsessiveness, "externally" determined by uncertainty about what the *examiner* might want to hear, not brought about by "internal" doubts.]

Score: 0-2

2. *What should you do if while sitting in the movies you were the first person to discover a fire (or see smoke and fire)?*

Report it to the manager if I could. I wouldn't let anyone else know. Let him take over. If I hollered "fire," it would probably cause a panic. [Once again, one can see the effort, via negation, to hold in check a temptation toward impulsivity.]

Score: 2

3. *Why should we keep away from bad company?*

Bad company? It's liable to get you into trouble that you can't get out of. It might affect your personality quite a bit, too. ("How's that?") It probably deflects you from right to wrong. If you go with the wrong crowd, you mightn't be liked by kids you like . . they wouldn't like you. ("Which answer would you choose?") That it would probably swing you from right to wrong. [The quality of this response seems obsessive in a "true," i.e., internally determined, sense. The response is interesting in that it contains both "hysterical" and "obsessive" features. Hysterical aspects include moralistic concerns about right and wrong and good and bad. The obsessive component can be noted in the choice of possibilities Wes offers.]

Score: 2

4. *Why should people pay taxes?*

Keep up the government and the armed forces, so they can fight for us and keep their men paid. We should be glad to pay them . . it's a privilege. (He speaks very fast, so that it is difficult to keep up.) I'll try to slow down. (He laughs.) [One can see that Wes needs to show himself on the side of law and order and of the "greater good." Siding unquestioningly with existing values is consistent with a hysterical character organization. Compare Wes's answer with Paul's, who, answering the same question, says, "Well, the government needs

Score: 1

No.	Question	Response and Comments	Score

money to keep going—to run the country. So people pay taxes to the government."]

5. *Why are shoes made of leather?*

It's the best kind of material they could find. It's pliable and workable. ("Any other reason?") No, that would be all.   **1**

6. *Why does land in the city cost more than land in the country?*

I imagine it all depends on how much it is by the lot. In the country, you pay by the acre, in town it's by the township. ("Why would it cost more in town?") It all depends on who you're buying from. In the country, you've got a lot more room. In the city, you only get one or two lots and you have to pay a pretty high price. ("Why does it cost more?") The location, I'd imagine. [Once again one sees Wes's vague circling about. At times his comments are grossly inaccurate—e.g., the idea that in town one pays for land by the "township."]   **0-1**

7. *If you were lost in a forest (woods) in the daytime, how would you go about finding your way out?*

Well, the sun comes up in the east and sets in the west. I wouldn't go by the moss on trees, because in our neck of the woods it grows on all sides. You could locate a river in your area and follow it . . pretty soon you'll hit a town or some kind of civilization. [Self-reference ("in our neck of the woods") is frequently noted in persons organized along hysterical lines.]   **2**

8. *Why are laws necessary?*

To protect people. ("How do you mean?") Well, like speeding laws . . If people drove just as fast as they wanted to . . On a day like this, they'd wipe out each other awfully fast. There are too many being killed as it is. [Again the moralistic identification of himself with the "proper" goals of society.]   **1**

9. *Why does the state require people to get a license in order to be married?*

. . . . . I wouldn' know that. I'd be afraid to take a guess at it. ("Take one anyway.") I'll just take a wild crack at it. So if you want to marry a certain person, you'd be sure that someone else couldn't horn in on it. In other words, you're legally bounded to that person. [Wes does not want to deal with this question, in all likelihood because (a) it has sexual implications and (b) it requires that he put himself into more adult shoes.]   **1**

10. *Why are people who are born deaf usually unable to talk?*

Well, they can't hear what's going on. Someone asks them a question, and they can't hear it, so they won't talk. It might be that they're afraid to talk . . afraid of what they might say. (He belches noisily.) Excuse me. ("How do you mean,   **0**

No.	Question	Response and Comments	Score

'afraid of what they might say'?") If they're in a conversation, you might say something that would hurt other people's feelings. You could think what they were going to say, but you wouldn't know how it would sound to others. [Here is an apparent paradox: Wes expresses concern about someone's speaking inappropriately but openly and noisily belches at the same time.]

RAW SCORE: ___10-13___

WEIGHTED SCORE: ___9-11___

DIGIT SPAN

(He correctly repeats seven Digits Forward and five Digits Backward. As he experiences difficulty, he exclaims "Gad!" or "Whew!" or "I really goofed up on that one.")

RAW SCORE: ___12___

WEIGHTED SCORE: ___10___

ARITHMETIC

I warn you on that. I haven't had any math. I never did like it. I had all D's in it at school. I'm going to save algebra, trig and geometry for college. [The "typical" apology of the hysterically organized person in response to the Arithmetic subtest.]

No.	Problem	Time	Response and Comments	Score
1.	How much is four dollars and five dollars?	10″	How do you mean? (I repeat the question.) Oh, I see what you mean—adding . . . nine! I was beginning to wonder how you meant them. [This is an example of Wes's need to present himself as helpless when confronted with a task which requires introspection. He has "warned" the examiner that he dislikes math, and it is therefore difficult to determine how much of his present confusion is motivated (i.e., how much it represents an indirect refusal to participate), and how much of his bewilderment represents a mild, temporary cognitive disorganization.]	1
2.	If a man buys six cents worth of stamps and gives the clerk ten cents, how much change should he get back?	1″	Four.	1

No.	Problem	Time	Response and Comments	Score
3.	*If a man buys eight cents worth of stamps and gives the clerk twenty-five cents, how much change should should he get back?*	3″	Eight and twenty-five. Is that it? . . . . Sixteen.	0
4.	*How many oranges can you buy for thirty-six cents if one orange costs four cents?*	2″	Nine.	1
5.	*How many hours will it take a man to walk twenty-four miles at the rate of three miles an hour?*	14″	Forty-eight minutes. ("How did you get that?") It may sound kind of stupid, but I took three into sixty. It went twice. I took that times twenty-four.	0
6.	*If a man buys seven two cent stamps and gives the clerk a half dollar, how much change should he he get back?*	13″	Forty-six . . no . . wait, thirty-six.	1
7.	*If seven pounds of sugar cost twenty-five cents, how many pounds can you get for a dollar?*	7″	Twenty-eight. [One is struck by the unpredictable pattern of Wes's successes and failures: easier examples of a type of problem are failed, while harder ones of the same type are passed. Such a pattern suggests the workings of motivational factors in the failures.]	1
8.	*A man bought a secondhand car for two-thirds of what it cost new. He paid $400 for it. How much did it cost new?*	—	You mean, how much did two-thirds cost him? (I repeat the problem.) Mm-mm. (Shakes head.) ("Do you have any idea how you'd start?") Mm-mm. (Shakes head again.)	0
9.	*If a train goes 150 yards in ten seconds, how many feet can it go in one fifth of a second?*	36″	It's somewhere either three or nine. I'm just taking a wild crack at it. I'm lousy on my math. I know that. ("Which would you choose as your answer?") Three. ("How did you do it?") I don't know. It just popped out. ("Try to explain how you might have gotten it.") I can't explain how I got it. [This is a striking example of how a person can achieve a correct response to a quite complicated problem without	0

No. Problem	Time	Response and Comments	Score

having any idea how the solution came about. Persons with repressive organizations tend to have answers "pop" into their minds; since they are reluctant to introspect, they often do not permit themselves to investigate how this could have happened. Such persons, when questioned, often prefer to give an incorrect solution, rather than thoughtfully to retrace the mental path which led to the correct one. Wes's almost correct answer is particularly impressive, in view of his failures on the much easier Problems 3 and 5.]

10. *Eight men can finish a job in six days. How many men will be needed to finish it in a half day?*

I got it for one day. Now, if I can cut it down (he smiles). It's about forty-eight (at 50″). Say forty-eight. That's the closest I can get. ("How did you get it?") Six times eight. ("How would you get half a day?") . . . You take twice that, I imagine. ("What would that be?") Ninety-six. [Wes demonstrates his striking passivity. Even though he knows how to arrive at the correct answer, he can do so only with prodding. He knows *how* to achieve the right solution, but his actual, or aggressively motivated, helplessness prevents him from following through.

[Arithmetic is typically a major stumbling block for hysterically organized persons. The looking-inward and concentration which arithmetical problem solving require imperil such persons' repressive, outward-looking orientation. Some variation of the comment, "I was never any good at arithmetic," is typically made by these externally (usually action) oriented persons when they are confronted by the Wechsler Arithmetic subtest.]

Score: 0

RAW SCORE: 5

WEIGHTED SCORE: 6

(On the Metropolitan Achievement Test, Wes achieves a score which puts him at the 5.9 grade equivalent level on Arithmetic Problems.) [This performance means his Arithmetic functioning is approximately six years below his actual school grade placement.]

SIMILARITIES

No. Items	Response and Comments	Score
1. *Orange-banana*	. . . . I'm afraid you've got me. I couldn't even take a guess on that one. (I give examples.) I was thinking along the line of citrus, but that wouldn't work. A banana is not a citrus fruit.	0
2. *Coat-dress*	Both are made of cloth . . could be the same kind.	1
3. *Dog-lion*	. . . . . Both got hair.	1
4. *Wagon-bicycle*	Wheels on both.	1
5. *Daily paper-radio*	Both carry the same kind of news. On the radio, you get it quicker. You usually get ahold of it first. [Wes's Similarities so far are based on extremely concrete likenesses. On this response, he even toys with a tendency to point to a difference, rather than a similarity. A question to be raised at this point is: does Wes's functional-concrete concept formation reflect a *preference,* or an *inability* to do anything else?]	1
6. *Air-water*	Air has moisture in it, and water *is* moisture. And water evaporates and collects in the form of clouds. Hot and cold air coming together condenses and comes down in the form of rain. [The tendency to wander off into concrete tangents is described as typical of persons who suffer some sort of "brain damage."]	0
7. *Wood-alcohol*	. . . . Both have a certain percentage of moisture in them. [Is this a mild form of the perseveration which is also characteristic of the "brain damaged"?]	0
8. *Eye-ear*	I'd say, sort of like the eye sees something . . like a train . . and it's making a lot of racket, and the ear can hear it. The eye can see what it is, and the ear can hear what it is . . on some things now. ("How would you say they're both alike?") The ear can't see, but it can tell; it can distinguish sound. [More and more, one feels that Wes's performance involves inability rather than preference.]	0
9. *Egg-seed*	This would be a wild guess, but in chemistry they talk about nuclei. Say both have a nucleus in them . . That I know.	1
10. *Poem-statue*	A statue can maybe . . A poem describes something . . a person or something. A statue can depict it, like a picture does. ("How would you sum that up?") Both can . . both show something.	0-1

No. Items	Response and Comments	Score
11. *Praise-punishment*	Both are for your own good. Too much praise can be harmful . . too little punishment, the same thing. [Once again, Wes presents himself as the champion of the culture's positive values. How can he reconcile being a spokesman for virtue and at the same time exhibit himself to latency girls? Can he succeed by keeping parts of himself isolated? Does he perhaps not try consciously to reconcile conflicting aspects of himself at all?]	0
12. *Fly-tree*	. . . . . . Mm-mm. I wouldn't know that one. ("Could you think of any way?") Well, they both grow. That would be about it.	1

RAW SCORE: ___6-7___

WEIGHTED SCORE: ___5-6___

[Wes's performance on the last two subtests is poor. One should certainly begin to consider the possibility that his low performance on both Arithmetic and Similarities is in part the result of an ("organically" determined?) disruption of the capacity to think abstractly and to manipulate symbols effectively.]

PICTURE COMPLETION

(We begin this subtest on the following day. Wes says:) I'm lucky to be here today. ("Why is that?") We're having aptitude tests in school. (He explains that he doesn't like these tests at all because he never does well on them. He has brought a model airplane magazine with him and shows me the airplane he plans to build.)

[Although it first seems as if Wes were reaching out, trying to make contact, his behavior actually has the quality of the obedient student who feels he ought to show his teacher what he is doing.]

(He completes this test fairly efficiently, although he starts by failing the first item: he says the woman's "ear," instead of her "nose," is missing.)

[Wes tends to have difficulty on the first item of any new test. It may well be that he has difficulty in "shifting" from one area to another, again a difficulty which might be consistent with the presence of a physiologic brain disorder.]

RAW SCORE: ___10___

WEIGHTED SCORE: ___9___

PICTURE ARRANGEMENT

(Wes completes the first four arrangements quickly and accurately. He receives no credit on the last two items, because of an unusual interpretation of *Taxi* and a careless sorting of *Fish*.

(On the *Taxi* item, after 40″, he sorts SALEMU and tells the following story:) I guess he's walking along the street there and had the thing that didn't look right. And he called a cab . . and . . and . . he . . uh . . didn't like it. It didn't look right for her to be sitting on the far side. So he pulled it over, so that it would look like man and wife. ("What is that thing called?") That's what they call a human

THE DOUBT-RIDDEN ADOLESCENT

head, isn't it? Just the upper part . . I think, I'm not sure. You're about to run out of space. I'll cut it down a bit. ("How do you mean, it didn't look right?") It wouldn't look right. He was embarrassed, probably. I would be. (He laughs.) [Wes shows his hyperpropriety, confusion and embarrassment when he deals with a situation which suggests a close relationship between the sexes.]

RAW SCORE: ___9___

WEIGHTED SCORE: ___8___

BLOCK DESIGN

(He says this test is similar to a game he has at home; he will bring it to show to me tomorrow.) [Again one sees Wes acting a good deal younger than his almost seventeen years.]

(When he sees how I mix up the blocks after he has correctly finished the first design, he always does the same after he says he has finished. He receives no credit on Design 5, because he destroys it too quickly, before he has an opportunity to look his construction over and correct the erroneous rotation at one corner. He makes a number of exclamations (e.g., "Eek!," "Wow!") when the designs look somewhat difficult.) [Wes's "helpfulness" does not lessen emotional distance. On the contrary, although he goes through the motions of pleasant cooperation, the examiner never has the feeling Wes wishes to demonstrate trust or to relax non-defensively.

[Wes's young way of relating himself to the examiner and the effeminate quality of some responses are apparent. It is rather startling to hear this tall, well-set-up young man say "Eek!"]

RAW SCORE: ___19___

WEIGHTED SCORE: ___9___

OBJECT ASSEMBLY

(He completes this test with little difficulty and obtains two time credits on the *Profile* item.)

RAW SCORE: ___20___

WEIGHTED SCORE: ___12___

DIGIT SYMBOL

(He loses some time because he erases whenever his symbols are not as neat as he wants them to be. Once he stops for 4″, searching for the correct symbol. He is apparently unaware that he skips one space altogether.) [Although, from a purely quantitative standpoint, Wes does not do badly here, some qualitative features of his performance raise certain diagnostic questions. Is Wes's mild graphomotor disorganization consistent with a diagnosis of "organic dysfunction," a question raised by his performances on some previous subtests?]

RAW SCORE: ___35___

WEIGHTED SCORE: ___8___

VOCABULARY

No. Word	Response and Comments	Score
1. *Apple*	You mean abbreviation? ("Tell what it means.") It's a fruit . . It has a red skin and the meat is white . . the fruit itself is white. ("How did you mean, 'abbreviation'?") When I'm working these, my mind wanders. I saw "app." on your sheet. I have a bad habit of letting my mind wander. He (the psychiatrist) found out in there. [The phenomenon of Wes's being at somewhat loose ends at the beginning of a new procedure is again evident. It is increasingly obvious that Wes experiences difficulty when he is required to shift from one type of task to another.]	1
2. *Donkey*	Animal.	1
3. *Join*	You join a club . . get together.	1
4. *Diamond*	It's one of the hardest stones . . on this earth . . ("Could you tell me some more?") It's hard to melt. It's made into rings. Jewelry . . Just put jewelry, that'll take care of it all. It cuts glass. (He gives a number of further industrial uses.) [Although he obtains full credit, Wes again circles around the area before he reaches its center.]	1
5. *Nuisance*	A bother.	1
6. *Fur*	A means of keeping warm . . used by animals. ("Would you tell me some more?") Animals use fur as a means of keeping warm. ("How do you mean?") Well, it's kind of their hair. [Only with help is Wes able to leave the periphery in order to reach the essential center.]	1
7. *Cushion*	Something soft. ("Could you tell me more about it?") It's used in chairs. You see it in model airplanes. They've got a plastic nose that'll cushion the crash, so that it won't wreck it.	1
8. *Shilling*	It's a term of money used in England.	1
9. *Gamble*	Well, one of the meanings . . One is, gamble . . means to gamble away . . lose . . like gamblers gamble. ("How is that?") Like when they play cards. ["One of the meanings" very often has obsessive implications.]	1
10. *Bacon*	It's pork . . It comes off a hog . . or pig . . and it's used to eat. [The phrasing "hog . . or pig" is a typical obsessive redundancy.]	1

No.	Word	Response and Comments	Score
11.	Nail	It's uh . . it can be either of three . . alunimum (sic), iron or steel. Most always it is used to help hold together structures. [Another hint of obsessiveness is seen in "it can be either of three."]	1
12.	Cedar	It's a tree.	1
13.	Tint	To color . . like . . like a tinted windshield in a car . . or plane. [Wes obsessively lists alternatives.]	1
14.	Armory	National Guard Armory. ("What is that?") A building in which . . building in which the National Guard keeps its supplies . . and rifles and such. ["Supplies . . and rifles and such."]	1
15.	Fable	A fairy tale.	1
16.	Brim	Like . . bring me this. (I show him the word.) Oh! It's the top of something . . like water has reached the brim of a cup.	1
17.	Guillotine	It's a large blade, usually of steel, which was used mostly in France. It's used as sort of kind of to execute people . . to cut off their heads (he laughs).	1
18.	Plural	Something . . that you add "es" or "s" to, to make two. Such as . . charities . . ies . . car . . that's it.	½
19.	Seclude	Lonely.	½
20.	Nitroglycerin	It is a . . powerful explosive used in the beginning for blasting purposes.	1
21.	Stanza	The stanza of music . . between the bar lines . . or a measure.	1
22.	Microscope	An instrument used to . . see . . small . . organisms. ("How do you mean?") It has a small lens which acts much like a telescope to enlarge things.	1
23.	Vesper	Vesper services. ("What are they?") It's combined with church. And that would be all I know of it.	1
24.	Belfry	It's a bell tower.	1
25.	Recede	The waters are receded . . that means to go down.	1
26.	Affliction	. . . . . Something like disease . . like . . "They have a strange affliction."	½
27.	Pewter	It's a drinking cup used in the old days.	0
28.	Ballast	Weights used in boats to keep an even keel.	1
29.	Catacomb	Caves used by the Christians under Rome.	1

No.	Word	Response and Comments	Score
30.	Spangle	Part of a name of a song . . *The Star-Spangled Banner.* [Such a superficial response stands in marked contrast to the preceding correct definition of *catacomb.*)	0
31.	Espionage	Come again? ("Espionage.") I'd say a spy.	½
32.	Imminent	It would go along with secluded . . lonely. [It is hard to know just what Wes has in mind here. Is he possibly thinking of the loneliness that goes with eminence?]	0
33.	Mantis	You mean m-a-n-t-i-s? ("That's right.") It's an animal . . nicknamed praying mantis because of the position in which it walks.	1
34.	Hara-kiri	A ceremony used by the Japanese before the suicide pilots would go on a mission.	0
35.	Chattel	I don't know that. I never even heard of it. (He laughs.)	0
36.	Dilatory	I don't know.	0
37.	Amanuensis	I don't know.	0
38.	Proselyte	I don't know.	0
39.	Moiety	I don't know.	0
40.	Aseptic	Wait . . would that be like . . no, never mind. ("What were you thinking?") Something like septic . . the tank, but I changed my mind.	0
41.	Flout	I don't know.	0
42.	Traduce	I don't know.	0

RAW SCORE: __28__

WEIGHTED SCORE: __12__

[The discrepancy between Wes's Vocabulary and Similarities scores becomes more explainable as it can be seen that he deals more than adequately with isolated elements which do not have to be combined into more complex concepts. So long as he is able to remain intellectually on a discrete basis, Wes functions fairly well (although he often finds it hard to get to the core of an idea). But when elements must be related to one another, when essences must be abstracted from them, and when the similarity of these essences must be understood and worked with, then Wes comes to grief. It still cannot be determined unequivocally whether Wes's lack of conceptual integration reflects preference or inability.

[One is struck by Wes's tendency to keep disparate aspects (e.g., verbal attitudes of high morality and exhibitionistic behavior) isolated from one another. Wes does not express shame or guilt in connection with his sexual symptom; he acts, in fact, as though it did not exist. Such an extreme isolating tendency raises the possibility that Wes's conceptual nonintegration is simply another aspect of the nonintegration so apparent in his everyday affective and symptomatic life, that it is Wes's style to isolate in *all* areas of functioning.]

STORY RECALL

IMMEDIATE RECALL

$+1$ $+1$ $+1$ $+1$ $+1$
December 6. / Last week / a river / overflowed / ten—in a small town /

$+1$ -1 $+1$ $+1$ $+1$
ten miles / south / of Albany / . . . . . . fourteen persons / were drowned /
$+1$ $+1$ $+1$ $+1$
and 600 / caught cold / because of the dampness / and cold weather. / While
$+1$ $+1$ $+1$ $+1$ $+1$ $+1$
rescuing / a boy / caught / under a bridge / a man / cut his hand. /

SCORE: $19-1(+4) = 22$

DELAYED RECALL

$+1$ $+1$ $+1$
December 6. / In a town / near—scratch out that "near" put / ten miles /
-1 $+1$ $+1$ $+1$ $+1$ $+1$
south / of Albany / a river / overflowed. / Water flowed in the streets / and into
$+1$ $+1$ $+1$ $+1$
houses. / Fourteen persons / were drowned / and 600 / caught cold / because of
$+1$ $+1$ $+1$ $+1$ $+1$
the damp / and cold weather. / While trying to rescue / a boy / caught / under
$+1$ $+1$ $+1$
a bridge / a man / cut his hand. /

SCORE: $20-1 = 19$

[Wes's nearly perfect scores on Immediate and Delayed Recall are consistent with the impression obtained so far, i.e., that he deals capably with discrete, in this case memorial, elements, When, as here, the elements need simply be repeated, without having to be recombined in any way, Wes does well.]

THE BENDER GESTALT TEST

PART A (PLATES 35 AND 36)

(Wes works very quickly and not very carefully. He numbers and circles most of his drawings. He makes guidelines to assure his drawing accuracy.) [Here again is the paradox: the apparent wish to be extra neat and orderly in a context that can only be described as sloppy. Although his guidelines are of some help when he draws Design 3, they do not help at all on Design 2. One wonders: Does Wes's quick "sloppiness" reflect lack of care or does he not *permit himself* to care for fear he might fail? In order words, does he generally only *seem* not to care, in order to disguise a probable lack of success?]

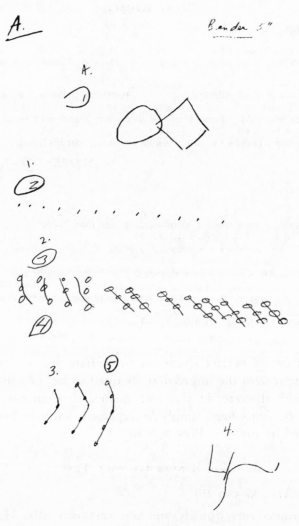

PLATE 35

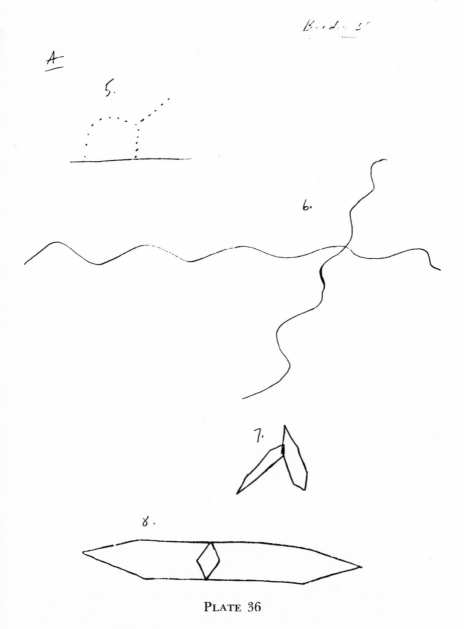

PLATE 36

PART B (PLATES 37 AND 38)

(He draws these more slowly and carefully; at one point he uses guidelines again.) [Although these designs are more slowly and carefully reproduced than those of Part A, one again observes rather

B

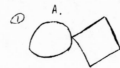

Bender - copy

② 1.

③ 2.

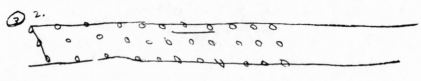

④ 3.

⑤ 4.

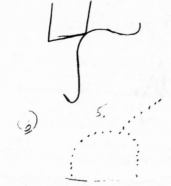

5.

PLATE 37

major inaccuracies. Wes draws dots of unequal size, and he tends to transform them into circles or dashes; his small circles are sometimes misshapen; his dots are perseveratively added to, and his straight lines are wavering and their pressure inconstant. One is reminded of the mild difficulties Wes experienced on Digit Symbol, and one wonders about the cause of his inaccuracies with these graphomotor tasks.

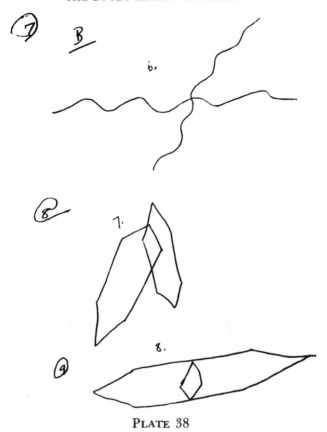

PLATE 38

[While Wes reproduces all the Seguin blocks correctly on the Tactual Form Test, he executes his drawings with the same speed as on the Bender, as though in this way he might be able to disguise the unsureness of his lines. He always knows what form he is drawing —e.g., a circle, a square, a star—but one never has the conviction that he feels at home with a pencil in his hand. His drawings are lightly and sketchily made, and they lack thrust and power.]

THE DRAW A PERSON TEST

PART I (PLATE 39)

(As he begins to draw, he says:) That's what gets me—figures. (He draws for about five minutes and then says:) Is there supposed to be a time limit on this? (He moves his pencil around in the air and makes various abortive strokes before he actually draws anything.

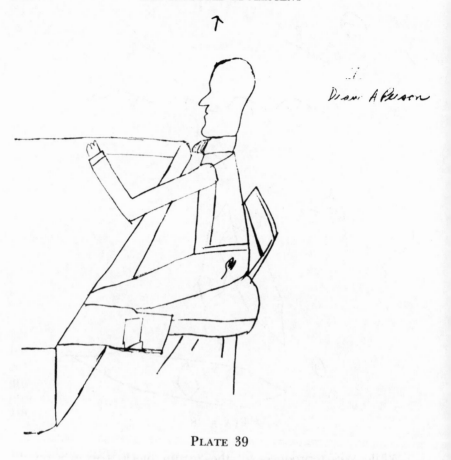

PLATE 39

(When I wonder who the drawing represents, he laughs and says:)
You. At least it's supposed to. (When I wonder about the meaning of
the arrow at the top of his drawing, he explains that this is the way
he wants the paper to face. The arrow is to remind him not to turn
the paper around. He adds:) I forget things quite easily sometimes.
(Keeping the paper in place has to do with my request, on the
Bender, that he try to make his drawings without turning the model
designs.)

PART II (PLATE 40)

(He pays great attention to the girl's skirt folds, but he first makes
her without a head. After much erasure and correction, he finally
adds a tiny head, although he has given her no arms. He says:) That's
the best I can do. I took one year of art. I was planning on being an

artist and then found out I couldn't draw, so I switched to another subject. (Asked further about this drawing, he explains:) It's more or less like some of the drawings I made in art class. I made about ten a week. Whenever I felt like sketching, I started in, sitting in the car . . sitting in the car or anywhere. ("What's that line coming from the head?") It's a feather.

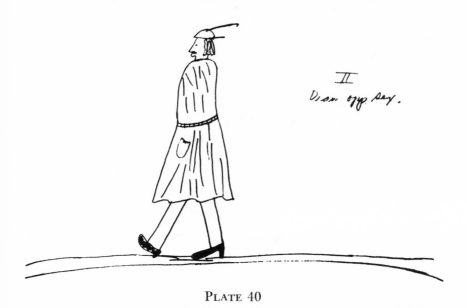

PLATE 40

[Several features are significant here. It seems incredible that Wes, with such an extraordinary lack of talent, should ever seriously have planned an artistic career for himself. Does such a major defect in judgment reflect an equally serious defect in other significant aspects of reality testing? If it does, does the unsound reality testing reflect a significant psychic disorganization or only the workings of repression and denial? Since Wes has shown very little disorganization otherwise, and since he has shown numerous examples of repressive blotting out, a hypothesis involving repression seems more fitting.

[Almost equally striking is the curiously paradoxical nature of the drawings themselves. Wes compulsively fills in minute lines and shadows (including a handkerchief peeking out of a pocket), but he completely omits much more significant aspects. Thus, while he draws the seams on the man's shirt and a small envelope on the side of his desk, he altogether neglects to draw in his facial features. Similarly, while he draws the folds of the woman's dress and the pocket in her skirt, he leaves out her arms. These contrasting tendencies—one toward detailing obsessively, the other toward blotting out hysterically—epitomize Wes's psychological organization.

[A third feature of the drawings relates to Wes's need to avoid self-determination. Not only is his "man" a copy of an actual person sitting next to him, but the man he draws leans upon his desk for support. The desk seems to serve the same use for Wes as the guidelines he drew for his Bender figures. Wes's "woman" is also given a stable line on which to walk. In this way Wes demonstrates his need to lean: on things, persons, opinions, commands. He is hardly able to strike out on his own. His symptom of exhibitionism may serve partly a dependency compromise, a way of satisfying both the demands of remaining a nonsexual, nonactive child, while trying out a more potent adult sexuality.

[Once again, Wes shows severe inability in graphomotor functioning. It will be important to see if this inability is reflected in the conceptual realm (as it seemed to be on the Wechsler Similarities subtest).]

THE BRL SORTING TEST

PART I

Stimulus	Patient's Sorting	Response and Comments	Score
1. Wes's choice: Toy hammer	You should have a pad there, so it (the hammer) doesn't dent up your desk. I'm picking one I'm familiar with because I got hit with one last night. (He describes almost having hit himself with a hammer as he was working on a project.) (Nails; wooden block with nail; pliers; screwdriver; toy screwdriver; lock; toy pliers.)	I think I catch on to what you mean. I'm not sure, though. ("Why do they belong together?") Well, a hammer hits the nails. (He puts the hammer to one side.) A hammer is a tool, so I picked out the rest of the tools to go with it. They make a kit. And the padlock *could* go on the kit to lock it. It's regarded sometimes as a tool. (He straightens up the items at the edge of the desk.) [Once more	Loose Chain Tend. Concrete Def. Narrow Conceptual Def.

Stimulus	Patient's Sorting	Response and Comments	Score
		Wes's difficulty in shifting is evident. Although he seems to have some concept, such as "tools," it has a strongly concrete and shifting quality to it. Again one feels Wes's lack of precision—his vagueness and nonspecificity. At the same time, he manifests the compulsive need to have things in physical order.]	
2. *Fork*	(Toy knife, fork and spoon; spoon; knife.) (He apparently wonders whether to add the sink stopper and asks:) Is it okay to pick it up and look at? (He picks up the sink stopper and adds it to the sorting. Then he adds the corks.)	These are eating utensils. They all belong in the same drawer. And this is a sink stopper as it says on there, and these are corks for Thermos bottles. ("Why did you add the sink stopper?") It's used in the kitchen. It's a kitchen utensil, like the others are. [Wes's concept is loose and tends toward the Concrete and Syncretistic. So far on the Sorting Test, Wes's nonabstract way of conceptualizing is consistent with his performance on the Similarities subtest.]	Syncretistic Def.
3. *Corncob pipe*	(Rubber cigar; cigar; cigarette; matches.)	Well, they're all .... These three—the cigars, the pipe and the cigarette, are all used for tobacco smoking purposes. And you use the matches to light it with.	Split-Narrow Tendency Functional Def. Concrete Def.

Stimulus	Patient's Sorting	Response and Comments	Score
4. *Bell*	You can't use the same one twice, can you? This is all alone. It's used on a bike for a warning. (No sorting.)	[This is a difficult item, but it is nevertheless significant that Wes can do nothing at all with it. His reluctance to use the same item twice (a matter which most people do not worry about) may in part be understood as growing out of his difficulty in shifting —that is, his difficulty in seeing a thing in more than one way.]	Failure
5. *Circle*	(Cardboard rectangle; file card.)	They're all paper. They're made out of the same . . paper material. (He replaces the items in the main pile.) [Except for slight "narrowing," this is Wes's first successful *conceptual* solution.]	Narrow Conceptual Def.
6. *Toy pliers*	Hm. That's already been in (pliers), but . . Shall I use it again? ("If you want to, go ahead." (Pliers; toy saw; toy hammer; toy screwdriver; screwdriver.)	They're all tools. [A completely successful solution.]	Conceptual Def.
7. *Ball*	(No sorting.)	It's alone. ("Would anything go with it?") No. [This is another of the more difficult items, but Wes is completely thrown by it. He does poorly on this portion of the test, not because he conceptualizes things	Failure

Stimulus	Patient's Sorting	Response and Comments	Score
		peculiarly, but because he is barely able to conceptualize them at all. It will be important to see how much more successful he is on Part II, where he is required to exert much less creative, synthesizing effort.]	

PART II

Examiner's Sorting	Explanation and Comments	Score
1. Red objects	All of these? Well, the sink stopper, eraser and ball all are made out of rubber. And the matches, circle and the square all have paper in them. And these (toy silverware) are all plastic. ("How would they *all* go together?") Well, they . . . . they all bend a little bit. (He bends the plastic.) Do you want them put back? (He does so.) [Once more, the almost inevitable disability that comes with a shift. Wes finds it so difficult to begin a new direction successfully that he gives a response which is inadequate and peculiar.]	Split-Narrow (Conceptual) Syncretistic Peculiar
2. Metal	They're all made out of metal . . steel probably. They've all got a purpose. [Wes spoils his good response with a global syncretism.]	Conceptual Def. Syncretistic
3. Round	It's probably the same as the last. They've all got a purpose. That would be my idea for all of them, I guess.	Syncretistic
4. Tools	They've all got some metal in them . . . and they're all tools. (He says the latter as I am taking the items away.) (He wipes off the table.) [Since *Tools* is such a simple concept, it would be a serious matter if Wes could not conceptualize it. He does so, but only after a false start.]	Conceptual Def.
5. Paper	They've all got paper in them. They're made out of paper or have paper in them.	Conceptual Def. (Split-Narrow Tendency)

Examiner's Sorting	Explanation and Comments	Score
6. *Double*	They're each in a pair. That would be my .. one of my guesses. [This excellent success is completely unexpected. The *Double* item is one of the most difficult, yet Wes grasps it immediately.]	Conceptual Def.
7. *White*	They're all white .. except for the cigarette, which has tobacco in it and dark printing. [Wes's tendency to get caught up in minutiae may reflect either an obsessive-compulsive *need* to focus on tiny details, or an *inability* to transcend concrete differences. Being immersed in the concrete is, of course, a frequent characteristic of persons with an organic impairment of the central nervous system.]	Conceptual Def. (Split-Narrow)
8. *Rubber*	All made of rubber.	Conceptual Def.
9. *Smoking*	The cigars and cigarette are for smoking, and you put tobacco in the pipe to smoke, and you use matches to light them with.	Concrete Def.
10. *Silverware*	Used for eating purposes.	Functional Def.
11. *Toys*	The hammer, screwdriver and pliers and saw are made out of steel, and they're used as tools. The spoon, fork and knife are made out of plastic and for eating purposes. And the rubber cigar and the ball are all made out of rubber. ("Can you think of a way they all belong together?") (He shakes his head.) ("Any way at all?") I couldn't say they all have a purpose.	Split-Narrow (Conceptual, Functional Defs.) Syncretistic Tend.
12. *Square*	Sometime during the makings they've all had some chemical treatment. ("How do you mean?") Well, the matches get treated for that color. The paper gets treated with chemicals .. to hold together .. with pulp. The wood gets dipped after the pulp. The nails (referring to the nail in the block of wood), if they are rustproof, they are dipped in something. And sugar is made out of a chemical. [This response is peculiar only because Wes is desperate to find some sort of binding concept. He does not ordinarily think in unusual ways, but he is apparently forced into a Peculiarity because of his cognitive helplessness. [Although Wes's performance on Part II	Syncretistic Peculiar

Examiner's Sorting	*Explanation and Comments*	*Score*

is somewhat better than on Part I, it is obvious that he finds it difficult to think abstractly, even when he can respond passively to concepts already sorted for him. It seems likely that Wes's remaining at a concrete level of organizing the world is based at least as much on his *inability* to do anything more as on a *preference* for the tangible here and now.]

THE STORY COMPLETION TEST

He was very angry, and was getting angrier by the minute.

(Wes writes the following completion:) He was very angry or mad also, he was getting madder every minute: He got very mad and finally blew his top.

(After he completes his story, I ask, "What was he mad about?") He didn't say. He just said he was getting mad. ("Make up something he might have been mad about.") He could have been mad at things not going his way. A lot of people are that way, including me. (He smiles.) ("How did he act when he was mad?") It's just a description .. a saying, you might say. He got a lot worse, and then finally he quieted down. ("How did he act?") Very angry. ("What did he do?") He got angrier by the minute. ("What did he actually do, how did he actually behave?") He could have sounded off. [Wes finds it immensely difficult to express anger, even indirectly, about a third person, in a make-believe situation.]

RORSCHACH TEST

[The Rorschach Scoring Sheet reflects Wes's tendency to be organized along both hyperideational (obsessive-compulsive) and hypoideational (repressive-hysterical) lines. As is true of many persons who depend primarily on repressive defenses, Wes tends to focus on large Details at the expense of Whole responses. His absence of any Movement response, together with a poorly controlled use of color, further reflects a repressive orientation that discourages ideational activity and prompts the expression of gross, poorly modulated affectivity. At the same time, Wes's tendencies to focus on quite small details, to organize percepts in unusual ways and to go "inside" and respond to shading nuances of the blots are more typical of the overideational, obsessive person. Other noteworthy features of the Scoring Sheet are the relatively low percentage of acceptable Form responses and the few Popular responses. These features, together with the noted Peculiarity and the relatively high number of Fabulized responses, cast some doubt on Wes's ability to deal adequately with aspects of formal reality. Also of interest is Wes's apparent preoccupation with the inanimate (e.g., geographical features, "coral," "nebula," "horizon," "sunset"), side by side with only one (partial) human percept, a profile. This de-emphasis of the human reflects the impoverishment of Wes's relation to other people. Such a de-emphasis goes along with his lack of genuine warmth, with his façade of pleasantness that disguises an avoidance of genuine human contact.]

RORSCHACH SCORING SHEET

Number of Responses: 20

Manner of Approach (Location)

W	2
D	12
Dd	0
De	0
Dr	6
Total	20

Location Percentages

W%	10
D%	60
Dr%	30
De%	0

Form, Movement, Color and Shading Determinants

F+	7		
F−	3		
F±	2		
F∓	3		
M	0		
FC+	1		
CF	1		
C	0		
F(C)−	1	F(C)+	1
C(C)F	1		
Total	20		

Groups of Contents

A	6
Ad	0
H	0
Hd	1
Obj.	1
Plane	1
Ats.	1
Pl.	2
Cloud	1
Geog.	3
Coral	1
Nebula	1
Horizon	1
Sunset	1

Determinant and Content Percentages

F%	75/90	Obj.%	10
F+%	60/61	At%	5
A%	30	P%	10
H%	5		

Qualitative Material

Popular	V VIII
Fabulation	4
Peculiar	1
Symmetry	1 (1)
Aggression	2

EXPERIENCE BALANCE: 0/2.5

RORSCHACH PROTOCOL

Card #	React. Time	Score	Protocol	Inquiry and Observations
I	18″	DrF+A	1. It could resemble a sort of spider-crab, in a way.	1. ("Tell me about the crab.") It had . . could I show you? ("Try to describe it without the card.") It had those little pincerlike things, like pinchers. (Upper half of central D.)
		WF∓A	2. And it could be sort of a Manta ray. It takes a sort of shape of one . . a sting ray. That'll be all.	2. ("How about the Manta ray?") It had like wings out there. And the things coming back (bottom Dr) looked like part of the tail . . the sting . stinger. (He vaguely outlines the entire blot.) [Wes's tentativeness—e.g., "sort of," "in a way," "like wings"—suggests his reluctance to commit himself.]
II	22″	DF∓ Nebula Fab.	1. It could resemble the Horse Nebula in space.	1. ("Tell me about the Horse Nebula.") The whole thing . just the one side (black side D) . . the right side. It resembled it in the shape of a horse's head. That's the reason I called it that. (His stomach growls.) Excuse me . . I didn't have any breakfast. ("How did it remind you of a nebula?") That's the name of it. Astronomers have given it that. ("But why a nebula?") Well, the shape of it . . sort of. [To what extent this response reflects a wish to demonstrate erudition, or represents an arbitrary imposition of a private preoccupation, or reflects both these tendencies, is not clear. In any case, the response is rather arbitrarily perceived and presented.]
		DF+A	2. This part down here (bottom center D) looks something like a monarch butterfly.	2. ("And the butterfly?") Well, there's a long slender part in the middle to represent the body, and then it branches out, sort of like wings. And then, the two spines coming

	React.		
Card #	Time Score	Protocol	Inquiry and Observations

Inquiry and Observations (continued):

back look like something like the back part of the wings. They don't use those. They're just decoration. ("Does anything else make it look like a monarch butterfly?") No, that'd be all. [Wes avoids mention of the vivid colors which are almost invariably described by persons who see this area as a butterfly. An avoidance of some color areas, together with an overreaction to others, is frequently observed among persons who rely on repressive defenses.]

DF∓Obj.
Fab.
Symm.

3. And this looks something like a shell of some sort (top red D) . . a sea shell, probably . . these two being just the same as the others. (He means the two D's are symmetrical.)

3. ("Tell me about the shell.") Sort of like a cockleshell in the South Pacific. The projections on the bottom made it look like a crab moves into it and occupies it until it gets too big and moves into another one. Those are the crab feelers . . the claws, sticking out. [Wes seems to have considerable knowledge about things connected with the sea.]

III   58″   DF+Ats

1. This is about all I can get . . This part looks something like the stomach (side red D). The esophagus and shape of the stomach (he yawns). That'd be all of it on that one.

1. [Wes's defensiveness here (i.e., avoiding the two Popular "persons") is additionally evidenced by his long reaction time and his yawn. In spite of some efforts by the examiner to test the limits after Card X has been administered, Wes declares an inability to see much more than the "stomach." A repressive scotoma of this degree is impressive.]

IV   92″   DrF—
Geog.
Fab.

1. This is not a hit. (He laughs, after 15″). This coming out here (light gray front portion of Popular "boot") cut off, right here I'd say .
it looks something

[Although this area is not usually seen as human (except for the "boot," which Wes interprets next), one is nevertheless impressed by the apparent preoccupation with nature as consisting of inanimate objects.

["The 38th" refers to the

Card #	React. Time	Score	Protocol	Inquiry and Observations
			like a peninsula of Korea. Cut it right here. (He draws an imaginary line across the center of this area.) And the 38th would go right through here.	38th Parallel, much in the news during the Korean War. Wes's response to Card IV is another example (cf. MacArthur at the beginning of the Wechsler-Bellevue) of his poor intellectual discipline—of his tendency to force an answer to fit any question.]
		DF± Geog.	2. And then, this looks something like the Italian boot (right side D).	[Geography again.]
V	13″	WF+AP	1. It resembles a bat. That's the whole thing.	
VI	34″	DrF(C)— horizon Pec. Fab.	1. This'll probably sound a bit stupid to you, but this long dark line along here (central dividing line) could be the far horizon.	1. ("Tell me about the horizon.") Well, it's a long ways off. It's small, pinched, like you're looking at it from a long distance. That's what makes it look so peculiar, because it looks like the clouds are too big (the "clouds" of response 2). ("How do you see the horizon?") Like I was standing over here, and it was sort of flat-looking. [If one interprets this as Wes's "personal" horizon—i.e., his future and his opportunity autonomously to make something of himself—then it is apparent that he feels trapped in the present: the small, pinched future is a long way off. The "clouds"—possibly his present familial situation—overpower the horizon and make it look "sort of flat."]
		DF— Cloud (Ch?) (C'?) Agg.	2. And this looks something like a cloud after an explosion or something. It could be a smoke cloud from a fire . . or an approaching	2. ("Is the cloud part of the horizon?") It could have been, but it should have been smaller if it was. It was slightly large. ("What made it look like a storm cloud?") The way it branched out. ("Anything

Card #	React. Time	Score	Protocol	Inquiry and Observations
			storm. The way it branches out, it sort of resembles an explosion. (Side D.) That's it.	else that made it look that way?") No. [The implication seems strong that the cloud, which follows an explosion or augurs an approaching storm, and which overwhelms the horizon, might well represent the father's explosive anger, which keeps Wes intimidated and which makes him fearful of expressing himself in direct ways. Again one sees repression operate in Wes's obvious avoidance of a description of the mottled and dark quality of the storm cloud.]
VII	28″	DF— Corral Symm. Tend.	1. Just pay no attention to the one side. It could look like a corral formation at the bottom of the ocean. (One half of the entire blot.)	1. ("What made it seem like that?") Well, I read a book just recently: *Half a Mile Down* by William Beebe. It showed a picture just like that —some even more balanced than that. [Wes achieves distance from the living present by creating vague forms, far away at the bottom of the ocean. More and more one becomes aware of the extent of Wes's isolation.]
VIII	24″	DF+AP	1. This part could resemble a dog . . or any animal like that, that's kind of low to the ground.	
				Some got some pretty pictures there, anyway.
		DFC Sunset	2. And this would be sort of like the sunset on the desert.	2. ("Tell me about the sunset.") Well, I read . . I was looking through a book about Arizona. They had clouds like that . . blue, pink, red and yellow, with a few orange scattered around . . They were pretty. When I see a picture of something pretty like that it just sticks in my mind. I remember it. (Bottom D.) [This percept combines several

React.			
Card #	*Time Score*	*Protocol*	*Inquiry and Observations*

things already touched on: Wes has moved from the bottom of the ocean to the Arizona desert, but he is still far away from other people. His familiarity with this particular scene is once more second-hand, through a book. Even though his interests are almost exclusively concerned with the inanimate, they nevertheless appear to be strong interests and suggest the restlessness he feels with his present situation. They point to his striving for something more beautiful and exciting. Wes's Rorschach interpretations, in other words, must be judged not only in terms of their "negative" (i.e., distant, inanimate) aspects, but in terms of their "constructive" ones as well.]

DF± Plane Agg.

3. This somehow strikes me as resembling a plane (top center D). The tail would be around here, and the center part would be the middle of that. The wheels would be coming up here. And farther up it looks like rockets or something under the wing. That'd be all. Do you want to know what that (central blue D) would be?

DrC(C)F Geog.

4. Yeah, wait a minute here. This side here . . it looks like it could be in a plane, looking down at mountains. There's a deep chasm here . . a valley.

4. ("And looking down at mountains?") It looks like you're looking down on top of it. The dark streak could be a chasm, the lighter one could be a valley . . a dip in the glaciers. The white spots on top look like the peak . . the top

Card #	React. Time Score	Protocol	Inquiry and Observations
			of it. (He sees this as it would be were one to look down from an airplane. The airplane itself is not visible.) If you're looking almost from on top of it, you'd naturally see that. The crevasses would be dark and the peaks would be light blue or white like that was. [It is striking to see these well-differentiated descriptions of color and shading nuances in someone who until this test appeared so organized around repressing this very sort of sensitivity. It is apparent now that Wes not only represses, but that he is also aware of and responsive to the subtleties which, on other occasions, he ignores.]
IX	75″ Dr tend. F(C)+ Hd	1. This part here could be . . what I was thinking of yesterday . . profile, instead of bust (referring to the preceding day's Picture Arrangement *Taxi*, item) . . The head, forehead, eye, mouth and chin. And this could be a shirt collar coming down. Leave that little part out (tiny Dr extension—the "mustache") and cut it off right here. (Half of bottom pink D.) That'd be all.	1. ("What kind of a profile?") A man. ("What made it look like that?") The way the face was built. You leave that projection off. [A human response! It is difficult to feel certain about the reason Wes makes a point of omitting that very portion (the "mustache") which gives the profile its masculinity.]
X	35″ DF+A	Ouch! (He laughs.) 1. This . . if you turn it around . . it looks sort of like a bug . . an insect. I caught it and went to my biology instructor with	1. ("Tell me about the insect.") I can tell you the color of it. It's got a gray body. (He means the one he has at home.) All I know about it, it's an insect. It's got an apparatus like

React. Card #	Time	Score	Protocol	Inquiry and Observations

it. He doesn't know what they are . . and I don't. I've got it at home, and I'm keeping it for reference until I find out what it is.

a stripe at the back end and feelers on the front. The way the body is, is sort of strange. Sort of a triangle with spines along the ridge. (Side D attached to outer yellow D.) [Once more Wes demonstrates his interest in natural phenomena. He invests himself quite vigorously in this sort of activity and is not content simply to sit back and wait to be stimulated by whatever comes along. His search for stimulation, in other words, takes an intellectual, as well as a symptomatic, impulse-expressive, form.]

DF+pl   2. I believe it's an elm tree. This doesn't resemble the elm tree, but it's that little helicopter thing that comes down. The seeds, you know, that twirls down. (Upper center D.)

DrFC+pl   3. Cut that off (the jutting portion of the outer central yellow D) and it looks something like a yellow rose, where the stem connects with the base of it. The petals are becoming undone. If you cut that projection off, it looks more like it. That'd be it.

3. [Another promontory is modified.]

Testing The Limits
("Could it look like anything else than what you saw before?")
1. This part right here (the black portion of the lower cen-

[In spite of the additional pressure to look, Wes still does not perceive the Popular human response. He prefers to focus on peripheral areas and ignore what most people find obvious.]

III

	React.		
Card #	*Time*	*Score*	*Protocol*

Inquiry and Observations

tral D) could resemble the heart.

2. These here (light gray portions of lower central D) could resemble stalactytes . . That's in the roof of an underground cave.

THEMATIC APPERCEPTION TEST

(Four of Wes's twelve TAT stories, two blandly unrevealing, and two moderately revealing, are presented here. These four stories are felt to be representative of the entire group of stories he tells.)

Card 2 (Country scene: in the foreground is a young woman with books in her hand; in the background a man is working in the fields, and an older woman is looking on.)

It looks like this woman on the left is coming home from school or is going into town to work, and the man's been plowing the fields, and from the looks of the land, it's been a drought. You got a house in the middle, barn on the right, what looks like a barn on the left, what looks like a lake on farther beyond. It's been a hot day because he's got his shirt off while he's plowing. ("Who is the other woman?") Well it could be his mother or the aunt of one of them. ("And what is she doing there?") Leaning against the tree, resting. ("What's this girl in front thinking about?") Wondering if the crops will come up. In dry weather they usually don't. She's probably thinking about her studies, too. [Wes presents very little more than description.]

Card 3 BM (On the floor against a couch is the huddled form of a boy with his head bowed on his right arm. Beside him on the floor is a revolver.)

It looks like here she has been badly upset by something, and she is laying there on the couch, and she could have been upset or purely tired and collapsed there. ("What's going to happen?") Well, after she has had a cry, she'll probably feel better. ("What had upset her?") Well, she could have maybe broke a date with a boy friend or quit going with him altogether, or someone in the family could have died, just anything. [Although Wes first seems to promise considerable drama, things come to a rather tepid conclusion. Not only does Wes resort to obsessive flight by offering a number of possibilities, but he "levels" what should be sharply discrepant, equating the serious (i.e., "someone in the family could have died") with the much more everyday ("she could have maybe broke a date with a boy friend"). In this way Wes tries to convey that everything is equally unimportant—i.e., equally unthreatening to him.]

Card 13 MF (A young man is standing with downcast head buried in his arm. Behind him is the figure of a woman lying in bed.)

I'd say this man could have done, something could have taken hold of him, he could have killed his wife or his girl friend there. It could have been that he felt that she was against him on things like his drinking maybe, for instance, and he just lost his temper and killed her. ("And what happened then?") I imagine, as always he'll probably get caught about it. Either that, or his conscience would bother him, and he confesses so he'd feel better. [This brief story shows the workings of sudden, deadly rage. Wes's history shows he has witnessed this type of rage in his father, but the story may also show what potentialities Wes fears in himself. Rage, with its inexplicable source ("something could have taken hold of him"), is almost immediately followed by contrition and by efforts to placate a nagging conscience. Only confession brings relief. But is confession alone a sufficient placating device? In the story, confession is not (need not be?) followed by punishment.]

Card 8 BM (An adolescent boy looks straight out of the picture. The barrel of a rifle is visible at one side, and in the background is the dim scene of a surgical operation, like a reverie-image.)

From the appearance of the gun there, and the look on the boy's face, the young one standing up there has evidently been in a hunting accident, and these are the doctors there, trying to work on the boy to get the bullet out, or pellets if it was a shotgun. The boy is evidently worried. He could have been the one that pulled the trigger or something, and it could be his relation or hunting partner on the table. ("And how does all that work out?") Well, it could have two endings. One, the guy might die and might not pull through it, and he could crack up—the boy; and he might, the other man might get well then. He'll probably get well again and go on with his way of life. I'll bet he'll be more careful about guns in the future. ("How do you mean, the boy might crack up?") Well, that's an expression used quite often .. by crack up, they mean he might go crazy in his head. ("If the patient gets better, how will he feel toward the boy?") He'll probably be a little bit sore at him and tell him to be careful next time. [Thinly disguised, Wes partially expresses the complex of feelings that may have attended the accidental death of his brother. This story, therefore, is a far cry from the descriptive level at which Wes needed to stay with Card 2. But as Wes reveals his feelings more openly, his language becomes more imprecise: first he says the doctors are trying to get the bullet out of the boy, but later it turns out that the boy, rather than being the victim of the shooting, seems to be its agent.[2] It is known that Wes, together with the rest of his family, feels vague guilt about the death of the brother; it is apparent that, under stress (e.g., of guilt), Wes's thinking becomes vague, confused and his logic difficult to pursue.

[On none of the other TAT stories does Wes's thinking become so loosely organized as on Card 8. Typically, his stories begin with a dramatic description which promises much. Afterwards, however, the initial impact becomes attenuated, and the point of the story becomes equivocal. Almost without exception, the story ends up tamely, nonspecifically, suggesting little more than potentialities. Although Wes does not always demonstrate this watering-down trend, he does so frequently enough to indicate a reliable pattern—his defensive mode, which initially permits feeling to come to awareness and expression, then involves a following up by work which inactivates spontaneity and buries it.

[The following story, told to TAT Card 5, demonstrates this process of gradual devitalization:]

Card 5 (A middle-aged woman is standing on the threshold of a half-opened door looking into a room.)
From the woman's expression who is opening the door, she looks like she's horrified at something in that room. From the looks of the room and furniture, it was quite a while back. She looks like an old lady, around seventy or eighty. ("What is she horrified about?") It

---

2 One wonders, of course, to what extent Wes is unconsciously confused about the degree to which his brother was agent and victim in his own death, as well as the degree to which Wes might have been responsible for the death himself.

could be, maybe someone in the room has died, or an accident in there, or she heard somebody yell like they needed help, and she came to investigate. ("Would you choose one of those situations and make up a story about it?") Well, if someone's had an accident, like maybe cutting their finger with a knife or something, she'll come in and get the first aid all together, give it to them, and that person will feel better afterwards, and she'll tell them not to yell so loud probably next time, and instead of yelling, tell her what's happening. ("Who could the other person be?") It could be her granddaughter, or if she is married her fa .. her husband. [The most significant feature of this story involves the enervation of its impact—the story begins with an old woman who is "horrified" by something in the room, but this "something" eventually turns out to be an inconsequential hurt. A steppingstone in Wes's attenuation procedure is his use of a temporal distance device, i.e., placing the event "quite a while back."]

WORD ASSOCIATION TEST

React. Time (In Secs.)	Stimulus	Response	Recall	Recall Time (In Secs.)	Inquiry and Comments
½	1. hat	coat	√		
1	2. lamp	light	√		
1½	3. love	marriage	√		
1½	4. book	reading	√		
½	5. father	mother	√		
2½	6. paper	ink	√		[This slight increase in reaction time may be a delayed reaction to father.]
3½	7. breast	body	√	3	[A "normal" reaction delay.]
1	8. curtains	window	√	2	
2	9. trunk	closet (His voice breaks.)	√		("What were you thinking of with 'trunk'?") We've got trunks in all of our closets. Every model I've ever built I've kept places for and

React. Time (In Secs.)	Stimulus	Response	Recall	Recall Time (In Secs.)	Inquiry and Comments
					put them in a box. Excuse me (he laughs), my stomach's growling. [Such collection tendencies are, of course, consistent with compulsive (over-ideational) character organizations. The "stomach growling" suggests that this is a sensitive area for some reason.]
2½	10. *drink*	milk (He laughs.)	√		
5½	11. *party*	food (He laughs.)	dance	6½	("Why do you think 'party' took so long?") Well, it just .. I remember going to parties before and trying to think of what to say. (He describes his always being first in line for food.) ("How do you like parties?") I like them .. they're okay. If they're the right kind. By right kind, I mean I don't like those wild things some people throw. About the only ones I've been to are church groups. ("How do you mean, 'wild'?") Like beer drinking— somebody pulls out a bottle of beer, and they get all liquored up and get in an accident. They always blame it on others, and it's

React. Time (In Secs.)	Stimulus	Response	Recall	Recall Time (In Secs.)	Inquiry and Comments
					the innocent people that get killed a lot of times. [Right-eousness seems to serve as a buffer against feeling left out. Wes is secure only in situations where moral sanc-tions prevent un-controlled expression of impulse.]
1	12. *spring*	water	√		
3	13. *bowel movement*	excretion	body	5	[Another "normal" delay.]
1	14. *rug*	carpet	√		
1	15. *boy friend*	girl friend	√		
5½	16. *chair*	couch	√		("Why do you think 'chair' took so long?") Should I rather put in "stool," or what? I didn't give the first word, "stool," that auto-matically came to my mind, but the most natural one. [The long delay here may be a delayed reaction from the preceding boy friend-girl friend combination.]
1½	17. *screen*	window	√		
6½	18. *penis*	body	√		[An understandable delay, considering Wes's presenting symptoms and his unconscious preoc-cupations with im-potence, castration and masculine lack.]
1	19. *radiator*	steam	√		

React. Time (In Secs.)		Stimulus	Response	Recall	Recall Time (In Secs.)	Inquiry and Comments
3½	20.	*frame*	frame? ("That's right.") window	√	3	[Wes's responses are beginning to have longer reaction times; the need to repress may be increasing as the word associations stimulate potentially disturbing thoughts.]
1	21.	*suicide*	death	√		
2	22.	*mountain*	hill	√		
2½	23.	*snake*	reptile	√		
2½	24.	*house*	building	√		
—	25.	*vagina*	What was that? ("Vagina.") I don't know that. (He laughs.)			[Once again, one can see evidence of repression.]
1	26.	*tobacco*	smoke	√		
3½	27.	*mouth*	throat	head	3	("Why did 'mouth' take longer?") It's practically the same thing again . . head, ears, eyes, nose. [Wes's oral conflicts stand out clearly on these tests. As he becomes psychologically uncomfortable, he brings obsessive mechanisms into play.]
½	28.	*horse*	cow	√		
28	29.	*masturbation*	I know it, but I can't define it. Dr. L. (the psychiatrist) defined it to me last hour. I	√		[Again one sees an apparent paradox: on the one hand, later on, Wes freely (and atypically) volunteers a mental image to the word *intercourse;* on the

React. Time (In Secs.)	Stimulus	Response	Recall	Recall Time (In Secs.)	Inquiry and Comments
		think it was the word, but I'm not sure (he laughs).			other, he is unable even distantly to respond to the word *masturbation*. Intellectualization, which has worked fairly adequately before, is not effective here. Repression is dominant once more.]
2½	30. *wife*	husband	√		
1	31. *table*	chair	√		
2½	32. *fight*	title	√		
1	33. *beef*	cow	√		
4	34. *stomach*	esophagus	√		("Why did 'stomach' take longer?") I just naturally thought of esophagus. I remembered in biology, studying about the body quite a bit.
3½	35. *farm*	acre	√	2	[The average reaction times have continued gradually to increase, possibly because Wes is more guarded in his responses, possibly because nonspecific tensions, and with them repressive tendencies, rise as he is asked to continue to react spontaneously.]
½	36. *man*	woman	√		
3	37. *taxes*	laws	√		
1	38. *nipple*	bottle	√	4	[This delay appears to be caused by oral conflicts.]
2½	39. *doctor*	dentist (he laughs).	√		

React. Time (In Secs.)	Stimulus	Response	Recall	Recall Time (In Secs.)	Inquiry and Comments
3	40. *dirt*	sod	clay	1½	
1½	41. *cut*	slice	√		
1	42. *movies*	shows	√	2	
3	43. *cockroach*	insect	animal	3	[The two 3″ reaction times to this word, and Wes's later report of a disgusting image and Scout (screen?) memory of a cockroach infestation, once again is consistent with a "hysterical" organization.]
2	44. *bite*	chew	√		
1	45. *dog*	cat	√		
1½	46. *dance*	waltz	√		("How do you like dancing?") I never did like it. Besides, I never did learn. Mom and Dad tried to teach me, but after a while, they saw I didn't like it, so they gave up. (He tells how he goes to school dances to watch the others and to put on records and drink Cokes.) ("Why don't you like to dance?") I associate dancing with dating, and somehow or other I just don't want to start dating. [Thus, vividly, Wes tells that he wants to remain the preadolescent, who watches the other boys and girls grow up, while he changes records,

React. Time (In Secs.)	Stimulus	Response	Recall	Recall Time (In Secs.)	Inquiry and Comments
					drinks Cokes and avoids growing into heterosexual maturity.
					[Inquiry with adolescents on "dance" almost invariably uncovers worthwhile diagnostic information.]
1½	47. *gun*	firearm	√		
2	48. *water*	H₂O .. formula	√		
1	49. *husband*	wife	√		
6	50. *mud*	clay	√		("What happened on 'mud'?") I was trying to think of whether to put water, clay, soil, sand, or sod. I finally put clay. [Once again, we see how too many choices keep Wes from being able to make a final commitment. *Mud* follows the stimulus word *husband,* a mature status which Wes is probably working to avoid.]
1	51. *woman*	man	√		
2	52. *fire*	flames	√		
9	53. *suck*	It means to suction on .. like a vacuum cleaner.	√		("Why do you think 'suck' took so long?") Well . . . . . there are several things that could be put on there. I watched a baby calf for a while, and there was sort of a sucking sound when I had

(In the water/H₂O cell: H_2O .. formula)

React. Time (In Secs.)	Stimulus	Response	Recall	Recall Time (In Secs.)	Inquiry and Comments
					the old car pulled out of a ditch. Then there's the vacuum cleaner . . more suction there, so I finally got it and picked *it* out. [The word *suck* almost always leads at least to mild disorganization. Considering Wes's oral conflicts, one is not surprised that he has problems with the word. Once again, one can see how obsessive-compulsive mechanisms serve an emergency function. They tend to be used whenever other defensive mechanisms do not hold anxiety effectively enough in check.]
5	54. *money*	dough, slang term	√		["What happened on 'money'?") Well, I was just thinking along the terms of the song. I had dough in there and bread. I said "slang term" so that you'd know which kind I meant.
1	55. *mother*	father	husband	4	("What happened the second time on 'mother'?") I thought the wrong thing. I should have said "father." I was trying to think what I said the last time. It took me quite a while, and I hit the

React. Time (In Secs.)	Stimulus	Response	Recall	Recall Time (In Secs.)	Inquiry and Comments
					wrong one. [Wes almost invariably finds his father difficult to deal with.]
5	56. *hospital*	veterinarian	√	2	("Why did 'hospital' take longer?") Well, it's an animal hospital. I took my cat there to have it patched up. I got it caught in the door. [Further reverberations of the brother's violent death? And of violence in general? And the word follows his association of "father."]
1	57. *girl friend*	boy friend	√		
2½	58. *taxi*	automobile	√		
1	59. *intercourse*	sexual	√		
2	60. *hunger*	food	√		

(After completion of the entire test, I ask about images Wes may have had to any of the words.) On "water," I was thinking along terms of chemistry. Different experiments we fooled around with. ("Any others?") Yes on "sexual intercourse" (*sic*) I found an image. ("What kind of an image?") Like what I thought it was. Then, on "party," I said, "dancing." I really said, "food." Every time I get to a party, I'm always in line first . . except a time a kid bigger than me got in there first. I wasn't going to argue with him. ("Any other images?") On "firearms" (*sic*) I automatically remember pulling the trigger of a gun, and it automatically blew up. That one I never will forget. On "cockroach," I thought of the time the Scouts went on a hike, and they got into everything. We had to shake them out. And on "fire," my dad can verify this, I mixed something up with something else, and it exploded. I got flash burns. I was a funny-looking kid for a while. If dynamite hadn't been invented, I would have been rich quick (he laughs). ("Any other images?") There was "mud." I thought of the time we had the old Dodge, and I got buried in a ditch. I was just learning to drive. There was a car coming down the road, and rather than having him hit us, I went into a ditch. [Wes tells of having a good many more images than are ordinarily reported. Image-thought is rarely found, or at least almost never reported, by persons who use repression to an unusual degree. The visualization of an image requires a capacity to bind tension similar to what is required for the "seeing" of a Movement response on the Rorschach. Since Wes gives no Rorschach Movement responses, it comes as a surprise when he reports Word-Association images, which require such a high degree of inwardly directed attention.

[As has already been suggested, this is a much richer, more revealing Word Association Test than one would have expected from Wes's rather bland Rorschach and Thematic Apperception Test performances. Perhaps the main reason for the difference in these performances lies in the fact that each word association requires only a relatively brief time to be expressed; hence, Wes never needs to maintain a self-revealing attitude for very long. Were the task to require much more time, then Wes might, as he does on the TAT, bury what he tells about himself under a multitude of defensive layers. The Word Association Test requires that he respond quickly, a situation which may not give him sufficient time to use repressive and suppressive defenses to becloud what is going on inside of him.]

SENTENCE COMPLETION TEST II

He hoped that when he grew up he could go to college and do what his mind told him to . . maybe in some sort of science research. ("How do you mean, 'What his mind told him to'?") He could go maybe into teaching, be a bank teller, a car racer. [The desire for greater independence and freedom to follow his own wishes, rather than having to do what his parents tell him, is a consistent theme throughout this test. At the same time, at least one of the careers he mentions (bank teller) hardly epitomizes independent functioning. The mixed (and in a sense contradictory) nature of Wes's character structure is nicely reflected in his choice of compulsive bank teller on the one hand, and action-oriented car racer on the other.]

His parents didn't like the idea of this because they were used to the idea of making up their minds for him . . his mind for him.

When he saw what the other kids were doing he realized it was wrong and quit . . left. For example, if they were drinking or driving fast, he was going to quit . . right there. [Wes's identification (except in his symptom) with his parents' moralism can hardly serve to make him popular among his peers.]

When he compared himself to his friends . . . . he thought he was pretty good.

He was sad whenever he thought of . . It could have been his mother dying.

When he was asked about his aches and pains he told the doctor . . if that was who asked him . . that it could probably have resulted from a bad accident. [Accidents of one sort or another are present throughout Wes's record. He has had a number of them, is afraid of them, and seems particularly vulnerable to them.]

The person he admired most was probably his father. ("Why was that?") Probably for things he'd done . . He'd gotten along well in the social world and had a good job. [Is this denial? Isolation?]

His brother . . . . probably had a fairly good paying job, but it could have been in a tavern, and his brother wanted the boy to work there, but he wouldn't because he was against that sort of stuff. [Could part of the guilt for the brother's death have arisen from differences concerning moral values?]

When the girl kissed him he asked her to maybe marry him. [In Wes's moralistic view of things, can a kiss lead only to marriage?]

When his father came into the room . . . . . . Let's see (he repeats the stem to himself). He was probably happy that the boy had asked the girl to marry him. [Father approves, too.]

When he was with his sister . . . . he was probably unhappy, because if it was like other kids in town, they don't like their sisters tagging along wherever they go.

At school he got pretty good grades, and he got along with the other kids.

When he looked at the work the other students were doing he felt that he himself could do better. That, by the way, is the way I've been feeling (he smiles).

He was very happy when he graduated from school.

The thing he found hardest to do was not to go along with the crowd . . with what the others were doing. ("Like what?") Well, if they said, "Let's go out to drink," and so on, he said he wasn't going. Maybe to set an example like that could help others. ("Would it be hard not to go along?") Yes, because they probably teased him quite

a bit about it. (He tells a story in which others called him "chicken.")
[This is the first time Wes shows that his armor of righteousness is
vulnerable. He occasionally finds it difficult to keep aloof from his
peers; yet he must keep aloof because he does not dare to take leave
of childhood.]

Whenever certain things really bothered him . . . . He
never let people know that he *was* bothered, so, as Dr. L. put it, they
couldn't rub it in. Or he wouldn't let them know there was a wound.
[Wes defensively needs to remain shut up inside of himself.]

His dreams were often happy.

When he saw that the man had left the money behind he would
try and find the person who had left it there and give it back. He
wouldn't keep it because it wasn't rightly his.

He thought that his mother had maybe disliked him. ("Why did
he think that?") If she made up his own mind for him quite a few
times, a person would evidently get that feeling.

Whenever he and his family disagreed there was probably an
argument.

When he was very little he could have had an accident . . either
in a car wreck or at home.

His best friend often comforted him when he was in trouble.

He was unhappy with his father when he disagreed with him
about maybe going to college. He started to make up his own mind,
and they didn't like it. [Wes feels that his parents put major obstacles
in the way of an independence he desires at least somewhat.]

When his mother asked about his girl friend he told her she was
a good person.

He never thought he would be able to ask her to marry him because sometimes it seems pretty hard to do.

He always hoped that he could grow up to be like his father.
[Father is a highly ambivalently held object. While he inspires fear
in Wes, Wes also feels a great deal of conscious admiration for him.]

What he liked best about himself was the way he got along with
others.

His mother was more likely than his father to agree with him on
subjects.

His sister often tried to tag along with him.

When he had nothing else to do . . . . . This may sound quite peculiar to you, but if he was like I was, our whole family often got
together to read the Bible. ("Like you *were*?") Like I am.

He thought that his intelligence was lacking in certain subjects. That refers back to me again, like in math. [The Sentence Completion Test often taps preconscious or conscious material and outright self-reference. The way the stems are worded (i.e., "He feels . . . ." versus "Bob feels . . . . .") seems largely to determine the degree of conscious self-awareness that the subject brings to the completion of the stems.]

What he liked best about school . . Could I sort of compare him with me? My favorite subject is chorus . . choral music.

When he couldn't see a way out of his problem he probably talked with his pastor to show him a way.

He saw the cockroach on the wall and swatted it with a newspaper (he laughs).

His teacher said he was a good kid. Scratch "kid" out and put "boy." [Propriety and conventionality are omnipresent.]

Whenever he got angry he let it be shown. ("How do you mean?") Well, like I came back to school, and this kid had been talking things on what I'd done, and it wasn't true, and I had a fight with him. I was determined to make him take it back, and he did (he laughs). [Wes is apparently referring to his symptom of exhibitionism. Rather than trying to deal with it by explaining, intellectualizing or isolating the behavior, he tries to deny that it ever happened at all.]

He remembered that when he was little he had an accident. ("What kind of an accident?") Like I had. I yanked a hot iron down on my arm. ("What happened then?") I don't remember. [Another accident.]

When the kids invited him to go with them to the hiding place, he thought that it was wrong . . that something wrong was going to take place. ("Like what?") They could have gone out and maybe stolen a car.

After school he usually took his books home for study.

He admired his father when he made a great decision. ("What kind of a decision?") Like my dad, when he decided to become a pastor and quit work at the plant. They started to manufacture something he didn't hold with. So he quit.

When the girl invited him to her party he assented.

When he and his brother were together they were quite happy.

He thought that his body . . Would you repeat that? (I repeat.) Had a bad disease. ("What kind of a disease?") Well, like cancer, or

TB, or polio. [Together with accident proneness, Wes is also concerned about the integrity of his body.]

When he had a lot of homework to do he did it and then played afterwards. By the way, don't refer that to me, because I don't.

What he disliked about school was what his teacher did, like one of mine did in math, when she told the other boy to hit me.

Whenever he spoke about his problems to someone they probably laughed at him. ("Why would they do that?") They didn't understand him. [One of Wes's reasons, or perhaps rationalizations, for maintaining distance from others is that they will not "understand."]

When he entered the haunted house he wasn't scared.

When the other fellow offered him a cigarette he refused it.

He didn't like his mother to make up his own mind for him. He felt he was big enough to do it himself.

When the baby arrived he felt that he had been deserted because it got more attention than he did. ("Did that happen when your brother was born?") No, that never happened to me. [Intense anger created by the brother's birth might have played a large role in the strength of Wes's guilt following the brother's accidental death.]

When the fellows asked him to join them in a rough game he shied away from it. ("Why was that?") Referring to me again, I'm sort of afraid of bodily contact. In football, I'll try going out of bounds when a guy comes at me. I don't like to get hit. [The repeated theme of contact avoidance.]

Whenever he didn't do what he was told he was punished. ("How?") It could be the old-fashioned way of spanking. Or maybe his privileges were taken away.

What would make him angriest . . Well, being accused of something he didn't do. [He continues to deny his symptom, although he never refers to the exhibitionism directly.]

In his spare time he worked with models . . referring that to me again.

What troubled him most were his problems that he had. ("Like what?") I can't tell you (he laughs).

When he was alone in his room at night he'd often lay down and listen to the radio.

What scared him most was possibly the thought of being in another wreck . . thinking that he mightn't be so lucky next time. [Might the "accidents" be partly motivated?]

He struck the match and (he gives a startled reaction to a cap pistol shot outside the office). That scared me. I wasn't expecting it. (I repeat the stem:) looked around the room. [Wes's reaction does not correspond to the stereotype of phlegmatic calm alleged to characterize persons of his size.]

He disliked his father when he wouldn't let him drive the car.

He thought that his looks were okay (he laughs). That was just an expression. I mean, you know, in the eyes of others, he was all right. [Wes has to excuse what an observer might consider to be his lack of humility.]

The thing he could do best . . . referring this to me . . singing. That's what I make the best grades in in school. In the A bracket.

He had no respect at all for certain people. Like this kid I had the mix-up with in school. ("What happened?") He *was* one of my best friends until that happened . . and that dissolved it quickly (he laughs). [The other person threatened Wes's denial-repression.]

He always enjoyed hunting and fishing. That's one of my favorite pastimes.

He had a very uncomfortable feeling when he talked to certain people. Shall I name one? ("Whatever you like.") They accused him of certain things. [The "certain things" remain unspecified, but it is rather obvious what "they" might be.]

He found it easiest to talk to . . I could say someone he knew, but don't refer that to me because . . well (he laughs) just because. ("How would you finish it?") Just leave that one blank. [Wes's need to keep his own counsel probably applies not only to adults, but to peers as well.]

THE PSYCHOLOGIST'S REPORT

Strong repressive tendencies exist with almost equally strong obsessive-compulsive ones in Wes, suggesting that his psychological organization can properly be described as "mixed."

Wes often succeeds in pushing both fact and feeling out of awareness. Although he is invariably pleasant and "good" during testing, one never feels genuine warmth from him. At most, he occasionally smiles anxiously or brings forth pseudoaffective exclamations, such as "Eek!" and "Ouch!" (e.g., when he is presented with some more complicated Block Designs). There are indications that Wes occasionally builds up feelings to a point where they finally emerge as explosions of rage, but he seems unable to express genuine emotions in a smoothly flowing, ongoing, well-modulated way. Repression of thought is suggested by such reactions as his forgetting what he is about to say while he is in the middle of a sentence. On the Rorschach he is unable to think creatively; even with encouragement, he can see no human Movement responses, and he shies away from serious introspection. On one of the more difficult Arithmetic problems he explains that the correct answer simply "popped" into his mind; he cannot explain how he obtained it. How repression is constantly reinstituted is seen in his Thematic Apperception Test performance. Frequently he begins telling a story dramatically and apparently revealingly, but as he realizes how he is about to give his feelings away, he covers up, and the story which originally promised so much drama ends blandly and equivocally. Inhibition and denial are also prominent defenses, sometimes difficult to separate from repressive tendencies.

Wes's obsessive-compulsive symptoms emerge in his preoccupation with numerous possibilities; in his concern about small detail; in his frequent difficulty with the making of an unequivocal choice; and in his preoccupation with saving, ordering and collecting. While he often tries to eliminate thought from awareness, he also occasionally permits himself vivid inner imagery. The "mixed" (hysterical and obsessive-compulsive) nature of his organization is epitomized by his reaction to the Sentence Completion stem, *He hoped that when he grew up——*. Here, he first stresses the importance of being able to have a free choice about one's future. The possible career choices Wes then proposes are: being a teacher, or a bank teller, or a car racer. These vocational possibilities reflect the "mixed" needs that characterize Wes.

It appears that Wes's obsessive-compulsive defenses do not occupy the same, almost constantly available, niche as the repressive ones; rather, the former are brought into operation whenever the latter cannot do their job adequately.

There are a number of suggestions, too, that Wes suffers from phobic (i.e., ideational-hysterical) symptoms. He is particularly concerned with the physical integrity of his body and is preoccupied with the many accidents and near accidents that have happened to him. (Either he has had many more accidents than most sixteen-year-olds, or he is more concerned about them—or he is both accident prone and accident preoccupied.)

Wes achieves a Wechsler-Bellevue Intelligence Quotient of 92-94 (Verbal Quotient 92-96; Performance Quotient 93). In some areas (e.g., Similarities) he does much less well than in others. He tends to be exceedingly concrete in his thinking, and although he has quite well-defined interests, the general impression he usually manages to convey is that of a rather unexciting person. He does relatively well when he is not required to relate isolated elements to each other (e.g., he does extremely well on Story Recall), but he is at a loss when he needs to combine individual elements into a new configuration. A wish to appear intellectual is often unsupported by actuality, and smacks, therefore, of pretentiousness. On the Rorschach, for example, he says he sees the Horse Nebula, but he can justify this unusual percept only by saying the area looks "something like a horse." While Wes refers to his reading of "scientific" books, his actual scientific knowledge is neither profound nor extensive. At the same time, his interest in nature seems genuine, and he has a capacity for appreciating and sensitively enjoying natural occurrences.

Although Wes tries to apply his obsessive-compulsive defenses as ways to intellectual achievement, these defenses are of little genuine usefulness in that regard. Frequently Wes focuses his attention on minute details and ignores what is most central. For example, when I ask him to draw a person, he copies me sitting at my desk. He shows the seams of my shirt, the pocket of my trousers, the paper lying on my desk, but he neglects to include my facial features. Similarly, in his drawing of a woman, he indicates folds of her dress but omits her arms. This type of missing the forest for the trees is typical of Wes's approach.

His omission of the obvious may be just another manifestation of Wes's difficulty in organizing effectively. Inability to organize and to think conceptually pervades Wes's protocol to such a degree that one cannot avoid entertaining the possibility that he suffers some sort of organic brain impairment. Wes's low performance in areas requiring symbolic and abstract thought, his marked need for external guideposts, his occasional perseverative tendency, the sloppiness of his motor performance in spite of compulsive efforts—these features raise a strong possibility that functional aspects are exacerbated by organic impairment.

On some (rather rare) occasions Wes's thinking becomes confused and difficult to follow. Such an occasion occurred when a TAT picture apparently triggered guilt feelings that Wes harbors about the sudden death of his younger brother. It seems unclear to Wes to what extent he himself was responsible for his brother's death. At the least, Wes appears to feel significant remorse for angry, competitive feelings he held toward his brother. In part, Wes seems to feel that he deserved to die in his brother's place. Although such strong feelings may occasionally cause Wes's thinking to become somewhat tangled, he usually thinks clearly and logically.

Wes's world is simply ordered into good and bad. He has at least superficially identified himself with expressed parental values, and he expresses righteous indignation at his peers' behavior. Largely for this reason, many of his peers probably tend to shun him and he them. Wes disapproves of smoking, drinking, swearing, racing cars, and he apparently makes no bones about his position. Because other young people tend not to like him much, he finds himself at the periphery of their activities (e.g., changing records at dances), or he withdraws totally to build airplane models. He very rarely admits his loneliness even to himself, but he makes it clear that he can permit himself to become part of the group only if the others accept his ascetic standards. Wes's disapproval of his peers' behavior hides severe anxiety about the free expression of his own impulses. In many ways he says that he would rather build his models and read his nature books than grow into heterosexual maturity.

Of special psychological danger to Wes is the area of sexuality. Thus, on Word Association, he either blocks on the sexual words, says he does not know what they mean, or cannot give an association to them at all. Even a kiss is compromising; on Sentence Completion it is (must be?) followed by marriage, which is in turn sanctioned by the family. Wes says he dislikes dancing because it is "too close to dating," for which he says he is not ready at all. He avoids any explicit discussion of his symptom of exhibitionism, although he occasionally refers to it in a roundabout way, mainly in order to create the impression that others have wrongly and unfairly accused him. Although Wes finds his exhibitionism impossible to integrate into his highly moral self-representation, it is not clear whether he has succeeded in actually convincing himself that he never behaved in the ways that the legal authorities claim.

Part of Wes's inhibition involves his inability to express overt aggression (except occasionally and explosively, as indicated previously). Although Wes speaks of someone "blowing his top" on the Story Completion Test, he is unable to say what specific behavior this might entail. Even though I exert considerable pressure to find out, I am unable to get beyond Wes's avoidance, evasion and repetition. Very often he expresses aggression passively: for example, he tells of holding grudges against people for long periods of time, and he seems willing to sacrifice a good friendship without making any effort to clear up a misunderstanding which is causing it to break up.

While Wes fears growing into adulthood, he nevertheless expresses the wish for increased independence. But although he resents his parents constantly telling him what to do and how to behave, he wishes to be independent as a boy, not as a man. He feels that his parents do not really love him, because they cannot relinquish planning for him, making decisions for him and, in general, running his life. He does not want to give up their surveillance altogether, however. For example, he tells a Thematic Apperception Test story of a boy who finds it difficult to leave a mother who is reluctant to let him go; the boy then visits her whenever he has a vacation. Wes's desire for continuing supervision is further emphasized by his story of a prisoner who, released from jail, immediately goes to his parson for life guidance. In other words, although Wes complains about not having enough freedom to decide matters for himself, he needs very much to lean on others in order to find out how he should behave.

Just as Wes divides the world simply into good and bad, so does he divide his parents. Although Wes seems unconsciously to fear and resent his father, he gives almost no conscious hint of the reaction one would ordinarily expect him to have toward a father who is so chronically irritable, impatient and explosive. Wes idealizes his father: he admires his religious zeal, his ability to get along with others, and his willingness to give up his means of livelihood for a principle. On the Thematic Apperception Test, Wes describes the father figure as helpful and supportive—someone who helps a young man over his distress. (Significantly, however, in these same stories, the father expresses love and longing for his son only after the son's death or near death.)

In contrast to this idealized paternal image, on the TAT Wes sees his mother as an ambitious person who achieves success vicariously through her son. She forces her will on him, and she unconcernedly disregards the needs of all men in order to achieve her own satisfactions. She is selfish and nagging. Still, Wes considers her superior to the father in her ability to be equal to an emergency—

she keeps her head and does the necessary, practical thing. While Wes thinks of his mother as usually able to maintain calm, he sees his father as the opposite—striking out quickly and murderously whenever he is sufficiently angered.

Although Wes seems to have confidence that help may develop out of his conception of therapy, it will be difficult for him to overcome his reluctance to establish a relationship in which he will be required to be open and to communicate genuine feelings. He is afraid that, as he permits others to see his real concerns, they will feel contempt for him.

Discussion

Wes is trying to resolve the tasks with which adolescence confronts him via two compromises. The first set of compromises involves the ways he deals with his thoughts and feelings. On the one hand, he tries to eliminate them through repression, and on the other, to enhance their importance through obsessive, intellectualizing mechanisms. His TAT performance furnishes the prototype of further efforts to go in the opposing directions of revealing and not revealing himself. First he openly expresses what is on his mind, but subsequently he tries to nullify it, to take the vigor out of it, to make it banal and irrelevant.

The second major compromise involves Wes's sexual (i.e., impulse) expression. Although he is rattling the bars of the psychic prison in which he has placed himself, he attempts to maintain the status quo of the younger child. His and his family's moral sanctions do not have enough suppressive strength to prevent the emergence of new sexual impulses. The impulses do emerge, but apparently they can do so only in distorted form, far short of optimal expression. The impulse compromise has two aspects: first, exhibitionism is itself a compromise between expression and inhibition; second, Wes's (conscious or unconscious) denial of the exhibitionism permits him, more or less successfully, to maintain a unified self-image.

Conclusion

We have examined the test protocols of two adolescents. One is trying to deal with his imminent adolescence almost exclusively by way of a well-established overideational process; the other is using a mixture of over- and underideational efforts to help him come to grips with wishes involving autonomy, dependency, impulse expression and identity.

Overideation represents one of various efforts to assure control of both the inner and the external world. By knowing everything, by organizing, planning and detailing one's life, the person hopes to avoid surprise and to anticipate all possibilities. Such a person's guiding principle is, "What I know can't hurt me."

As is obvious, particularly from Wes's material, this defensive mode can be quite inadequate to the task of dealing with strengthened impulses which appear at the time of adolescence. "Knowing" alone is not effective, so its opposite, "not knowing," may be tried. While the person who is at the extreme of the overideational distribution may spend all his time in (often pointless) rumination at the expense of productive action, the underideational one may spend almost all his time in (occasionally destructive) action at the expense of reflective thought.

The next chapter contains test protocols of adolescents whose underideational (repressive) defenses are excessively prominent. The young people to be discussed live almost exclusively in nonreflective action.

6

The Nonreflective Adolescent

So far we have attempted to demonstrate how both the *quality* of thought organization and the *quantitative* role which thought plays in the adolescent's over-all personality organization influence not only the way he appears at the moment, but the way he solves the major task of making a successful transition from childhood to adulthood.

Joan and Helen continue the sequence of persons whose emphasis (in these two cases, *de-emphasis*) on thought reflects their idiosyncratic ways of dealing both with various internal forces and with external realities. The preceding chapter deals with adolescents who tend to overemphasize thinking; this chapter contains the test protocols of two adolescent girls who shun serious thought, or at least relegate it to a position of unimportance. It will be seen how these adolescents depend on motoric activity or inactivity as primary (if not sole) agents of accomplishment.

It may well be an overabstraction to speak of thought in isolation from other psychological functions, particularly in isolation from motor activity. Certainly thought and action are interdependent, and what is done with one invariably affects the other. Optimally, thought and action intertwine so that neither is conspicuous at the expense of the other, either because of inadequate or hypertrophied representation in the psychological organization. In Chapter 5 we saw how *too much* emphasis on thought interfered with well-planned action, and in this chapter it can be seen how *too little* emphasis on differentiated thinking processes has similar results. Action, of course, may take various forms. It may be impulsive, vigorous, destructive action (Helen); or it may be passive, withholding, stubborn action (Joan).[1]

1 "Doing nothing" is considered to be a form of action.

With "action" (or "inaction") such as Joan's it is difficult to draw clear lines between "passivity," "repression," "constriction," and "stubborn withholding." These characteristics (each conceptualized at a different level of abstraction; some more, others less, descriptive) all contain aspects of the others. An inhibited person may be inhibited in either thought or action; a person who makes strong use of repression may utilize this device with thoughts or affects; an obdurate, ungiving person may withhold thought, affect or gross action; and he may do so consciously or unconsciously.

Prior to the present examination, Joan was described by persons who saw her as "stubborn," "constricted," or "highly repressive." It is difficult to know to what extent these characteristics actually constitute only somewhat different aspects of a single syndrome; nor is it easy to know to what degree one is dealing with conscious withholding on the one hand, or with unconsciously determined mental impotence on the other. While Helen offers a psychological picture which, certainly at first glance, seems dramatically different from Joan's, they share a major psychological characteristic: the degradation of reflective thought and the consequent substitution of more or less ill-considered action.

CLINICAL SUMMARY: Joan

Joan is fifteen years old and has a brother aged ten. She has been doing failing work in school, has been refusing to attend school for a year and has been tearful and rebellious at home.

Joan's mother got in touch with the Children's Service of the Menninger Clinic when Joan was twelve. At that time the mother said that Joan was doing inadequate school work and that she seemed to be an unhappy child who suffered from constipation and poor eating habits. The mother did not bring Joan for an examination at that time, however.

Although Joan had done poorly in school since the first grade and had always been described as very shy and as not mixing well with other children, her first really severe school difficulty occurred one and a half years ago. At that time, Joan threatened to quit school and was persuaded to continue only after her teachers reduced their expectations of her. As a result of this episode, the parents took Joan to see a psychiatrist, but they did not find this one interview helpful. A year later, Joan complained of competition in the school band; she said she felt ill and again refused to attend school. She attended school irregularly for a brief time thereafter, but dropped out of school altogether two months later. She had become markedly irritable a year and a half previously, when she began to menstruate, but this irritability decreased after she left school. In addition to the school problem, the parents complain of Joan's negativism, her poor appetite and constipation. They feel that nothing they do pleases Joan. After Joan stopped attending school, she began to sleep until noon, and did very little during the rest of the day. Her mother complains of how difficult it is to get Joan to clean up after herself. The mother has continued to do things for Joan rather than waiting for Joan's slow, inadequate and unwilling work. Although the parents wish that Joan would finish high school, they have told her that they do not care whether she finishes or not. The high school reports that, educationally, Joan is three or four years behind her age group.

Joan's friendships have always been limited to a very few persons, but she cut herself off from even those few when she stopped going to school. She told her friends that she was going to attend another school somewhere else. She ignores boys and feels they dislike her.

The mother's pregnancy with Joan, planned contrary to the father's wishes, was her first, and it was uneventful. Joan's motor and speech development were normal. She did not, however, gain adequately on breast feeding and later refused vegetables when these were added to the diet. Joan's eating problem has persisted until the present. The father says that his wife nags Joan at least once each meal about her insufficient eating. Joan's toilet training, begun at the age of one, was rigid. She withheld from the very beginning, and her mother used laxatives and suppositories during bowel training. Constipation continues to be a severe problem. By the age of two, Joan was already thought of as an extremely stubborn child. The mother complains of Joan's inability to take responsibility but seems to infantalize her.

Physical and Laboratory Findings: The physical, neurological and laboratory examinations were all within normal limits.

THE PSYCHOLOGIST'S DESCRIPTION

One is immediately struck by Joan's extraordinary passivity and by her inability and unwillingness to initiate action. She sits almost immobile, waiting for whatever may happen. When she comes to a partly open door, she stands in front of it, waiting for someone else to finish opening it for her. When an object drops to the floor near her, she makes no move to pick it up. She almost never makes a spontaneous comment or asks a question about what is going on. Only three times during our five hours together did she initiate any behavior: once she began to put the cards from a Picture Arrangement sequence together; once she volunteered that some dolls she was making, about which I had shown interest, were outside in the car; and at the end of the Story Completion Test, she asked, "Am I a pretty good storyteller? Did I do just like the others did?"

Joan's passivity is not to be confused with affective blandness, however. She expresses considerable tension throughout the testing and almost constantly shakes her foot and picks at her fingernail polish. It is difficult, however, to know exactly how she is consciously feeling at any particular moment. At times she seems sullen and uninvolved; at other times she seems on the point of bursting into depressed and angry tears. She always denies having an unhappy feeling, however, and it is possible that she is unaware of affects which appear obvious to others.

THE WECHSLER-BELLEVUE SCALE

Name: Joan   Age: 15-8

	RS	WTS	0 1 2 3 4 5 6 7 8 9 10 11 12 13 14 15 16 17 18 19 20
COMPR.	13-14	11-12	
INFOR.	7	6	
DIG.	10	7	
ARITH.	3-4	3-4	
SIMIL.	10	8	
VOCAB.	12	6	
P. A.	6	6	
P. C.	9	8	
B. D.	19-22	9-10	
O. A.	17	9	
D. S.	43	10	

TOT. VERB.	34-36	
TOT. PERF.	42-43	
TOT. SCALE	76-79	

VERBAL I.Q.:   84-87   LEVEL: Dull Normal

PERFORMANCE I.Q.:   89-90   LEVEL: Dull Normal→Average

TOTAL I.Q.:   85-87   LEVEL: Dull Normal

[Although Joan obtains a Total Verbal I.Q. in no more than the Dull Normal range, she is nevertheless able to achieve a Comprehension score above that normally expected of her age, with even a somewhat higher alternate score. The scatter of eight points between Comprehension and Arithmetic reflects not only the major unevenness of Joan's performance, it also suggests that a motivational factor may play a prominent part in keeping her total performance at its relatively low level. Joan's weighted score of 3 on Arithmetic is very poor, and the alternate score of 4 hardly helps it. Were her Arithmetic score on approximately the same level as most other verbal ones, one might be justified in thinking that Joan simply lacks ability in many areas. The fact that Arithmetic stands in such isolation, however, makes one strongly suspect that Joan's disability is specifically related to a requirement for introspection.

[Her Performance scores are bunched more closely together (at about 9) than her widely ranging Verbal ones. This Verbal-Performance discrepancy suggests that Joan functions practically at a normal intellectual level in tasks which require her to respond primarily with action. When tasks require verbal competence, however, the situation is different. Here Joan's repression, constriction, passivity and negativism exert their influence fully and combine to make her abilities emerge erratically.

[The Comprehension-Information reversal is typically seen in persons organized along "hysterical" dimensions (persons who depend on conventional models as guides to their behavior). Information of the type tapped by the Information subtest tends to be less easily available to persons organized in this way.]

INFORMATION

(She speaks in a very low, soft voice and appears to be quite tense.)

No. Question	Response and Comments	Score
1. Who is the President of the United States?	...... Ike. ("Can you think of his regular name?") No. ("Who was the president before him?") (She shakes her head.) [It is evident from Joan's first response that her approach to the world, particularly to knowledge, tends to be naïve and impoverished. She does not know that "Ike's" name is Eisenhower and does not seem to care that there was a president before him. This lack of awareness, not to say interest, in what is going on in the world is typical of the person who relies on ideational repression.]	—

No.	Question	Response and Comments	Score
2.	*What is a thermometer?*	An instrument to tell the temperature of the body, I guess. [The "I guess" reflects Joan's lack of commitment to knowledge. In part she seems to be saying not only that the information is not of great importance, but also that she does not have the skill, knowledge, or general know-how to make a proper response.]	+
3.	*What does rubber come from?*	Tree.	+
4.	*Where is London?*	In England.	+
5.	*How many pints make a quart?*	Four. ("Are you sure?") I don't know. [Here Joan announces her helplessness, and possibly her unwillingness to become involved.]	−
6.	*How many weeks are there in a year?*	Fifty-two.	+
7.	*What is the capital of Italy?*	I don't know. ("Can you think of any Italian city?") No. [Such lack of knowledge (and presumably lack of interest) in the composition of the world is typical of the person organized primarily around repression. Such persons find it important to keep life as constricted as possible. For this reason, the world seems to consist of a circumscribed local area, which contains only family, friends and the daily round of activity—interest is primarily in the here and now, only very rarely in the abstract and distant.]	−
8.	*What is the capital of Japan?*	I don't know. [For Joan, Japan is far away from the here and now.]	−
9.	*How tall is the average American woman?*	Five feet four inches.	+
10.	*Who invented the airplane?*	Wright brothers.	+
11.	*Where is Brazil?*	. . . . I don't know. ("Do you know what continent it's on?") Uh-uh. [Still another piece of nonavailable world information.]	−
12.	*How far is it from Paris to New York?*	Oh my! (She gives a very small smile.) One thousand.	−
13.	*What does the heart do?*	It beats. ("Can you tell me any more?") It keeps us alive. ("Any more about what it does?") No, I don't know. [Joan approaches this problem naïvely and "functionally."]	−

No.	Question	Response and Comments	Score
14.	Who wrote Hamlet?	What is that? [Joan cannot be said to be widely read.]	—
15.	What is the population of the United States?	I don't know. ("Take a guess.") Four million?	—
16.	When is Washington's birthday?	February 22. [The fact that Joan has this piece of information available comes as a surprise after five failures. The birthday of "The Father of Our Country" (apart from being a school holiday) may carry very special affective connotations, however.]	+

(Joan did not know the answers to the remaining questions.)

RAW SCORE: 7

WEIGHTED SCORE: 6

COMPREHENSION

No.	Question	Response and Comments	Score
1.	What is the thing to do if you find an envelope in the street, that is sealed, and addressed and has a new stamp?	(She smiles.) I guess I'd mail it.	2
2.	What should you do if while sitting in the movies you were the first person to discover a fire (or see smoke and fire?)	I'd call the fire department.	1
3.	Why should we keep away from bad company?	We wouldn't have very good friends. ("How do you mean?") We'd get the wrong ideas about different things. [Joan clearly seems to be making a point about "bad influence."]	2
4.	Why should people pay taxes?	Help the schools. ("Can you think of any other reasons?") And the roads. [Joan's tendency to conceptualize "functionally" and in an isolated, fragmented way is becoming increasingly clear. Only rarely does she conceptualize in an inclusive way.]	0-1
5.	Why are shoes made of leather?	They stand up in all kinds of weather. ("Can you think of any other reasons?") They're more comfortable.	1

No.	Question	Response and Comments	Score
6.	Why does land in the city cost more than land in the country?	Cause more people want it in the city. [This precisely formulated response demonstrates Joan's ability to think in fairly abstract terms. It seems likely, therefore, that her concrete attitude represents preference more than inability.]	2
7.	If you were lost in a forest (woods) in the daytime, how would you go about finding your way out?	Walk till I come somewhere (she smiles). [This response somehow epitomizes Joan's helpless inability to think of planful, productive steps which will help her get out of difficult situations.]	0
8.	Why are laws necessary?	To guide people in what to do.	1
9.	Why does the state require people to get a license in order to be married?	So they can tell that they *have* been married. ("So who can tell?") The government, I guess.	2
10.	Why are people who are born deaf usually unable to talk?	Cause they can't hear you talk. [Again Joan gets to the crux of the matter right away.]	2

RAW SCORE: _____13-14_____

WEIGHTED SCORE: _____11-12_____

[Joan's style of verbal response is by now fairly clear. She wastes no words, indulges in no verbal frills and speaks laconically. On occasion her brief answer is accurate and to the point. More often, however, it reflects the absence of both knowledge and interest in matters that she does not consider of particular relevance. When she is intellectually unsure, she does not offer a great variety of alternatives, as Paul does; instead, she almost invariably says, "I don't know." This difference between Paul's and Joan's reactions to intellectual challenge is dramatic.]

DIGIT SPAN

(She repeats five Digits Forward and five Digits Backward. As soon as she goes above her comfortable memory limit, particularly on Digits Backward, her response becomes confused. Asked, for example, to repeat the sequence *539418* backward, she says, "*81345*.") [Joan's ability to memorize meaningless material is about on a par with her ability to memorize and integrate the type of meaningful factual material required for a successful performance on the Information subtest.]

RAW SCORE: _____10_____

WEIGHTED SCORE: _____7_____

ARITHMETIC

No.	Problem	Time	Response and Comments	Score
1.	How much is four dollars and five dollars?	½"	Nine.	1
2.	If a man buys six cents worth of stamps and gives the clerk ten cents, how much change should he get back?	1"	Four.	1
3.	If a man buys eight cents worth of stamps and gives the clerk twenty-five cents, how much change should he get back?	17"	What did you say? (I repeat the problem.) Seventeen. [It is difficult to know what makes Joan's mind wander at this point. Possibly her not hearing the problem is a way of evading the type of task which she finds so unpleasant.]	0-1
4.	How many oranges can you buy for thirty-six cents if one orange costs four cents?	3"	Nine. [A quick arithmetical success, but the last.]	1
5.	How many hours will it take a man to walk twenty-four miles at the rate of three miles an hour?	21"	What did you say? (I repeat the problem.) Eighty-four. ("It took eighty-four hours?") I don't know (she smiles). ("What did you do to get the answer?") I multiplied. [Joan seems helpless in the face of this problem. Her answer is vague and naïve, and she expresses no concern about not understanding the logical arithmetical steps that are required for a proper solution.]	0
6.	If a man buys seven two cent stamps and gives the clerk a half dollar, how much change should he get back?	26"	Now, what did you say? (I repeat the problem.) Forty-six. [This is the third time Joan appears not to have heard the problem. One wonders to what degree this is a conscious delaying and avoiding mechanism, or (and?) an unconscious, repressive blocking out of the unpleasant.]	0
7.	If seven pounds of sugar cost twenty-five cents, how many pounds can you get for a dollar?	—	I don't know. ("How would you do it?") . . . . ("Do you know how you might begin?") No. [The examiner should not have left Joan such an easy opportunity to say "No." For example, he might have asked, "How would you begin?" She	0

No.	Problem	Time	Response and Comments	Score

obviously welcomes any chance to avoid dealing with these problems, particularly once they require her to exert a greater degree of intellectual effort.]

(Joan cannot do anything with the last three problems.)

RAW SCORE: ___3-4___

WEIGHTED SCORE: ___3-4___

SIMILARITIES

No.	Items	Response and Comments	Score
1.	Orange-banana	They're about the same color. ("Can you think of any other ways?") I don't guess so. (I give examples of how else they might be considered alike, one example from each level of abstraction.) [It is apparent again that Joan avoids thinking either in conceptual or in precise terms. Also evident again is how easily she gives up.]	0
2.	Coat-dress	Both clothes. [Once she realizes what is expected, she does a good deal better.]	2
3.	Dog-lion	Both animals.	2
4.	Wagon-bicycle	Both have wheels. [Now she begins to become more concrete.]	1
5.	Daily paper-radio	They tell the news.	1
6.	Air-water	You use it to keep alive. [Although this response receives a score of 2, it is doubtful that Joan makes use of a genuinely abstract conceptualizing process.]	2
7.	Wood-alcohol	. . . . . You use it to make a fire.	1
8.	Eye-ear	They're both in the body.	1
9.	Egg-seed	They're both food.	0
10.	Poem-statue	. . . . I don't know. ("Can you think of any way?") (She shakes her head.) [As the items become increasingly difficult to reconcile conceptually, the abstraction effort becomes too great for Joan.]	0
11.	Praise-punishment	Uh-uh.	0
12.	Fly-tree	. . . . (She shakes her head.) ("Any way at all?") No.	0

RAW SCORE: ___10___

WEIGHTED SCORE: ___8___

PICTURE COMPLETION

(Joan answers nine of the fifteen items correctly. She misses Items 5, 7, 11, 13, 14, and 15. Reaction times on the items she solves correctly are brief—1" to 3". When she does not know an answer right away, she keeps looking at the card and eventually says, "I don't know." Sometimes, when I ask her to try a little longer, she merely shakes her head.) [It is apparent how difficult it is for Joan to apply herself to a problem-solving process for any extended period. At any early sign of difficulty, she gives up.]

RAW SCORE: 9

WEIGHTED SCORE: 8

PICTURE ARRANGEMENT

No.	Item	Correct Order	Time	Arranged Order	Story and Comments	Score
1.	House	PAT	3"	PAT	He was building a house.	2
2.	Holdup	ABCD	23"	ABCD	(She gives the cards a long puzzled look before she even touches them. She yawns.) He held someone up, and he was in jail. [Apparent is Joan's inhibition about involving herself before she is altogether sure of what way to take.]	2
3.	Elevator	LMNO	8"	LMNO	He's coming up in the elevator. (She puts the cards together for me after she has sorted them.) [This is the first even slight movement in the direction of Joan's wanting to establish somewhat closer, helpful, contact. It is also the first time Joan has shown some initiative.]	2
4.	Flirt	JANET	35"	NJAET	They're in the right order, aren't they? ("Do you think they are?") I guess. ("What's the story?") They got in the car and pulled up to the curb. He saw this woman. He got out and started walking with her. [Joan misses the point, not to mention the humor, of the sequence.]	0
5.	Taxi	SAMUEL	32"	SAMELU	("What was the story?") Walking along with this	0

No.	Item	Correct Order	Time	Arranged Order	Story and Comments	Score
					dummy, I guess. And he got in this car. He was riding ... ("What happened?") She was close to him, and she got farther away and got back close to him. ("Why was that?") I don't know. [Joan is not concerned about having missed the point of this story, too.]	
6.	Fish	EFGHIJ	29″	EFHIGJ	He went fishing and caught a fish, and he left. ("Was there anything else to the story?") I don't guess so. ("What was that thing coming out of the water?") (She smiles.) I don't know. [Joan seems unaware of, and uninvolved with, what is going on around her. The weighted score of 6, which she obtains on Picture Arrangement, is the lowest of her Performance scores. Since this test is said to require interest in the activities of others, her low performance is not surprising.]	0

RAW SCORE: 6

WEIGHTED SCORE: 6

BLOCK DESIGN

No.	Time	Accur.	Description of Behavior and Comments	Score
A.	6″	Yes	(No difficulties.)	—
B.	47″	Yes	(Considerable trial and error, but she eventually solves the design after she first says, "It doesn't work," and I encourage her to continue to try.)	—
1.	9″	Yes	(No difficulty.)	5
2.	12″	Yes	(No difficulty; immediate analysis and solution.)	4
3.	13″	Yes	(No difficulty.)	3
4.	22″	Yes	(Very slight trial and error, but essentially a good analysis and solution.)	4

No.	Time	Accur.	*Description of Behavior and Comments*	*Score*
5.	51″	Yes	(No real difficulty. Her approach is quite systematic.) [Until this point, Joan experiences hardly any problems with the solutions of this type of task. Although she does not usually make her constructions quickly, she analyzes the designs well and seems to have no major problems in going ahead correctly. Things seem a good deal easier for Joan so long as she can proceed without having to interact with another person (as she must on the Verbal subtests).]	3
6.		No	(She begins by trying to make the design with full reds and whites. Then she adds some half-red, half-white blocks. After 1′ 10″ she shrugs and says, "I can't figure it out." I encourage her to keep trying, and at 2′ 15″ she begins to make stripes correctly. At 2′ 48″ she has the design almost done but still has included some full reds and whites. She keeps working but is never able to complete the design correctly. She says, "It didn't work though, did it?") [One can see again that Joan is ready to give up after she experiences some difficulty, but that she can continue once she is encouraged. Her failure here does not seem entirely genuine, since she understands how to make the stripes. Does she need to avoid total success?]	0
7.	3′ 30″	Yes	(She immediately does the top row correctly but then experiences some difficulty with the side. She discards the side and puts in the center rectangle correctly. Then she again finds herself unable correctly to continue with the sides, adding whole red blocks. She keeps trying but eventually says, "I can't." After I encourage her to continue, she correctly does so, first completing the right side, then the left. The bottom side remains undone, and there is some more trial-and-error behavior here. She seems unable to see that all sides should be constructed in essentially the same way. She eventually completes the entire design correctly, although she is slightly overtime.) [Joan's behavior here seems based, in part at least, on her constricted approach, which prevents her from making the cognitive generalization that all sides are to be constructed in the same way. It is likely that, at least unconsciously, she avoids total success on such a complex design. She apparently finds it important to avoid appearing better than (or even as good as) others.]	0-3

RAW SCORE: 19-22

WEIGHTED SCORE: 9-10

OBJECT ASSEMBLY

Item	Time	Accur.	Description of Behavior and Comments	Score
Manikin	18″	Yes	(She shows some initial trial-and-error behavior and at first tries to fit the leg pieces into the wrong—opposite—sockets.)	6
Profile	1′ 10″	Yes	(There is some trial-and-error behavior with the nose and mouth pieces, but she seems generally to know what she is doing.)	6
Hand	53″	Partial	(She immediately places the thumb correctly and follows it with the wrist piece. She studies the problem a while and then puts the remaining pieces together quickly. Two fingers are reversed.) [The speed with which Joan does this difficult item once more suggests that her native abilities are more developed than she can allow to let be known. The reversal of two fingers is almost like an afterthought, a kind of last minute spoiling of what would otherwise have resulted in a weighted score of 11 on Object Assembly. A similar situation can be observed on the preceding Block Design. Had Joan continued in the correct directions she started on, she would have obtained a weighted score of approximately 12 on Block Design. On the next test, Digit Symbol, were Joan to avoid certain careless errors, she would achieve a weighted score of at least 11. In other words, one must entertain the thought that Joan is at least unconsciously motivated to avoid showing how well she could function. On Verbal items she only has to say, "I don't know" to demonstrate "ignorance"; on Performance items, however, this approach does not work. She does well almost in spite of herself; apparently she then requires herself to undo what she has done successfully, either by making careless errors or by becoming "confused" by problems that previously she had not found confusing.]	5

RAW SCORE: <u>17</u>

WEIGHTED SCORE: <u>9</u>

DIGIT SYMBOL

(Joan changes each of the seven   symbols into an N and loses $3\frac{1}{2}$ credits because of it. She makes an additional incorrect substitution.) [In spite of her eight errors, Joan is able to achieve an average weighted score. It is by now difficult to avoid the conclusion that Joan is, through one means or another, trying to avoid more than average success (or even just average success). It is additionally possible, of course, that some of her errors result from her lack of involvement with what she is doing. Were she eager to demonstrate her ability, however, she would not have to avoid involvement in the way she does.]

RAW SCORE: 43

WEIGHTED SCORE: 10

VOCABULARY

No.	Word	Response and Comments	Score
1.	*Apple*	Fruit.	1
2.	*Donkey*	Animal.	1
3.	*Join*	To put together.	1
4.	*Diamond*	A stone. ("Would you tell me a little more?") It's white. ("Could you tell me some more?") It has carats. ("What does that mean?") Uh-uh. [An almost sixteen-year-old girl should have no problem in defining "diamond." It is questionable that Joan obtains only half credit because she is at a cognitive loss; the culprit, much more probably, is her lack of motivation to do well.]	½
5.	*Nuisance*	To bother someone.	1
6.	*Fur*	Animal skin.	1
7.	*Cushion*	Soft place to sit down.	1
8.	*Shilling*	I don't know. ("Have you ever heard it?") Uh-uh. [Joan's ignorance about foreign currency is not surprising. It is consistent with her constricted approach to all things outside her immediate area of activity.]	0
9.	*Gamble*	Throw your money away, I guess. ("Could you tell me a little more?") I don't guess so. ("Any more about 'gamble' at all?") Play cards, I guess. [This response reflects Joan's naïve, moralistic view. It also reflects her unwillingness to give information (and probably anything else) freely, and usually only after she is pushed.]	½
10.	*Bacon*	Food. ("Could you tell me some more?") Breakfast food. ("What kind of breakfast food?") Fat. ("Where does it come from?") Pig. [This is an extreme example of Joan's unwillingness to "give" freely. Although she knows the answer, she responds in bits and pieces, adding one little morsel each time she is prodded.]	1

No.	Word	Response and Comments	Score
11.	*Nail*	I don't know. ("You know what a nail is!") I don't know. ("What is it used for?") To put things together, I guess. ("What does it look like?") A pin. [This represents the apex of Joan's negativism, which began with her response to *gamble*. It is not clear why Joan closes herself up in this way now. It seems that her negativism appears cyclically— periods of cooperation are followed by periods of noncooperation, and openness is followed by closedness. It almost seems that whenever Joan senses approval from others, she needs to seal herself in further.]	½
12.	*Cedar*	Tree, I guess.	1
13.	*Tint*	I don't know.	0
14.	*Armory*	I don't know.	0
15.	*Fable*	I don't know. ("Have you ever heard that word?") Uh-uh.	0
16.	*Brim*	I don't know.	0
17.	*Guillotine*	I don't know.	0
18.	*Plural*	More than one.	1
19.	*Seclude*	I don't know.	0
20.	*Nitroglycerin*	I don't know.	0
21.	*Stanza*	Something in music. ("What kind of thing in music?") I don't know.	0
22.	*Microscope*	An instrument to make things look bigger.	1
23.	*Vesper*	I don't know.	0
24.	*Belfry*	I don't know.	0
25.	*Recede*	I don't know.	0
26.	*Affliction*	I don't know.	0

(The remaining words were not administered.)

[It seems doubtful that these definitions reflect Joan's genuine ability or knowledge, particularly since she obtains a weighted score of 11-12 on Comprehension. It is difficult to know how much of Joan's unresponsiveness one should attribute to constriction, how much to negativism, and how much to repression. Whatever the cause or causes, her intellectual activity is crippled as a result.]

RAW SCORE: 12

WEIGHTED SCORE: 6

STORY RECALL

IMMEDIATE RECALL

$+1$ $+1$ $+1$ $+1$
December 6 . . . / It was a flood . . . . . / fourteen were / . . . . . drowned, I guess.
$+1$ $+1$ $+1$ $+1$ $+1$
/ And 600 / had a cold / from dampness / . . . . A man / trying to save / a
$+1$ $+1$
boy / cut his hand. /

SCORE: <u>11+4 = 15</u>

DELAYED RECALL

$+1$ $+1$ $+1$ $+1$
December 6 / A river overflowed / and went in the streets / and some of the
          $+1$ $+1$ $+1$ $+1$ $+1$
houses. / And fourteen / drownded / and 600 / caught a cold / from the dampness.
$+1$ $+1$ $+1$ $+1$
/ In trying to save / a boy / a man / cut his hand. /

SCORE: <u>13</u>

[Joan's scores on this memory test are consistent with her obtained Intelligence Quotient. She omits certain elements from both Immediate and Delayed Recall; some elements are repeated somwhat vaguely (e.g., "There was a flood," instead of, "A river overflowed"). It is important, however, to note that Joan never distorts, fabulizes or otherwise modifies the basic meaning of the paragraph. In other words, Joan's memory functioning presents no evidence of disorganized thinking.]

THE BRL SORTING TEST

PART I

Stimulus	Patient's Sorting	Response and Comments	Score
1. Joan's choice: *Ball*	(None.)	I don't know of anything that goes with it. [This is the first of a number of responses on this portion of the test that are defective in one way or another. Once again, it is difficult to decide what is most responsible for Joan's inadequate reactions: her constriction, her lack of energy, her negativism, or her relatively limited ability.]	Failure
2. *Fork*	(Spoon; knife.)	So you can eat your food. [A narrowed (constricted) response, organized along functional lines, is what one expects of Joan.]	(Narrow) Functional Def.

Stimulus	Patient's Sorting	Response and Comments	Score
3. Corncob pipe	(Matches.)	It's to light your pipe, I guess. [Constriction and concretism are more marked here.]	(Narrow) Concrete
4. Bell	(None.)	I don't know of anything that *goes* with it. ("Try to figure out something that might go.") (She shakes her head.)	Failure
5. Red paper circle	(Red cardboard rectangle.)	I guess because they're the same color. [Is this sorting made on a *con*ceptual or a *per*ceptual basis?]	(Narrow) Conceptual Def.
6. Toy pliers	(Toy screwdriver; toy hammer.)	Because you can build something. [Although she sorts on a "miniature" basis, she makes no explicit mention of this fact.]	(Narrow) Functional Def.

PART II

Examiner's Sorting	Explanation and Comments	Score
1. Red objects	Same color.	Conceptual Def.
2. Metal	Cause they're made of metal.	Conceptual Def.
3. Round	I don't know. ("Can you think of any reason?") Maybe cause they're all round. [When a concept is already formed in deed, though not in words, Joan is rather easily able to complete the verbal abstraction process; it is surprising to see her experience so little difficulty with it. The discrepancy between Joan's performances on Parts I and II of the BRL make one feel that she has the intellectual capacity to think abstractly, but that her lack of motivation and energy for the task inhibit her.]	Conceptual Def.
4. Tools	They're tools for building purposes.	Conceptual Def.
5. Paper	All paper.	Conceptual Def.
6. Double	All in pairs. [This item is usually difficult to solve.]	Conceptual Def.
7. White	They're all the same color. [On this item, too, people often fail.] (Filled with honest surprise, I tell her how well she has been doing.)	Conceptual Def.

Examiner's Sorting	Explanation and Comments	Score
8. *Rubber*	Cause they're round. ("How about the eraser?") I don't know. They're the same color as the others. ("How about the cigar?") . . . . ("Can you think of a way that they're all alike?") No. [It is apparent how self-defeatingly Joan immediately reacts as soon as she is praised. Following my comment about how well she has been doing, she achieves no more Conceptual definitions and fails three of the remaining five items. It is apparent that Joan tries to avoid being considered competent. When her ability is recognized, she proceeds to demonstrate right away that she really is not able at all.]	Split Narrow Failure
9. *Smoking*	You use the cigarette to light the pipe. ("You use the cigarette?") No (she smiles). You use the matches to light the others.	Concrete Def.
10. *Silverware*	Eating purposes.	Functional Def.
11. *Toys*	I don't know. ("Can you think of any way they might go together?") (She shakes her head.) ("Try to think of some way they all might belong together.") (She shakes her head again.) [Something has obviously happened to Joan's ability to conceptualize since her "white" abstraction.]	Failure
12. *Square*	I don't know. ("Can you think of any way?") (She shakes her head and looks away.) (She says "I don't know" immediately after she sees the sorting. Once she has expressed her inability to conceptualize the items, she will not look at them any longer.)	Failure

[Joan's performance on this test emphasizes the effects of a strong motivational component. She is apparently unable to accept her own and others' awareness that she can do well; once her success is explicitly recognized, she needs to nullify it quickly.]

The Bender Gestalt Test

(Joan's forms, both on the 5″ Exposure and the Copy, are rather accurately drawn. The drawings are not badly constricted, although they are somewhat smaller than the originals.

(She reacts in an extremely passive manner while she is taking this test. For example, even though she is seated at some distance from the table, she never moves her chair forward in order to draw more comfortably. I have the feeling that she will stay wherever she is put, without making the smallest effort to adjust her position. Often Joan looks as though she were on the point of tears.

(She makes her drawings without hesitating or obsessing. At no time does she manifest any particular need to be accurate; when something is not exactly right, she simply lets it be. On the Copy, she counts the dots, but she still works speedily and without hesitation.) [Most apparent on this test is the degree of Joan's passivity. This characteristic shows itself particularly in her extremely limited (really almost absent) tendency to initiate even a very minor independent action such as moving her chair to the table in order to be able to work more effectively. It is apparent, in other words, that Joan's constriction takes primarily the form of passivity (or how her passivity takes primarily the form of constriction).]

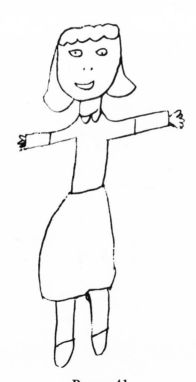

PLATE 41

The Draw a Person Test

PART I (PLATE 41, p. 441)

(At first Joan draws only the head of the girl and considers her drawing finished. She completes the rest of the drawing when I encourage her.) [Striking again is Joan's constriction, evident this time in her drawing. Joan originally leaves out everything except the head and places the entire drawing on the left-hand side of the page. Although she adds very few details, she puts in a little collar which effectively cuts off everything below the head. Her pencil pressure, as one would expect, is exceedingly light.]

PART II (PLATE 42)

[The boy she draws has strangely foreshortened arms, and trousers which do not reach the ground. He seems to have hoofs rather than

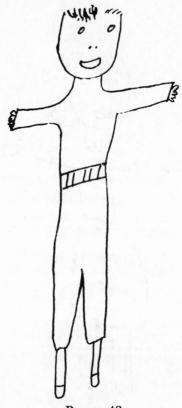

PLATE 42

feet. The only sartorial adornment she gives this figure is a belt. Thus, while the male in some ways seems to have more freedom than the female (e.g., he has no choking collar), he appears to be even less adequate. Both drawings certainly reflect a much younger self-image than is consistent with Joan's chronological age.]

RORSCHACH TEST

[Since Joan gives only two Rorschach responses, no formal Psychogram is shown.]

Card #	React. Time	Score	Protocol	Inquiry and Observations
I	4″	WF∓A Vague	1. A bug, I guess. ("Anything else?")	1. ("Would you tell me about the bug?") It might have wings. ("Anything else?") And little hands. It was wide. ("Anything else about it you remember?") No, that's all. [Joan's inclusion of "little hands" in her description of a bug reflects the uncritical way she approaches reality. A bug, of course, is one of the least differentiated responses possible on the Rorschach. By and large, "bug" is on about the same level of differentiation as "a cloud."]
		DF+H Vague	2. Maybe a body. ("Anything else?") (She wiggles her leg tensely.) I don't know.	2. ("Could you tell me about the body?") In between the wings. ("What kind of a body was it?") Little. ("What sort of body?") I don't know. Narrow. ("Was it a human or an animal body?") A bug. ("Was it the same or a different bug than the one you saw just before that?") What do you mean? (I explain what I mean.) I don't know. (She smiles.) ("Were the body and the bug the same thing?") I don't know what you mean. ("Tell me what kind of body you saw.") Maybe it was the body of a human. ("Could you tell me more about it?") It was just a regular body. ("Was it a man or

Card #	React. Time	Score	Protocol	Inquiry and Observations
				woman?") A woman. ("Was the body dressed?") I don't know. [Joan's extreme reluctance (inability?) to offer her own ideas without being urged, probed, or pushed, is again markedly evident. Joan's passivity requires others to become extremely active. While others are working so hard in this way, Joan stands quietly by and produces as little as she can. It is increasingly apparent that Joan's passivity contains not too subtly aggressive, depriving components.]
II	3′	Failure	I don't know. ("Look at it a little while longer.") I don't know. ("Does any part look like anything?") She shakes her head.) (Joan is unable to see a single other response. Her main reaction to my questions is to say, "I don't know" or, "I don't see anything." She sits silently and shakes her head. Although her expression is bland, her foot is shaking furiously.)	
X	3′	Failure	"I don't see anything." ("Do different parts look like anything?") (She shakes her head.) ("Can you see a wishbone?") (She shakes her head.) ("Can you see a rabbit's head?") Uh-uh. (I point out the area others often see as a rabbit's head, and I wonder how it seems to her.) It	[Persons who depend strongly on repression nevertheless often acknowledge an area as looking like something when it is pointed out. Joan's not recognizing what most people can eventually identify, even after it is pointed out and suggested to her, suggests the workings of a strong negativism. Neither repression alone nor negativism alone is responsible for Joan's lack of productivity; but together they

React.				
Card #	*Time*	*Score*	*Protocol*	*Inquiry and Observations*
			doesn't look like one to me. ("Why not?") I don't know. It just doesn't look like it.	prevent Joan from being "normally" productive and spontaneous.]

THE STORY COMPLETION TEST

He was very angry, and was getting angrier by the minute.

(She writes the following:) He and his wife had had a very serious disagreement. They want a devoirse, but a girl friend toll them thats not the answer so they stay together and live happyily ever after and they were good to each other.

("How do they act?") They threw a fit, I guess (she smiles). ("What was that like?") Oh, they broke several things. He hit her and jumped up and down (she laughs). Am I a pretty good storyteller? Did I do just like the others did? ("You did just fine. Do you sometimes wonder how you compare to the others?") What's that white thing? (Referring to a Christmas tree star I have lying on the table. She admires it.) [While one almost expects an undifferentiated story and poor spelling and sentence construction from Joan, one does not expect to hear her wonder whether she is a "good storyteller." Judging from Joan's Rorschach performance, for example, one does not think she will permit herself to be sufficiently involved in Story Completion to let herself care how well she does. Her "caring" is a good sign; it indicates that she is aware that others also deal with problems, and she is eager to compare herself favorably to her peers. Joan's negativism, in other words, does not always override other characteristics. Still, she is unable to answer questions about aspects that show her caring how she fits into a more general, less overwhelmingly self-centered, negativistic and constricted picture.]

THEMATIC APPERCEPTION TEST

Card 1 (A young boy is contemplating a violin which rests on a table in front of him.)

Am I supposed to just make up a story? ("That's right. Just make one up.") . . . . How long is it supposed to be? ("However long you want to make it.") . . . . I guess he wishes he could play the violin. And he is too young. So he'll have to wait until he's older. I guess that's all. ("How does he happen to have the violin?") It might be his father's. [This story emphasizes, among other things, that Joan does not feel grown up. Once she is older, she can do thing that grownups do. In the meantime, she has to wait.]

Card 2 (Country scene: in the foreground is a young woman with books in her hand; in the background a man is working in the fields, and an older woman is looking on.)

I guess she wished she could be that lady. So she can have a home of her own instead of going to school. I guess that's all. ("What about him?") He is working in the fields. ("Who is he?") A slave, I guess. ("Who is the woman leaning against the tree?") I guess she's the woman that owns the place. ("Who is the girl?") She wants to be like her, I guess. ("Are the girl and the woman related?") I don't know. ("How does the story turn out?") She'll have to wait until she's older. [Again, the theme of having to wait until one can grow up. The implication is strong that Joan thinks she has to wait until she can become "free" instead of enslaved (e.g., going to school). Adulthood, for Joan, does not involve responsibility nearly so much as freedom from the childhood chores under which she frets.]

Card 3 GF (A young woman is standing with downcast head, her face covered with her right hand. Her left arm is stretched forward against a wooden door.)

She's crying because she was kicked out of her house . . . . because she hasn't done what she was supposed to. I guess that's all. ("What was she supposed to do?") Maybe she had different chores to do. ("Who threw her out?") I guess, her . . . maybe the maid. ("How does the story end?") She'll have to find someplace else to live. Maybe a relative or something. ("What will her parents do when they find out?") They'll probably get another maid. [This story illustrates Joan's view of the severe disadvantages, not to say the hazards, of not being grown up. Unless you do your chores, you can be thrown out of the home. You are appreciated for what you do, rather than for what you are. Joan does not explain why she does not do the chores, but it seems most likely that angry resentment keeps her from doing what she is told. She illustrates her (at least partially realistic) awareness that her resistant position may result in the loss of her security. It seems fairly obvious that Joan was about to say the girl's mother or father, rather than the maid, threw her out of the home.]

Card 4 (A woman is clutching the shoulders of a man whose face and body are averted as if he were trying to pull away from her.)
    I guess he's trying to leave her, and she doesn't want him to ... Cause they disagree on all their problems and have quarrels all the time. I guess that's all. ("Who are they?") Man and wife. ("How does it all end?") She tries to find a way of bringing him back. ("Then what happens?") I guess he comes back. ("How does she do it?) She promises that they won't have fights and start agreeing on things. ("What do they argue about most?") Oh, the bills and . . . . . other problems. [As on the Story Completion Test, Joan presents a theme involving marital conflict. As before, the conflict is resolved, this time when the wife offers to start agreeing on things and promises to avoid fighting with her husband.]

Card 5 (A middle-aged woman is standing on the threshold of a half-opened door looking into a room.)
    I guess she came downstairs, trying to find her daughter who had not been in bed when she looked. I guess that's all. ("What happened?") I guess the girl ran away. ("Why?") Because she wasn't being treated right. ("In what way?") She couldn't make any decisions for herself or buy her own clothes for herself or anything. ("How does it come out?") They decide she should have more freedom, and she comes back. [Adolescent TAT themes frequently involve complaints about parental unfairness and restriction. Until this point, Joan's marked lack of initiative has been stressed, but now she complains that her parents do not permit her the initiative that she feels she should have. One wonders to what degree Joan's passivity is parentally induced or encouraged, and to what degree Joan's parents simply respond to characteristics which they find present in her. The fantasy of running away from "unfair" parents is often seen among adolescents. Once again, the situation is saved by the one side's giving in, thus avoiding a "divorce" between parents and child. One feels quite certain by now that there is considerable turmoil going on within Joan's family, turmoil to which Joan responds primarily through negativism and fantasied wish fulfillments.]

Card 6 GF (A young woman, sitting on the edge of a sofa, looks back over her shoulder at an older man with a pipe in his mouth who seems to be addressing her.)

I guess he's asking her to marry him, but she doesn't want to. Cause she feels they have nothing in common. Guess that's all. ("What happens then?") He decides that she isn't the right one for him, and they don't get married. ("What don't they have in common?") They have completely different jobs. They don't agree on anything. [Once again Joan presents the theme of a basic incompatibility between an adult man and woman.]

Card 7 GF (An older woman is sitting on a sofa beside a girl, speaking or reading to her. The girl, who holds a doll in her lap, is looking away.)

(She sighs.) I guess it's getting close to Christmas, and she wishes she had a new doll, but her mother and father can't afford it ... because they're such poor people and don't have much to give away. I guess that's all. ("How does it end?") The neighbors get together and chip in and buy her a beautiful doll. [This time the theme of deprivation is somewhat differently put. The little girl's parents do not give to her, even though they apparently wish they could. The daughter is able to gain her wish through the intervention of well-intentioned persons outside her immediate family.]

Card 10 (A young woman's head against a man's shoulder.)

They're sad because their son's been kidnapped ... and was not found in his bed that morning. So they call the police, and after days and days they finally find him. That's all. ("How did all that happen?") He went to bed, and this woman wanted a little boy, so she broke in and took him. ("What happened to her?") She was put in jail. ("Why did she want him?") Cause she couldn't have any children, and she'd lost her little boy. [Parents (i.e., Joan's) will be sorry when they lose their child to a woman who really wants him (her).]

Card 12 F (The portrait of a young woman. A weird old woman with a shawl over her head is grimacing in the background.)

This old lady put some wicked ideas in this young girl's mind, and she almost committed murder, but her friend stopped her. I guess that's all. ("What was the murder all about?") This lady wanted to get rid of this young lady, and the only way she could do it was to have her put in jail or something. ("Why did she want to get rid of her?") So she could be in the house alone. ("What are they to one another?") Grandmother and granddaughter. ("Why does the grandmother want to be alone?") So she could do things for herself. ("What happens to the grandmother?") She gets taken away to an old persons' home. [The theme of mother-daughter antagonism comes out clearly. Joan seems to feel that her mother wants to be rid of her, so that the mother can rule the home without interference. "Her friend stopped her" again suggests how helpless Joan feels about controlling herself.]

Card 12 M (A young man is lying on a couch with his eyes closed. Leaning over him is a gaunt form of an elderly man, his hand stretched out above the face of the reclining figure.)

This is a wicked doctor, and he doesn't want his patient to get well because this young fellow knows that he is a wicked doctor and would tell the police. That's all. ("What's happening right now?") He's trying to make him die, I guess. ("How does the story end?") He thinks he's dead, but when he leaves, the boy goes and tells the police, and the wicked doctor is put in jail. ("How is the doctor wicked?") He doesn't cure people. He makes them worse. [This seems to be a fairly clear transference reference: i.e., Joan thinks the testing procedure does not and cannot help her. The "wicked doctor," probably, is not only the examining psychologist and psychiatrist, but Joan's father as well. After all, under the guise of helping her, the father is responsible for exposing her to this unpleasant examining procedure. She and her father are probably not at all agreed about the things the father claims will be of help to Joan.]

Card 13 MF (A young man is standing with downcast head buried in his arm. Behind him is the figure of a woman lying in bed.)

This is a man and his wife. And he has just killed her because they can't get along together, and he wants to be free from her without getting a divorce. Guess that's all. ("What happens then?") He gets caught and taken away by the police. ("What was the trouble between them?") They always have fights and can't get along together, and she wanted a divorce, and he didn't, so he killed her. ("Why didn't he want a divorce?") Because it would have caused too much trouble. [Striking are both the grossness of Joan's solution to the couple's marital problem and the naïveté with which she describes their differences. It is apparent what violent things can happen when reflective thought is relatively absent and when personal problems can be sketched out in only the most primitive fashion. Almost no reflection is described as taking place in this situation, and vague feelings are immediately translated into explosive, irrevocable acts. Since Joan has hardly any action-attenuating reflection available to her, it seems likely that she resorts too easily to thoughtless, gross actions whose consequences she does not consider beforehand. Here is an extreme example of marital disharmony.]

Card 18 GF (A woman has her hands squeezed around the throat of another woman whom she appears to be pushing backwards across the banister of a stairway.)

This is a mother and her daughter, and the daughter is very ill. And she (mother) wants to get her to a hospital as soon as possible. Soon after that she (daughter) gets well and comes home again. ("What's happening now?") She has had another attack. ("What kind of an attack?") Her heart. ("What happens eventually?") She comes home. ("And then?") That's all. [Although Joan talks about physical aggression between man and woman (i.e., husband and wife, mother and father), she evades describing the blatantly pictured aggression between a mother and her daughter. On the contrary, she transforms into helpfulness what is most often interpreted as violence.]

Card 16 (Blank card.)

There is a man and his wife. And they have a child, and this child has cancer. And after three months, it dies . . . . . . And they adopt another child to replace the one they lost. That's all. ("How did they feel about all that?") Just—okay. [It is surprising to see that Joan can make up a story when she has practically no external stimulation to encourage fantasy. Although her story is brief, she is nevertheless able to tell about what seems to be on her mind: the replacement of one child (her present self?), by another, ideal, healthier person, who will give her parents pleasure and who also will derive more pleasure from her life.]

SENTENCE COMPLETION TEST II

(She speaks in a very low voice.)

She hoped that when she grew up she would be a good person.

Her parents loved her very much. [Does Joan truly feel this way?]

When she saw what the other kids were doing she went and joined them.

When she compared herself to her friends she was different in all ways. [Joan apparently sees herself as different, not only from her parents and other adults, but from her peers as well.]

She was sad whenever she thought of leaving her parents. [While, on the one hand, she has TAT fantasies of runing away from home, she thinks, on the other, how lost she would feel without her parents.]

When she was asked about her aches and pains . . . . she was embarrassed.

The person she admired most was her mother. ("Why was that?") I don't know. [The preconscious denial may be too brittle to handle specifics.]

Her brother annoyed her. ("Why was that?") I don't know. [Joan's "I don't know" repudiates the impulsive first revelations she makes about feelings she has toward her intimate family.]

When the boy kissed her she was happy.

When her father came into the room it lit up.

When she was her sister . . . I don't know. ("Finish it in some way.") She was angry. ("Why was that?") I don't know.

At school she had to work.

When she looked at the work the other students were doing she also went to work.

She was very happy when she went on a trip.

The thing she found hardest to do was to study.

Whenever certain things really bothered her she went for help. [It is much more likely that Joan sits quietly and waits for help to come to her.]

Her dreams came true. ("What were they?") I don't know. [The omnibus "I don't know" allows Joan to maintain a closed front to the surroundings.]

When she saw that the man had left the money behind she picked it up. ("And?") And returned it.

She thought that her mother was going to town. [This evasive ending suggests that Joan, even consciously, does not always think of her mother as "the person she admired most."]

Whenever she and her family disagreed she went in her room. [This probably is not a rare occurrence.]

When she was very little she played in the sand pile.

Her best friend stayed on out with her. ("Stayed on out where?") All night. ("What were they doing?") I don't know. [Although such semi-"delinquent" behavior may take place only in fantasy, one would not be much surprised if it actually happened. Joan has so little awareness about the consequences of her actions that she can make others very concerned about her and have no realization that anything is amiss.]

She was unhappy with her father when he disagreed with her.

When her mother asked about her boy friend she changed the subject. [Or said, "I don't know"?]

She never thought she would be able to have a career. ("Why is that?") I don't know. [The ubiquitous "I don't know."]

She always hoped that she could have a dog one day. [A modest wish.]

What she liked best about herself . . . . I don't know. [Joan probably likes almost nothing about herself.]

Her mother was more likely than her father to tell her off.

Her sister got into her jewelry.

When she had nothing else to do she rode around. ("How do you mean?") In the car.

She thought that her intelligence was not very good.

What she liked best about school . . . . . was history class.

When she couldn't see a way out of her problem she turned to someone else.

She saw the cockroach on the wall and ran away. [This is a very unusual response and suggests that Joan may suffer from phobic concerns.]

Her teacher punished her. ("Why was that?") I don't know (she smiles).

Whenever she got angry she went to her room. [This is the second time on this test that Joan says that an angry atmosphere causes her to withdraw.]

She remembered that when she was little she was liked very much. [This ending suggests Joan feels that a long time ago things were a great deal better than they are now. Rather than remain in her present unpleasant situation, Joan may try to turn time back to an earlier, happier era; or, realizing she cannot recapture the past this way, she may try to skip the remainder of her adolescence and leap prematurely into adulthood. Considering her unproductive efforts so far, it is doubtful that Joan's "adolescent solution" will involve optimal maturation. Most likely, she will try to push headlong into adulthood by continuing to close herself off to most inner (and external) experience.]

After school she usually . . . . went to The Fairy Land. ("What's that?") A drug store. [Joan's assumption that the examiner knows what she means by this private reference once again reflects her naïveté.]

She admired her father when he settled his problems.

When the boy invited her to his party she went.

When she and her brother were together . . . . . I don't know (she whispers). [Joan is exceedingly protective about revealing most aspects of her relationship with her brother.]

She thought that her body was not right. ("In what way?") I don't know.

When she had a lot of homework to do she did it.

What she disliked about school was algebra.

Whenever she spoke about her problems to someone they ignored her. [Although it initially appears that Joan is explaining the reason for her not telling her problems to others, her "reason" is probably a rationalization. Even if she were not "ignored," it is difficult to think of Joan's revealing herself to the point of speaking to any "strange" adult about what troubles her.]

When she entered the haunted house she was scared.

When the other girl offered her a cigarette she refused.

She didn't like her mother to tell on her. ("How do you mean?") . . . . ("Tell who?") Other people. [The examining team?]

When the baby arrived she was glad.

Whenever she didn't do what she was told . . . . . she went riding. [Avoidance again.]

What would make her angriest . . . . . I don't know. [Some more avoidance.]

In her spare time she played records.

What troubled her most was going to school.

When she was alone in her room at night she would make monkeys. ("How was that?") Out of socks.

What scared her most was when she left home. [Joan once again tells how frightened she is of entering adulthood.]

She struck the match and blew it out. [Impulse is quickly curbed.]

She disliked her father when he told her to go to her room.

She thought that her looks were not so good. [In many ways Joan tells about the low opinion she has of herself. She has already mentioned that she thinks her body is "not right," that her intelligence is "not very good," that she does not know what she likes about herself, and that she does not think she will ever be able to have "a career."]

The thing she could do best was making friends.

She had no respect at all for her brother. [Negative feelings toward her brother are being spoken about more openly now.]

She always enjoyed dancing.

She had a very uncomfortable feeling when she went to a picnic. ("Why was that?") I don't know.

She found it easiest to talk to her friend.

Word Association Test

(While she is taking this test, she is tensely peeling her fingernail polish.)

React. Time (in Secs.)	Stimulus	Response	Recall	Recall Time (In Secs.)	Inquiry and Comments
18	1. *hat*	I don't understand. (I explain the task again.) You said "hat?" ("That's right.") Girl.	man	6	[Patients whose personality is organized along a repressive dimension frequently "don't understand" what they are supposed to do on this test. Their not understanding is usually a way of expressing reluctance to respond speedily and spontaneously, reluctance to enter a situation which gives them relatively little opportunity to guard against self-revelation.]

React. Time (in Secs.)	Stimulus	Response	Recall	Recall Time (In Secs.)	Inquiry and Comments
1	2. lamp	shade	√		
1½	3. love	boy	√	2	
1½	4. book	teacher	√	4½	[Joan reacts fairly quickly on the first portion of the test, but an increasing tendency to block is apparent on Recall. After the word "stomach" on the Recall section (No. 34, below), it can be seen both how Joan's reaction times tend to be longer and how she has greater difficulty recalling the word she gave before. While Joan's proneness to repress makes efficient recall difficult for her, it is also probable that her less efficient performance on the Recall section is related to gradually mounting tension. Joan's tension rises as she continues to be asked to respond to fuzzily structured (i.e., projective) material. She finds her defenses less effective than usual when she must deal with this sort of assignment, and as her defenses lose effectiveness, her tension mounts.]
1	5. father	mother	√		
1	6. paper	book	√	2½	[The sporadic rise and fall of reaction times, occurring

React. Time (in Secs.)	Stimulus	Response	Recall	Recall Time (In Secs.)	Inquiry and Comments
					without obvious reason, is often a sign of rather significant underlying disorganization. In Joan's case, the unpredictable reaction times may well reflect the sporadic ebb and flow of her repressive process.]
	7. breast (omitted)				[Most words with outright sexual denotations were omitted. It was felt that such words would be too disorganizing for Joan.]
1½	8. curtains	window	√		
2	9. trunk	car	√	2	
2½	10. drink	coke	√	2½	
1	11. party	dress	√		("Do you like parties?") M'hm. ("What do you like best about them?") Oh, I don't know. ("What do you think?") . . . Dancing, I guess. ("Are you a pretty good dancer?") Fairly, I guess.
1	12. spring	time	√		[This type of "phrase completion" is typical of persons who wish to avoid the spontaneity of "true" association.]
	13. bowel movement (omitted)				
1	14. rug	floor	√	3	
1	15. boy friend	girl	girl friend	2	

React. Time (in Secs.)	Stimulus	Response	Recall	Recall Time (In Secs.)	Inquiry and Comments
1	16. *chair*	table	√	2	
1½	17. *screen*	door	√		[Another "phrase completion."]
	18. *penis* (omitted)				
4	19. *radiator*	house	√		[Here is an example of a rather extreme and quite unaccountable increase in initial reaction time. Joan could not see the omitted word, *penis,* and therefore was not reacting to it.]
2½	20. *frame*	picture	What? ("Frame.") √	7	[The sudden mishearing or not hearing of a word is another hallmark of a "hysterical" organization.]
1	21. *suicide*	girl	√		("What were you thinking of with 'suicide'?") Oh, a girl committed suicide. ("Did you know her?") No. ("How did it happen?") Oh, I don't know. ("How did you find out about it?") Our Home Ec. teacher told us about it. ("Do you know why the girl did it?") Yes. ("Why was it?") Oh, she had a baby, and she got married, and she couldn't stand it, so she committed suicide.
2½	22. *mountain*	tree	√	9	[Is this a delayed reaction to suicide?]

React. Time (in Secs.)		Stimulus	Response	Recall	Recall Time (In Secs.)	Inquiry and Comments
1	23.	*snake*	bite	√	2½	("Are snakes kind of scary?") Yeah. ("Have you ever seen any?") Yes. ("Poisonous ones?") Uh-huh. (She tells how, in the countryside, she saw snakes roaming around in the open.)
1½	24.	*house*	yard	√	3	
	25.	*vagina* (omitted)				
1½	26.	*tobacco*	purse	√		("What was your thought on 'tobacco'?") Lots of men have a little purse where they keep their tobacco.
1½	27.	*mouth*	lips	√		
1½	28.	*horse*	cow	√		
	29.	*masturbation* (omitted)				
1	30.	*wife*	husband	√		
½	31.	*table*	chair	√		
1	32.	*fight*	boys	√		("What was your thought on 'fight-boys'?") They usually fight.
1	33.	*beef*	cow	√		
2	34.	*stomach*	boy	√	9	("What happened on 'stomach'?") I don't know.
1½	35.	*farm*	animal	√	2½	
1½	36.	*man*	wife	What? ("Man.") Women.		
1½	37.	*taxes*	paper	√	5	("What did you have in mind on 'taxes'?")

React. Time (in Secs.)	Stimulus	Response	Recall	Recall Time (In Secs.)	Inquiry and Comments
					I don't know. [It is becoming increasingly clear that inquiry with Joan leads to very little.]
1	38. nipple	bottle	√		
1	39. doctor	nurse	√		
1	40. dirt	clean	mud	16	("What happened on 'dirt'?") (She laughs.) I don't know (she laughs again). ("Why do you laugh?") I don't know. [Neither the Recall delay nor the reason for Joan's laughter become apparent.]
2	41. cut	heal	What did you say? ("Cut.") Hand.	13	[Joan's question apparently attempts to disguise the reason for her delay—a reason which seems somehow associated with the preceding word, dirt.]
2	42. movies	seat	pictures	2	
1	43. cockroach	bite	√		
6	44. bite	Huh? ("Bite.") Oh—snake.	√		
½	45. dog	cat	√		
1	46. dance	boy	√		
1	47. gun	bang	√	3	[This is a rather primitively conceptualized association.]
1	48. water	cup	dirt	2	
½	49. husband	wife	√		
1½	50. mud	dirt	√	3½	

React. Time (In Secs.)	Stimulus	Response	Recall	Recall Time (In Secs.)	Inquiry and Comments
2	51. woman	girl	man	2	
1	52. fire	house	√	4	("What happened on 'fire'?") I was thinking of firehouse.
5	53. suck	sucker	√	1	
1½	54. money	dollars	bag	3	("What happened on 'money'?") Bag, that's where you usually keep money. [Inquiry continues to be not particularly revealing.]
1½	55. mother	father	√	2	
1	56. hospital	bed	√		
1	57. girl friend	boy friend	√		
2	58. taxi	man	cab	4	("What happened on 'taxi'?") A man drives a taxi.
	59. intercourse (omitted)				
1½	60. hunger	children	√	2	("What were you thinking about with 'hunger'?") Children are hungry. [It is apparent that Joan understands inquiry in only the most literal sense. For her, inquiry is not a way to try to understand psychological phenomena connected with a response. Joan interprets whatever she says at face value; in that sense, she is not in the least psychologically minded.]

THE PSYCHOLOGIST'S REPORT

Joan's ways of thinking indicate that she is exceedingly constricted and severely repressive. Sometimes these two ways of functioning are complicated by a conscious, stubborn withholding, but it would be an oversimplification to dismiss her unresponsiveness primarily as conscious willfulness. It seems that Joan rarely starts out being purposely resistant; rather, this attitude unfolds as she finds herself in difficulties because repression permits so few thoughts to enter her mind. The extent of Joan's repressiveness makes it very difficult, occasionally impossible, for her to deal with whatever thinking task she is asked to perform. Typically, when she is required to look within herself, particularly at her feelings and motivations, Joan finds herself unable to proceed. She dismisses questions which require her to introspect with an almost automatic, "I don't know."

The combination of constriction, repression and conscious withholding is dramatically evident in Joan's Rorschach performance. The Rorschach, of course, threatens repression to a major degree, so that defenses which are ordinarily depended on become particularly emphasized. Joan gives two weak responses (i.e., "a bug," "a body") to the first card of the Rorschach and is almost unable to describe these during the inquiry. She cannot (does not?) produce a single additional response on any of the subsequent cards. Even when Popular areas are pointed out and named, her reaction is, "Well, it doesn't look that way to *me*." She responds with somewhat more freedom to the Thematic Apperception Test, perhaps because this task is more structured, or perhaps because the TAT was administered the last day, when she knew the entire examination would soon be over. Joan's nongivingness obviously can and does make others angry, but the degree to which her withholding involves *primarily* motivated aggression is still an open question.

Although both conscious and unconscious negativism play some role, the major part in Joan's constriction seems to be attributable to intense repression. Such an inference is partly borne out by Joan's Wechsler-Bellevue, on which she achieves a score in the Dull Normal range (Verbal Intelligence Quotient 84-87; Performance Quotient 89-90; Total Quotient 85-87). The consequences of her repressive needs to eliminate or shut out may be seen in her gaps of information, as well as in the naïveté with which she approaches problem situations. She has no idea who was president of the United States before Eisenhower (to whom, by the way, she refers as "Ike"). She knows the names of no Italian or Japanese cities and has never heard of *Hamlet*. Asked what the heart does, she replies, "Beats"; further questioning elicits only that "It keeps us alive." She knows no intellectual curiosity and gives no evidence that she has a need to derive or understand any sorts of meaning. Her contentment with superficial appearances is exemplified in the story she tells to her incorrect sorting of the *Taxi* sequence on Picture Arrangement: "Walking along with this dummy, I guess. And he gets in this car. He was riding . . . . . ('what happened?') She was close to him, and she got further away and got back close to him. ('What was that all about?') I don't know." Not only does she not know; it is quite clear that she does not particularly care, either.

Her reluctance to go below the psychological surface of things, and her use of conventional, "good," socially approved standards as a way to judge events, can be seen in her Story Completion: *He was angry and getting angrier by the minute.* (She then writes:) "He and his wife had a very serious disagreement. They want a devoirse, but a girl friend toll them thats not the answer so they stay together and live happyily ever after and they were good to each other." This brief story is like a child's tale, based on wish fulfillment rather than on psychological truth. While her dependence on conventional (external) guideposts allows Joan to achieve a higher than average score on the Comprehension subtest, her inability to look inward causes her to obtain a weighted score of only 3 on the Arithmetic subtest.

Joan's lack of intellectual drive and creative energy is reflected in her BRL performance. Her "active" sortings on Part I are marked by major constriction on almost every item. Sometimes Joan adds only a single object, when she experiences two failures. On the "passive" (Part II) section, where she has to find the concept that unites items which have been sorted for her, she is able to give seven excellent conceptual definitions in a row. That more than uncomplicated repression interferes with Joan's optimal performance is suggested by the fact that, once I praise her good performance, she immediately fails three items and gives two less adequate definitions. Such behavior makes it apparent that Joan fears being successful; when she inadvertently permits success to come her way, the fact must not be stated in so many words. If anyone should happen to become aware of her competence, she must quickly reaffirm her inadequacy.

That she is potentially able to do better than average work is suggested by her behavior on several of the Wechsler subtests. She misses *a better than average* score on these by a hair's breadth— because of some careless errors, or because of a tendency to spoil what she has already completed successfully. It seems clear that Joan finds it necessary to avoid appearing capable. Whenever others (and she herself) might be tempted to consider her adequate, she is impelled quickly to undo such an impression.

Regarding Joan's conflicts with her parents, an apparent paradox is evident. Consciously she describes intimacy, love and admiration. For example, she offers the following Sentence Completions:

Her parents loved her very much.
What scared her most was when she left home.
She was sad whenever she thought of leaving her parents.
The person she admired most was her mother.
When her father came into the room it lit up.

While conscious feelings toward her parents are stated in this positive way, more hidden feelings, which emerge on the Thematic Apperception Test, are of quite another sort. On the TAT, Joan seems to express much resentment and anger toward her parents who, she feels, take initiative away from her, so that they do not permit her even to choose her own clothes. Joan's stories describe family relationships which are always marked by the family members' inability to get along with each other. In these stories (i.e., in fantasy), Joan solves the problem of escaping from the argumentative family atmosphere by running away from home. In order to get back a child who has run away, or a husband who is thinking of leaving, the story parents or wife promise to change their ways and to stop arguing, so that all ends happily. Withdrawal and running away are Joan's most common ways of dealing with unpleasant emotional situations at home. But often this kind of avoidance still does not manage the trick of making her situation better. When withdrawal and running away do not work, more extreme measures are required. For example, Joan's test material suggests that she sometimes considers the solution to her unhappy lot to lie in magically starting everything over again—remaking her parents, her brother, herself, everything.

Joan expresses conscious anger toward her brother quite freely, and one reason for Joan's hidden anger toward her mother may have to do with the unwanted appearance of this younger brother. In Joan's stories, the kidnapping of a baby son appears with impressive frequency. It may well be that the antagonism Joan feels toward her brother serves, in part at least, as the paradigm of all relations between the sexes, relations which consist primarily of fights that are resolved only after the woman gives in to the man. The models for this sort of relationship may, of course, also very well be Joan's parents.

In summary, Joan manifests a hysterical organization, marked particularly by affective and intellectual constriction, repression, passivity and negativism. She functions intellectually in the Dull Normal range, but there seems little doubt that her intellectual functions are considerably affected by the repressive and withholding defenses, as well as by her need to avoid appearing adequate.

Although Joan might well be helped through a psychotherapeutic process, a therapist will encounter immense resistances, certainly at the beginning. Joan's view of therapy as a destructive process is suggested by her Thematic Apperception story to the "Hypnosis" card. Here, she tells of a "wicked doctor" who is trying to kill a boy who knows the doctor's secret—i.e., that the doctor makes people worse. The boy can avoid destruction only by having the doctor put away.

DISCUSSION

Joan's protocol exemplifies the effects of constriction, repression, inhibition and negativism. At times one feels most unprofessionally tempted to shake her in order to force her to respond in the ways one is (erroneously) convinced she "actually can." One is never altogether sure to what extent Joan (a) is genuinely helpless because of the attenuating effects of the repression, or (b) willfully holds back what one is convinced she knows or is capable of doing. One finds oneself in the continual dilemma of trying to understand Joan's not doing more than what she is doing, while at the same time trying to understand and deal effectively with one's own angry reaction to her apparent unwillingness to cooperate.

How will Joan deal with the task of growing into adulthood? At the moment she partly handles it by rejecting her adolescence. Childhood, she tells us, was a fine time, during which she was surrounded by love. Adulthood will be a fine time again; she will be her own mistress, will have her own house and possessions, and she will no longer have to do the chores which she finds so unpleasant. Joan is shunning the psychological work required for dealing with adolescence. When she does halfheartedly try to face the problems of growing up, she finds herself up against the equally unsatisfactory quasi solutions of throwing herself either back into the "remembered" happiness of childhood, or forward into the imagined joys of adulthood. Whichever of these possibilities she chooses, she avoids dealing with the essential-to-solve stresses of the present. In other words, she avoids the painful period when feelings, impulses, values are unstable and insecure, when a variety of solutions should be experimented with, when she would have to experience pain as she left herself vulnerable to the violent psychological eruptions which inevitably characterize this period. If she persists in her present course, she will continue to stand apart, to avoid involving herself in the essentials of ongoing life experiences about which she could reflect, accepting those she found suitable and rejecting those that would not substantially add to her life or that could disrupt it.

Helen's protocol, which follows, reflects a psychological organization which, although similar to Joan's in significant ways, has a number of dissimilar features. Like Joan, Helen has a tendency to avoid both serious thought and serious self-contemplation. But while Joan is behaviorally constricted, Helen is the opposite: she is highly active, both verbally and in other behavior, and relates herself "intrusively" to others. Unlike Joan, Helen rarely takes an interpersonal back seat. She almost always assumes the initiative with others and does much more than simply react to whatever or whomever she comes (or brings herself) face-to-face with. It is once again apparent that similar internal propensities can be modified by other mechanisms in ways that create an apparently different final organization.

CLINICAL SUMMARY: Helen

Helen is fourteen years old and an only child. The referring physician indicates that, while Helen has always been "difficult," she has lately become openly and actively resentful of her mother. She has been physically abusive and a severe management problem.

Helen's parents were delighted when the mother became pregnant, and they very much looked forward to having a child. Except for some edema and calcium deficiency which required medical attention, the pregnancy was normal. The mother knows nothing about the delivery, but it appears to have taken place without difficulty. In early infancy, Helen is described as having been sickly and anemic; she had many colds and some violent allergies. At the age of three months, she had severe vomiting and diarrhea, and was lethargic. Following this difficult start, Helen seemed to develop well, and she is now described as "always on the go."

Helen has always required a good deal of supervision. Early in life she began to have tantrums whenever she could not get her way; in retrospect, her mother feels that Helen was "spoiled rotten." Helen often held her breath while she screamed and kicked the floor; she broke things and banged her head. Although her temper outbursts were not frequent, they were extremely severe. When Helen was between four and five, the family doctor suggested that the mother throw water in her face whenever she held her breath. The mother did this, but Helen's behavior only became more disorganized.

At three-and-a-half, Helen attended nursery school. She seemed to enjoy the experience and to get along well with the other children. From the first grade on, she received additional help at home with her school work. She always brought home A's and B's on her report cards. She was talented in music, although she was unable to maintain attention long enough to learn anything well. Gradually, she began to show a lack of interest in various activities, and her attention span became increasingly short.

At about the age of ten, Helen began to develop physically and to menstruate. She hated menstruation and even now still screams and becomes angry at the onset of each period.

Her behavior over the past year has become increasingly more impulsive, hostile and uncontrollable. She has been opposing her parents at home, and her behavior has embarrassed them in the community. For example, when they did not allow her and a girl friend to go to an all-night picture show, Helen bought sleeping pills and threatened to commit suicide, "because you are so mean to me." She became increasingly difficult to control: occasionally she ran away from home and once, in a fit of anger, she drew a butcher knife on her father, who had to wrestle with her to get the knife away. Another time, while riding with her mother, she became so angry that she threw her mother's shoes from the car and then hit her, so that her mother had to stop by the edge of the road and have a friend drag Helen home. Once, in a fit of rage, Helen threw two gallons of milk around the kitchen, tore down the kitchen racks and ran from the house in panic. On another occasion, Helen hit another car when she was driving (although she was not legally of age to drive), and then left the scene of the accident. Most recently, she ran away with an adolescent boy and was gone for three days. The couple first stole gasoline for a new convertible and later were involved in an accident and wrecked the car.

Helen threatened to "boycott" the diagnostic examination. She said there was nothing wrong with her that could not be cured by her parents' giving her the freedom to do what she wanted.

Physical, Neurological and Laboratory Examinations: Physical examination, serology and urinalysis were not done because of Helen's objections. All other examinations were within normal limits.

THE PSYCHOLOGIST'S DESCRIPTION

Helen attempted to establish control from the moment she first laid eyes on me. She used every bit of seductive charm she could muster, and I was surprised to see so much laughter and teasing blandishment, instead of the angry defiance which her clinical history had led me to expect. After our first meeting, she consistently came dressed in shorts and in other ways that displayed her considerable physical charms. She frequently touched me and gave me playful pats on the arm; occasionally she leaned on me to see what I might be writing; once she stroked my arm in what seemed intended as an absent-minded gesture. Her warehouse of seductive devices also included flattery, pleading, cajolery and an attitude of wishing to please in all matters. Whenever she wanted something, she pursued the quest with great insistence, and I vividly experienced how difficult Helen's parents must find it to deal with her insistent wishes.

Helen's relationship to the tests and to me was affective, hyperemotional and histrionic, rather than objective, thoughtful and intellectual. Her language was filled with exaggerations and with self-directed verbal attacks. Throughout the interviews she often announced how "dumb" she was, thereby indirectly requesting my reassurance that this low self-conception was without foundation. She continually questioned me about her Intelligence Quotient and indicated that she doubted that I would treat what she was telling me as confidential. In spite of my efforts to deal with her worries about such matters, her fears never seemed to abate. It became increasingly evident that Helen did not ask her many questions because she was interested in any objective answers; instead, she was trying to establish an interaction in which she could be the little girl who demanded reassurance from a male on whom she had projected "masterful" qualities.

Helen displayed great concern about my verbatim recording. She constantly checked to see what I was writing and just as constantly expressed fear that I would share her test material with her parents. She (correctly) thought that her TAT stories, for example, would present me with insights into her thoughts, and concluded that it would therefore be best not to tell me certain portions of her stories. Were I to note what was on her mind, I would surely suggest that she be sent to an "insane hospital." Her reluctance to let me know what she was thinking was particularly marked on TAT pictures which could be even vaguely endowed with sexual meaning. Whenever such a picture appeared, Helen would laugh, flush, and turn the card over, saying, "I don't know."

THE WECHSLER-BELLEVUE SCALE

[The first noteworthy feature of Helen's Scattergram is that her Performance I.Q. is approximately ten points higher than the Verbal (although this relationship is due primarily to Helen's high Picture Arrangement performance). Verbal-Performance relationships of this type are most usually found in persons who tend to rely on activity rather than on thought to accomplish their purposes in day-to-day living. Picture Arrangement stands out from Helen's other fairly homogeneously distributed subtest performances. As will become more and more apparent, this higher Picture Arrangement score probably reflects Helen's alertness to situations that involve the behavior of others. In order to manage people in the way she wishes, Helen is sensitive to their motivations and is aware of how one action leads to the next. Significant, too, is Helen's Comprehension-Information pattern. Although Helen achieves an equally low score on both these subtests, her alternate score on Comprehension places this performance three points above Information. Such a pattern is consistent with that of persons who depend primarily on a repressive personality organization for defensive purposes. One of Helen's high scores is on Digit Span, a subtest which is ordinarily rather sensitive to felt tension. The fact that she does relatively well here suggests that she permits herself to feel little tension, and from what can be seen later, it seems likely that much of Helen's tension is dissipated in activity. With the exception of Picture Arrangement, Helen's subtest performance seems well integrated. Seven of her eleven subtest scores fall within three points of one another. Such a stable configuration suggests an absence of the impairing effects of internalized conflict.

[It is difficult to pin down to what extent Helen's Dull Normal→Average Verbal Quotient is the result of her tendency to repress, and to what extent the relatively low quotient finds a repressive organization most congenial to it. In any case, as is often true, Helen's repressive orientation is associated with a fairly low Verbal intelligence.]

Name: Helen   Age: 14-7

	RS	WTS	0 1 2 3 4 5 6 7 8 9 10 11 12 13 14 15 16 17 18 19 20
COMPR.	7-10	6-9	
INFOR.	8	6	
DIG.	12	10	
ARITH.	6	7	
SIMIL.	11	9	
VOCAB.	16	7	
P. A.	16	14	
P. C.	8-9	7-8	
B. D.	17	8	
O. A.	17	9	
D. S.	35	8	

TOT. VERB.	35-38
TOT. PERF.	46-47
TOT. SCALE	81-85

VERBAL I.Q.:   86-90   LEVEL: Dull Normal→Average

PERFORMANCE I.Q.:   97-98   LEVEL: Average

TOTAL I.Q.:   90-93   LEVEL: Dull Normal→Average

INFORMATION

No.	Question	Response and Comments	Score
1.	Who is the President of the United States?	President Eisenhower. ("And who was president before him?") Golly! Truman, I think . . Oh no! ("And who was president before that?") No, I'm telling you, I don't know any of that. That's proof of how smart I am in the world. (She seems quite tense.) [With this first response, Helen tells a good deal about herself. She reacts histrionically as she finds herself in intellectual difficulty, and she shows how quickly she gives up in the face of a relatively minor obstacle. She is quick to disclaim even everyday knowledge and promptly sets out to demonstrate how "dumb" she is. She makes no effort to think who might have been president before the one preceding the incumbent. She conveys, instead, that answering this type of question represents more of a demand on her than should rightfully be expected.]	+
2.	What is a thermometer?	It's a thing that reads the weather . . Or your temperature? ("Which do you think?") Well, it reads the degrees. [Available knowledge is vaguely and fuzzily organized.]	+
3.	What does rubber come from?	Trees, doesn't it? Trees and plants. [The "doesn't it?" reflects the helplessness Helen wishes to convey.]	+
4.	Where is London?	France. [This answer, given without hesitation, shows how uncritically Helen's knowledge is organized.]	—
5.	How many pints make a quart?	(She laughs.) I don't know. I should, gosh! ("What would you guess?") Six, I think. [Helen continues to demonstrate how uninformed she is about elementary matters. Is she as concerned to do well with this type of problem as her, "I should, gosh!" suggests?]	—
6.	How many weeks are there in a year?	I think . . Gosh, I'm so dumb. There's 365 days, I know that. There's twelve weeks in a year, isn't there? ("How many months are there?") Four. ("Four months in a year?") Twelve. ("How many weeks are there in a year?") Let's see . . forty-eight. Is that right? [Comments referring to her "dumbness" are possibly not altogether genuine; they may well represent a request that I deny that she is "dumb." She may be willing to think herself "dumb" in areas which she considers "unimportant."]	—

No.	Question	Response and Comments	Score
7.	What is the capital of Italy?	I don't know. I haven't any idea. ("Could you give me the name of any Italian city?") No . . Uh-uh. [Outside her personal sphere of operations, the world has little, if any, significance.]	−
8.	What is the capital of Japan?	I don't know (she smiles). We didn't study those. We studied about voting and all that. Congress and all that. Maybe I had it before. It proves how well it sinks in. ["Voting" and "Congress" have nothing to do, of course, with the capital of Japan.]	−
9.	How tall is the average American woman?	Oh . . about five feet five inches. [As questions touch on areas nearer Helen's own concerns, she is able to give a correct answer again.]	+
10.	Who invented the airplane?	Oh . . the Wright brothers.	+
11.	Where is Brazil?	In South America . . I think. South or North. I don't know which. I think it's South, though. [It can hardly be said that Helen's information is rigorously ordered.]	+
12.	How far is it from Paris to New York?	Oh gosh! About 2,000. [It is surprising suddenly to see this correct answer to a geographical question.]	+
13.	What does the heart do?	It sends blood through the rest of your body and keeps your body circulating. ("Keeps your body circulating?") Uh-huh. You know, because it pumps. It sends blood in the rest of the parts and keeps it circulating. [Although vaguely conceptualized and fuzzily worded, this response is probably more correct than not.]	+
14.	Who wrote Hamlet?	I don't know.	−
15.	What is the population of the United States?	Oh . . gosh! I just don't know. ("What would you guess?") Oh, about . . that would be dumber than anything. I guess about six or seven million.	−
16.	When is Washington's birthday?	Washington? Uh . . oh golly! Gee, I don't remember. I know we had that day off and everything. ("Do you remember what month it is?") I think it's either January or February. Probably it isn't either one. [Even referring to a situation which involved her personally and directly does not help this time.]	−
17.	Who discovered the North Pole?	I sure don't know.	−

No.	Question	Response and Comments	Score
18.	*Where is Egypt?*	..... I can't think of it. I know where it is. ("Could you give the continent?") What do you mean, continent? (I explain.) The north continent, I think. Is that right? (I list the continents.) I think Australia, isn't it? I don't know. I have no idea.	—
19.	*Who wrote Huckleberry Finn?*	I sure don't know.	—

(She does not know the remaining answers.)

RAW SCORE: ___8___

WEIGHTED SCORE: ___6___

COMPREHENSION

No.	Question	Response and Comments	Score
1.	*What is the thing to do if you find an envelope in the street, that is sealed, and addressed and has a new stamp?*	Uh .. if it had a return address, I'd try to return it, and if it didn't I'd take it to the post office.	0-1
2.	*What should you do if while sitting in the movies you were the first person to discover a fire (or see smoke and fire)?*	*Would* or *should?* (She underlines the distinction between "would" and "should" histrionically. I repeat the question.) Gosh .. Oh! .. I don't know. I'd go down, I guess. You shouldn't get everybody excited. Go down and call the fire department and those fire extinguidshers (*sic*) .. You use them .. if they had any .. and if they weren't too big. That's what I *should* do. But actually I'd probably sit there and yell "Fire! Fire!" (She laughs.) [Helen is aware of her tendency to resort to thoughtless, and therefore frequently destructive, action and of her inability to do much about this tendency.]	1
3.	*Why should we keep away from bad company?*	Oh .. because .. uh .. people consider you .. If they don't have a good reputation, people consider you what they consider them (i.e., the bad company). And if you're easily influenced, they might influence you. ("Which of those two answers would you choose?") People might think of you as they think of them .. because if you're strong enough, you won't be influenced (she yawns). [Helen may be telling how she defends herself against parental accusations.]	1-2
4.	*Why should people pay taxes?*	Well .. uh .. to support the government. [It is difficult to know whether this well-expressed response is thoroughly thought through.]	2

No.	Question	Response and Comments	Score
5.	Why are shoes made of leather?	(She laughs.) Well, I don't know .. ("Why do you think?") Let's see .. Well, wouldn't it be because .. uh .. They're warm .. I don't know. That's dumber than anything.	0
6.	Why does land in the city cost more than land in the country?	Land in the city is more valuable. ("Could you tell me some more?") You can build buildings on it .. and .. uh .. You can price it for higher. [Although Helen seems to have a valid idea in mind, she is unable to express it in scorable terms.]	0
7.	If you were lost in a forest (woods) in the daytime, how would you go about finding your way out?	Well I'd .. find my footprint and follow my way back.	0
8.	Why are laws necessary?	Well .. uh .. if there wasn't any laws, people would just run by .. wild. ("Why is that?") Because .. uh .. I mean, there'd be all sorts of things. No one would mind anything. There wouldn't be schools .. there wouldn't be uncivilized (sic). Do you have to write down everything I tell you? (She asks this anxiously.) ("I try to write down everything.") Gosh, it must be tiring. [Helen describes her anxiety about not being adequately controlled from outside. If there were no one to say "No," anything could happen. This is the second time on this subtest that she reveals a problem with using words correctly. She expresses anxiety about my writing down comments which, it later turns out, she fears I may convey to her parents.]	1
9.	Why does the state require people to get a license in order to be married?	I don't know. ("Why do you think?") Well, I mean! (She laughs.) Because of .. hm .. to .. to .. let's see .. Well, men .. There wouldn't be any divorces. Men might marry over and over, and women might marry over and over, and children would never know who their parents were. [Once Helen is able to get beyond the question's sexual implications which seem to trigger so much disturbing affect, she finds herself at a loss. The portion of her answer dealing with parentless children may reflect easily aroused feelings of helplessness.]	0-1
10.	Why are people who are born deaf usually unable to talk?	Because they never hear anyone else speak, and that's how you learn. [Another unexpectedly successful answer.]	2

RAW SCORE: 7-10

WEIGHTED SCORE: 6-9

DIGIT SPAN

(She correctly repeats seven Digits Forward and five Digits Backward. While she misses eight Digits Forward by a hair's breadth, she obviously finds six Digits Backward too difficult.) [Helen's perfectly adequate performance on this subtest suggests, as was already mentioned, either that she does not experience significant tension or that she dissipates tension by constantly expressing it in action.]

RAW SCORE: __12__

WEIGHTED SCORE: __10__

ARITHMETIC

(Helen achieves credit on the first seven problems, with the exception of Problem 3:)

No.	Problem	Time	Response and Comments	Score
3.	If a man buys eight cents worth of stamps and gives the clerk twenty-five cents, how much change should he get back?	15″	Oh .. let's see .. about nineteen? I'm just guessing. I'm dumb. Poor guy, he has to write down what I say. (I readminister this problem after Problem 8. She says:) Seventeen (12″). No! Seven .. wait! .. no, seventeen!	0
7.	If seven pounds of sugar cost twenty-five cents, how many pounds can you get for a dollar?	15″	Twenty-eight? Oh golly! ... yeah, I guess ..... Is that right? You can't tell me, can you? ["Oh golly" is Helen's typical declaration of helplessness. Her frequent need to ask whether she is "right" represents one of her ways of seeking approval (i.e., she gives the impression of caring how well she does). She knows the examiner cannot tell her if she is right or not, and she does not expect a literal answer.]	1
8.	A man bought a second-hand car for two-thirds of what it cost new. He paid $400 for it. How much did it cost new?	—	Do I have to work it out in my head? I can't. Let's see .. (First she tries to do the problem mentally; then she uses pencil and paper and figures out the wrong answer of 267.) I can't work problems in my head at all. [This is a "typical" helpless reaction of the overly repressive ("hysterical") person who is required to concentrate seriously. Helen knows she is supposed to work this problem in her head, as she did the others. Rather than do this more difficult mental work, however, she assumes an inept, incapable attitude, in this way justifying her use of pencil and paper. One can see that Helen bends the rules when existing ones do not fit her needs or desires.]	0

(She is unable to do the last two problems and declares her inability even to make a stab at them.)

RAW SCORE:	6
WEIGHTED SCORE:	7

SIMILARITIES

No.	Items	Response and Comments	Score
1.	Orange-banana	Both thruit (sic).	2
2.	Coat-dress	Clothes.	2
3.	Dog-lion	Animals. [This is Helen's last score of 2 on this subtest.]	2
4.	Wagon-bicycle	You can ride 'em . . ride in 'em, I should say. Ride on 'em.	1
5.	Daily paper-radio	They've got news.	1
6.	Air-water	Uh . . they're God-made things.	0
7.	Wood-alcohol	I don't know. ("Can you think of any way?") Uh-uh. [Helen's ability to think in abstract conceptual terms becomes increasingly ineffectual, beginning with the fourth response (i.e., as the two ideas are less easily integrated, because the differences between them become more pronounced). Only a brief reversal of Helen's difficulty with effective abstraction capacity is noted below.]	0
8.	Eye-ear	Oh . . they're things on you. [This response is crudely conceptualized and actually represents no great improvement over the two preceding ones. Still, the response is technically good enough to merit a score of 1.]	1
9.	Egg-seed	Uh . . You can . . uh . . They're born things. ("Would you explain what you mean?") Yeah . . If you're having . . A plant has a seed and then it has . . You know, it grows some more . . like plants. And a chicken can hatch an egg, and it grows into . . well . . a kind of plant, you know. They both develop into other things . . into things . . into animals . . into plants and animals . . Is a plant an animal? ("Do you think it is?") Oh, I'm dumb. [Helen's reaction reflects the lack of precision which characterizes her approach to somewhat more intellectually complex material. Although her answer is confusedly conceptualized, it merits a score of 1, from a purely formal standpoint.]	1
10.	Poem-statue	(Between the last item and this, she asks, "Do you think I'm dumb?") A statue brings back memories	1

No. Items	Response and Comments	Score
	of someone, maybe. And so does a poem. Don't let mother see this. She won't let me do anything. Do you think I'm dumb? [Even though Helen hopes I will contradict her, her real fear that she may be dumb is becoming increasingly obvious. She is trying to enlist my help in her fight against her mother.]	
11. *Praise-punishment*	They're alike because to praise someone you're telling them how good they are ... Gee, they're just the opposite! And to punish them, you're telling them how bad they are. ("Can you tell me a way they're alike?") Yeah, cause you're telling them. [Only after Helen has begun to answer the question do all its implications seem to sink in. It is as if Helen proceeded to this point without reflecting about the question. She responds immediately, quasi-automatically, almost without first thinking.]	0
12. *Fly-tree*	I don't know. ("Can you think of any way?") Uh-uh.	0

RAW SCORE: __11__

WEIGHTED SCORE: __9__

PICTURE COMPLETION

No. Item	Time	Missing	Response and comments	Score
1. *Girl*	2″	nose	The bones of her nose. [A peculiar formulation.]	1
2. *Face*	1″	mustache	Half a mustache (she laughs).	1
3. *Profile*	1″	ear	Ear.	1
4. *Card*	13″	diamond	There should be a five here (on one side). No, there shouldn't (she laughs). I don't know. [Although this error is understandable and occurs fairly frequently, it nevertheless comes about because of a nonthinking through of the available data.]	0
5. *Crab*	3″	leg	His head, I guess. I don't know. I've never seen that. It's a crab, isn't it? [Even though Helen does not recognize the animal—and many persons with a hysterical organization do not—a thoughtful viewing makes the crab's asymmetry obvious.]	0
6. *Pig*	8″	tail	(She laughs) I don't know .. Oh! His tail.	1

No.	Item	Time	Missing	Response and comments	Score
7.	Boat	10″	stacks	Part of the ship? ("What part?") The top, I guess. I don't know what you call it. ("What might it be?") I don't know. I'm just guessing. [Again and again the vagueness of Helen's perceptual organization is apparent.]	0
8.	Door	2″	knob	I don't know.	0
9.	Watch	15″	hand	The minute hand. ("Where would that be?") Right here (points incorrectly). No, it should be a second hand. (She means a sweep second hand.) No, right here, in this little thing (points correctly).	0-1
10.	Pitcher	9″	water	The rest of . . The stuff pouring down into the glass.	1
11.	Mirror	8″	reflection of arm	Her hand with the powder puff should be in the mirror. [This item is often failed. Perhaps because of her preoccupation with self-beautification, Helen is able to pass it. Once again, she does adequately in areas that are personally important to her, while she does much less well with tasks (such as the *Card*, the *Crab* and the *Boat*) which are of less personal relevance.]	1
12.	Man	10″	tie	His tie. Are you timing these? [This item, too, is often failed, but men are important to Helen.]	1
13.	Bulb	5″	thread (or prong)	The rest of the light bulb . . up here (she points to the top of the bulb).	0
14.	Girl	5″	eyebrow	The rest of her body . . the back of her neck. [In line with Item 11 and its discussion, one would expect Helen to solve this item correctly.]	0
15.	Sun	3″	shadow of man	His shadow. [This is a difficult item, but Helen solves it quickly. She seems to be more alert to pictures of people than to pictures of objects. With the exception of Item 14, she correctly completes all pictures that involve people.]	1

RAW SCORE: 8-9

WEIGHTED SCORE: 7-8

PICTURE ARRANGEMENT

No.	Item	Correct Order	Arranged Time Order		Story and Comments	Score
1.	House	PAT	4″	PAT	He was building a house.	2
2.	Holdup	ABCD	10″ 15″	ACBD ABDC	He pulled a holdup and got arrested. [Since Helen solves all the remaining arrangements correctly, her Picture Arrangement score would be even higher than it is, had she received credit for this item. Inquiry should have been made to find out why she arranged the pictures so that the criminal was in jail before he was brought before the judge. Not infrequently, however, persons working on this sequence understand the accused to be waiting for his trial in jail. If Helen sees the sequence in this way, her error may not be a serious one.]	0
3.	Elevator	LMNO	13″	LMNO	He was coming up the elevator.	2
4.	Flirt	JANET	20″	JANET	First this King was driving by . . the Little King. Then he saw this lady carrying something on her head. Then he stopped. Then he pointed back to them to stop. And then he asked her if she wanted a ride. And she said "No," so he got out and walked with her. [Helen fabulizes elements of the story, apparently in order to make matters clear to herself.]	3
5.	Taxi	SAMUEL	28″	SAMUEL	Gosh! Well, this man was carrying a statue down the street, and he called to this car to come and stop and pick him up. And when he got in, he was holding this statue, and it looked like they were . . uh . . they had their heads together. I guess	5

No.	Item	Correct Order	Arranged Time	Order	Story and Comments	Score
					someone teased him, so he got embarrassed. So then he moved her over a little ways. And then he moved her clear to the other side of the car. I like to do these tests. The kind I put together.	
6.	*Fish*	EFGHIJ	46″	EFGHIJ	The little fish . . I mean the Little King went fishing and pulled himself out a fine fish and stuck it in the hat . . I guess what you'd call it. Like, and then he stuck his pole in again and he got a second fish. Then he put *it* in the hat. And then he called to the man who was handing him a fish. [Even though the cards are no longer in front of her to help Helen check the precise details of her story, it is nevertheless a fairly significant distortion to say the King put the caught fish in his "hat," particularly since he is wearing his crown at the time. This distortion represents another example of Helen's somewhat cavalier attitude toward the way things actually are. Helen's better than average (and much better than *her* average) performance on Picture Arrangement reflects both her concern with the attitudes, thoughts and behaviors of people—i.e., her other-directedness—and her proneness to modify situations (not enough to distort reality too severely, but just enough to show she is not overly concerned with its "true" nature).]	4

RAW SCORE: 16

WEIGHTED SCORE: 14

(She asks many questions about the coming EEG examination. She wonders whether it will hurt her or mess up her hair. She says she thinks her mother should have an EEG.)

BLOCK DESIGN

No.	Time	Accur.	Description of Behavior and Comments	Score
A.	11″	Yes	(She does this easily.)	—
B.	29″	Yes	(Considerable trial and error, with some unusually conceived initial attempts to solve the problem.) Do you always have to put down what I ask you? I think I'm dumb. I am (she laughs). [Although she uses comments about being "dumb" as a sort of game, it is increasingly apparent how concerned she is about how intelligent she appears not only to others, but probably to herself as well. She wants to make sure the examiner will note how low an opinion of herself she says she has; she probably feels that she can negate the low opinion he might form of her by anticipating him. Whether she consciously thinks as badly of herself as she says is unclear.]	—
1.	11″	Yes	(No problems.)	4
2.	14″	Yes	(No significant problems.) I bet you could put these together fast. [Helen uses rather obvious flattery, probably so that the examiner will be kindly disposed and think well of her.]	4
3.	19″	Yes	(No significant problems.) Is there a trick to it? [Here is a trace of suspicious thinking. Helen is on guard against others' trickery.]	3
4.	40″	Yes	(Here she shows considerable doubt, hesitation and confusion.) What should be the time it takes you? What does AC (on the scoring sheet, the notation to check accuracy) stand for? [As Helen finds the going more difficult, she becomes increasingly alert to "irrelevancies" in the surroundings.]	3
5.	1′ 28″	Yes	(Initially she has all corners rotated but then realizes the corners are wrong and corrects them.) What is that you're writing? Read it, please. (She is very concerned about my notations.) [Helen is extremely alert to the examiner's writing. She is fearful, among other things, that he might use this sort of information about her to give a negative report to her parents.]	3
6.		No	(She tries out different ways to make the stripes but does not realize she has found the right way when she has. She finally heaves a big sigh and says:) It won't go. I can't do it! Look . . see? I'm too dumb. (She hesitates to continue even when I offer help.	0

No.	Time	Accur.	Description of Behavior and Comments	Score
			She expresses much concern about being "dumb." She wants to know whether I'll tell her how stupid she really is.)	
7.		No	(She has a great deal of difficulty here.) Are you dumb if you can't get these together? Oh (she whispers), I'm so dumb. Is any of this right? (Actually, at 2′ she has almost nothing right. She finally puts the design together in a planless, helter-skelter fashion.) Is that right? ("What do you think?") No (she laughs). [It is often difficult to separate Helen's real inability from pseudo inability. For example, she can easily recognize that her copy is not at all like its model, yet she asks with apparent sincerity whether her construction is correct. When she is asked to reflect on her question, however, she easily gives it up. Does she really initially not know whether what she has done is accurate?]	0

RAW SCORE: 17

WEIGHTED SCORE: 8

OBJECT ASSEMBLY

Item	Time	Accur.	Description of Behavior and Comments	Score
Manikin	22″	Yes	(She approaches this task impulsively, first putting the wrong arm pieces in the sockets, but then correcting these wrong placements.) [Helen does not act on the basis of an initial internal plan. Action comes first and is corrected only after it is found to be inadequate or inappropriate. In an almost literal sense, Helen leaps before she looks.]	6
Profile	1′ 3″ 1′ 30″	Yes	(Although she knows vaguely where to place the pieces, she does not fit them exactly and sometimes rotates them. She makes such comments as:) Does that go there? *You* know if it does or not (she laughs). (When one piece is still rotated, she says she is finished and asks:) Did I get that accurate? ("Almost.") What did I get wrong? ("Look at it a while.") (She sees her error and corrects it. She tells how worried she is about the "brain wave" test and wonders if "they" can read her mind. She says she thinks her mother is the one who is nuts and should have the test. She worries that her parents may see her Wechsler-Bellevue and watches closely to see what I write.) [Helen's reaction to this item nicely epitomizes her real and mock helplessness, her flirtatiousness, her impulsivity, her pseudo naïveté, her suspiciousness and her anger toward her mother.]	5

Item	*Time*	*Accur.*	*Description of Behavior and Comments*	*Score*
Hand	1' 28"	Yes	What is it? (Through apparent trial and error, she suddenly sees that she is putting together a hand. Once she sees what the pieces are supposed to make, she completes the item with little difficulty.) [Helen uses speech primarily as a space filler, as an outlet for tension. She does not seriously expect me to answer such questions as, "What is it?"]	6

RAW SCORE: _17_

WEIGHTED SCORE: _9_

DIGIT SYMBOL

(She draws the symbols fairly neatly and accurately, although she distorts one so that the gestalt is significantly different from its model.)

RAW SCORE: _35_

WEIGHTED SCORE: _8_

VOCABULARY

No.	Word	*Response and Comments*	*Score*
1.	*Apple*	A fruit.	1
2.	*Donkey*	A mule (she laughs).	1
3.	*Join*	To join together in a crowd . . to get together.	1
4.	*Diamond*	Something that's worth a lot of money. ("Would you tell me some more about it?") You find 'em in rings and in mines.	1
5.	*Nuisance*	A pest.	1
6.	*Fur*	Oh . . something on an animal . . that coats are made of.	1
7.	*Cushion*	Something to sit on. ("Could you tell me some more about it?") No (she laughs). ("Try to tell me something more about it.") Well, it's a pillow . . sometimes it's padded. [It hardly seems necessary to comment again on Helen's action orientation and on her unwillingness to reflect. As part of her wish to disarm through humor, she sometimes becomes somewhat aggressive.]	1
8.	*Shilling*	I don't know. ("Have you heard the word?") No, I haven't.	0
9.	*Gamble*	Oh . . to . . throw away something . . or make bets.	1
10.	*Bacon*	A meat (she laughs) . . a pig. Meat of a pig . . Is it? Is it a meat of a pig? Please tell me. [Helen's emphatic, high-pressure style makes it difficult for the	1

No.	Word	Response and Comments	Score
		examiner to maintain a casual approach, either to her or to the tests.]	
11.	Nail	Oh . . hm . . it's a long thing (she laughs) that you use to hold things together. [Her laughter is sexually suggestive, showing how easily Helen's sexual pre-occupations are aroused.]	1
12.	Cedar	Wood.	1
13.	Tint	To change color. [The usual tendency is to define this word as a noun; Helen's definition of it as a verb is consistent with her action orientation.]	1
14.	Armory	A building. ("Would you tell me some more?") Well, we've got an armory building in Tucson. Or else, you'll see trucks, and say "Oh, that belongs to the armory." I don't know what it is really.	0
15.	Fable	I don't know.	0
16.	Brim	Brim of a hat. ("What is that?") A thing of the hat (she motions correctly). A wide thing (she laughs). [Helen simply does not have sufficient words available to her, so she resorts to vaguely descriptive actions to help convey an idea.]	1
17.	Guillotine	I don't know.	0
18.	Plural	More than one.	1
19.	Seclude	I don't know.	0
20.	Nitroglycerin	I don't know. [This word ought to be at least somewhat familiar.]	0
21.	Stanza	I've heard of that. I don't know. I thought it was something in a phrase. ("What do you mean?") A sentence.	½
22.	Microscope	Something that makes things bigger. ("How do you mean?") Maggerfies (sic) them . . something. That's not what it's for, is it? So dumb.	1

(Helen can not define the remaining words.)

RAW SCORE: 15½

WEIGHTED SCORE: 7

[Helen's typical functioning on the Wechsler-Bellevue Scale provides enough diagnostic information for the clinician to gain a vivid picture of her personality organization. The remaining tests do little more than highlight aspects which so far may have remained relatively subdued, and suggest variations on themes which have already been outlined.]

THE BRL SORTING TEST

PART I

Stimulus	Patient's Sorting	Response and Comments	Score
1. Helen's choice: Ball	(See adjoining column.)	Why didn't you tell me I had to do that? (I.e., sort other items with the ball.) I would have picked something easier. You mean what it's made from, or what? What do you mean? (I repeat the instructions, "Any way you think they might go together.") I mean, an eraser is rubber, the cigar is rubber. (She adds the eraser; rubber cigar; red paper circle; file card; chalk; sink stopper.) (She picks up the bell, rings it and then adds the red circle; red plastic toy knife; fork and spoon.) I'll put this (toy knife) because it's red. I'll cut you apart with it (she smiles). The ball is for little children, so I'll put these little play toys. This is a little boy's or little girl's ball. And you know how little kids like to play with that. She might have been trying to draw a ball, and this is what she drew (red paper circle). Now, the rubber. We were at the manufacturing place, and a ball is made from rubber, isn't it? And this (rubber cigar) is rubber I think, and the eraser is rubber, I think, and this (sink stopper) is rubber. So they might all go together as being in a manufacturing place. So, now we're at school. And here's a ball a little child might play with. And the teacher might write with chalk. [Helen's sorting and description reflect her severe	Fabulized

Stimulus	*Patient's Sorting*	*Response and Comments*	*Score*
		lack of intellectual discipline, which has already been noted on the Wechsler-Bellevue. Her putting together (it can hardly be described as "sorting") of objects shows how little control she exerts over her activity, how little focus there is to it. Her "sortings" are make-believes which have almost no relation to what can be described as objective stability. Helen proceeds willy-nilly, now in this direction and now in that, wherever a particular impulse happens to push her.]	
2. *Fork*	(Spoon; knife; file card; sink stopper.) Could this (file card) be used for a napkin? Well, I'll pretend it is. ("Use it for what you think it really is.") You mean, it *has* to be this? It can't go into the fireworks with the rest?	Here they are set at the table. And then I wash them. We're eating in the kitchen tonight, so all this is in the sink. [So far on this test Helen underlines how she lacks concern for formal intellectual boundaries: her sortings are based almost exclusively on affective, "playlike," self-centered criteria. It seems almost as if, for Helen, the world has no formal reality except as it directly impinges on her in some way.]	Fabulized
3. *Corncob pipe*	(Rubber cigar; cigar; cigarette; matches.)	You smoke this, and smoke this, and this is the play cigar and you smoke it, or you pretend. And they have to be lighted, so you need matches. (She blows through the empty pipe. She expresses more of her concern about the EEG and playfully taps my elbow.)	Concrete Def.
4. *Bell*	(Lock; pliers; toy pliers.)	This is a bicycle bell on a bicycle. This is a lock .. You know, that you put on a bicycle. And these (pliers)	Concrete Def.

Stimulus	Patient's Sorting	Response and Comments	Score
		are things that you took in case you need to tighten it up or something. [The last two definitions share their concreteness and self-centeredness with the first two fabulized ones. Although the scores may be different, the sortings and their descriptions are highly similar for all four sortings.]	
5. *Circle*	(Cardboard square; file card.)	You're just cutting things out at school.	Concrete Def. (Fabulized)
6. *Toy pliers*	(Toy hammer; toy screwdriver; toy saw.) And this, I guess: (square block of wood with nail in it.)	They're toy tools, and this might be something to hammer in at school with your toy tools (she hammers on the nail placed in the wooden block).	Conceptual Def. Concrete Def.

PART II

Examiner's Sorting	Explanation and Comments	Score
1. *Red objects*	All red.	Conceptual Def.
2. *Metal*	(As I am putting them in front of her:) Because they're all (she peeks at the test sheet on which I'm writing) metal (she laughs). Don't put down that I'm a cheater. I won't do it anymore .. honest (she plays with hammering the nail into the block of wood). ("Please don't hammer that nail.") Are you mad at me? [Helen's "cheating" is done teasingly, but her tendency constantly to test the limits of what is acceptable becomes irritating. One soon becomes weary of Helen's persistent kittenishness. One feels that her integrity often falls below a desirable level.]	—
3. *Round*	A child might use them all. [Helen often refers to childhood.]	Syncretistic
4. *Tools*	They're all tools. And I didn't look. Aren't they all tools? [Helen's seductive efforts contain strong elements of "little girlishness." How much of her very young appearance is genuine and how	Conceptual Def.

Examiner's Sorting	Explanation and Comments	Score
	much represents her understanding of what it means to be coquettish?]	
5. *Paper*	Because it's all paper. Well, *you* can tell that, can't you? Do you think I'm cheating? I'm not. Honest. Have you ever had the brain test? ("No, I haven't.") How do you know you're all there? [Helen's comment, "*You* can tell that, can't you?," suggests that she is either extremely naïve and believes the material is as new to the examiner as it is to her, or, much more likely, she is expressing her by now familiar pseudo naïveté. "Cheating" has come to occupy a prominent place in her relationship to the examiner; she takes great pains to convince him that she is not a "cheater." Once again, it is difficult to determine how many of her concerns are genuine—her manner is so histrionic that one is tempted almost automatically to discount the sincerity of what she says. Is she, for example, truly worried about the EEG? And if so, how strong is her worry? Or is the EEG question something she uses to demonstrate her helplessness and fearfulness? One could easily slip into error and dismiss Helen's worries as "only histrionics," when actually the histrionics might disguise or exaggerate real anxieties.]	Conceptual Def.
6. *Double*	All usable.	Syncretistic
7. *White*	All white.	Conceptual Def.
8. *Rubber*	I don't know. Would it be because they are rubber? Would it?	Conceptual Def.
9. *Smoking*	Because you can all smoke 'em.	Functional Def.
10. *Silverware*	All silverware. Not silverware. All forks and knives. They're spoons and forks and knives. [Apparently Helen feels "silverware" does not cover the conceptual realm adequately because the toy silverware is made of red plastic.]	Conceptual Def.
11. *Toys*	Because they're all play toys.	Conceptual Def.
12. *Square*	I don't know this. Because I don't know what that thing (block of wood with nail) is, and you won't tell me. They're	Syncretistic

Examiner's Sorting	*Explanation and Comments*	*Score*
	all made. Put that down. They're all made. What is that? ("What do you think it is?") It looks like a block of wood with a nail in it. [Helen's efforts to manipulate (e.g., "... and you won't tell me") seem to mask her inability to solve the problem. In this way Helen throws out decoys which draw attention away from her limitations. Helen's Part II performance illustrates the degree to which she benefits when boundaries are imposed *for* her. At such times (i.e., when she need not set her own limits) she can function much more effectively.]	

The Bender Gestalt Test

PART A (PLATES 43 AND 44)

(She makes some sort of comment about almost every design she draws. Before she begins, she says:) Is there any special way you want me to do each?

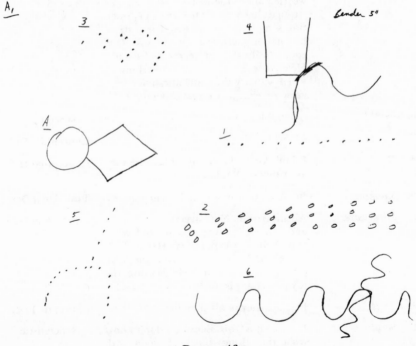

PLATE 43

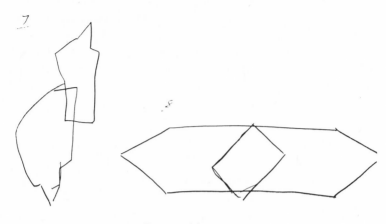

PLATE 44

(On subsequent drawings she says the following:)

Design A. (After she has finished:) I tried.

Design 1. (Before she begins:) Shall I put them all on one paper?

Design 2. I guess that's right. I didn't count the dots.

Design 4. Would it be all right if I started to draw it before you took it away?

Design 5. I can draw it better than dot it.

Design 7. I can't! (After she has completed it.)

Design 8. Oh, I didn't even get to see it because I was looking at what you were writing. (After she completes the drawing:) Or something like that.

(In a very obvious manner she looks at what I have been writing. She wants to know the purpose of the Bender and makes a derogatory comment about her examining psychiatrist.)

[Although Helen gives an appearance of cooperating, she tries constantly to manipulate explicit and implicit rules. Her drawings on Part A are fairly accurately made, but they are executed in a characteristically uncontrolled and impulsive fashion. Although she realizes she will be asked to draw quite a few more designs, she places her first drawing in the middle of the page and after that proceeds in a rather haphazard fashion. If lines do not meet as they ought, she unconcernedly erases them and casually patches them up with other lines. Sometimes the lines are simply left hanging and do not meet. Dots, which often are unevenly spaced, easily become circles. Sizes are occasionally expanded out of all proportion. Design 7 is particularly poorly drawn, its form elements severely distorted.

[Does Helen's performance here reflect perceptual-motor interference, or is her performance an expression of flighty attention? Do the intersecting forms that supposedly represent Design 7 indicate a significant perceptual-motor disturbance, or are they another example of Helen's tendency to fabulize in order to avoid meeting the demands of a more complex reality?]

PART B (PLATES 45 AND 46)

(She takes more time as she draws these designs; again she keeps up a fairly constant commentary:)

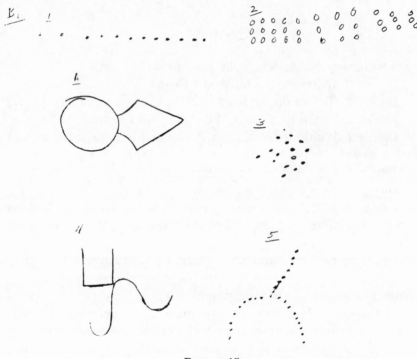

PLATE 45

Design A. I can't even draw a circle.

Design 1. Are those (tiny, adventitiously made pencil marks on the test cards) meant to be there, or did somebody just do it by accident?

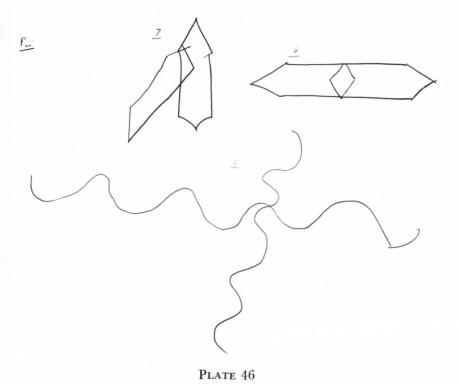

PLATE 46

Design 2. (She counts the circles.) I sure messed that one up last time.

Design 3. (She rotates the design and her paper as she copies it. While drawing, she tells how angry she is with the psychiatrist because he would not answer one of her questions.)

Design 5. (She counts all the dots but does not plan sufficiently well, so that the diagonal line and semicircle do not meet as they are supposed to.) Oh heck! This is supposed to be down farther. What shall I do? (She erases and corrects.)

Design 6. (She counts the "waves" to locate the point of intersection.) This is real dumb. There I go, using "dumb" again. (She laughs. I had mentioned her frequent use of the word.) Did you talk to that lady (the social worker) about me? ("Did I talk to her about what?") What she said to my parents. What'll you do with me? Will you tell us to go on vacation? ("I don't know yet what we'll say.") Please don't tell us to go on vacation because I can't stand to be with my parents that long.

[As Helen has more time and feels under less pressure, she becomes better organized. Nevertheless, her drawings still reflect her difficulty with assuming a general overview: although individual lines, dots, rows and other elements may be accurately reproduced, the total gestalt often is not. Helen's lack of restraint is again evident on Design 6, which is highly out of proportion. Design 7 is a good deal more accurately drawn this time; it does not reveal nearly as many of the peculiar, fabulized aspects as were present on the 5″ Exposure.

[Although Helen's Copy drawings are much more self-disciplined than those in her 5″ Exposure series, one can still see how much of a problem she has with self-restraint.]

THE DRAW A PERSON TEST

PART I (PLATE 47)

(After I give the instructions, she says:) I can't. ("Just do the best you can.") I'll make a stick figure. ("No. Draw a real person.")

(She produces a quick, careless drawing. She pays considerable attention to the face, but the rest of the figure is drawn rapidly and impressionistically. After she has finished, she says:) Now, this isn't what I think a person looks like. You promise you won't think so?

(She points out the examining psychiatrist's lack of understanding in comparison to my attempts "really" to get to know her. But her expressions of trust in me are almost immediately followed by her mentioning how worried she is that the examining team might tell her parents "bad things" about her and that her parents, in turn, might tell the team even "worse things" about her. After she tells me this, she looks to see what I am writing.)

Are you mad? I'm just playing around. I can't draw. Some people just can't.

(She first labels her drawing, "My Mother," but then crosses this designation out.)

PART II (PLATE 48)

(Following my instructions, she says:) Honest, I can't draw it! Can you? My father can't.

(As she draws, she says:) Are you mad? ("Mad about what?") Cause I'm doing this. Why am I? ("Why are you?") Because I can't draw. I just want to be dumb. Don't put that down. I don't really think I'm dumb.

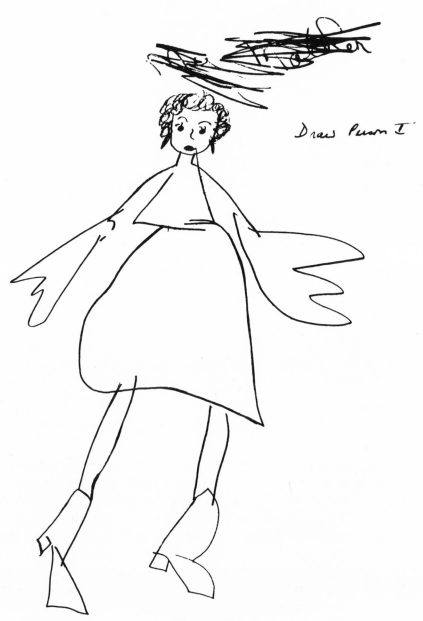

PLATE 47

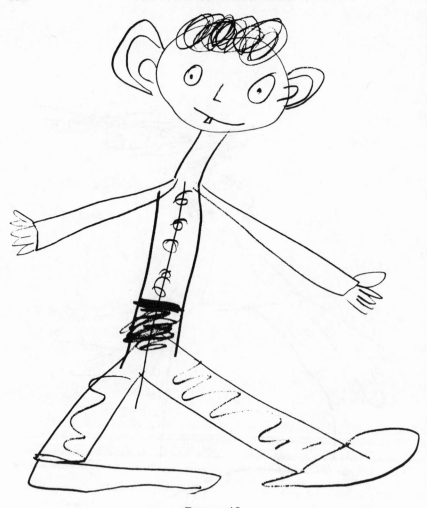

PLATE 48

[It is striking to see the discrepancy between Helen's drawings of the woman and the man. Although both are carelessly drawn, the woman's face has a great deal more care given it than either the rest of her body or any part of the man. Although the man is, in some respects, more carefully drawn than the woman, Helen's male drawing suggests she has a rather profound disrespect for men and sees them as not particularly intelligent. Although the female ("My Mother") is so carelessly and aggressively drawn, the doll-like face is relatively (and significantly) attractive, if empty. Thus, while Helen otherwise tries to make her mother into an ogress, she also conveys her conviction that her mother is an attractive woman whom, as will become apparent, she experiences as an imposing competitor. With her comment, "I just want to be dumb," Helen conveys that she herself believes there may well be a strong motivational component to her "stupidity."]

RORSCHACH TEST

RORSCHACH SCORING SHEET

Number of Responses: 17

Manner of Approach (Location)

W	6
D	7
Dd	0
DoS	1
Dr	3
De	0
Total	17

Location Percentages

W%	35
D%	41
DR%	24
De%	0

Form, Movement, Color and Shading Determinants

F+	6	M	0
F−	4		
F±	2		
F∓	1		
FC	0		
CF	0	CC′	1
C/F	1	C	2
Total	17		

Color Denom.   1

Groups of Contents

A	6
Ad	2
At.	1 (1)
Ats.	2
Pl.	1
Blood	3
Painting	1
Geol.	1
Total:	17 (18)

Determinant and Content Percentages

F%	76/76	Obj.%	0
F+%	62/47	At%	18 (24)
A%	47	P%	18 (24)
H%	0		

Qualitative Material

Failure	VI
Popular	I (IV) V VIII
Combination	VIII
Fabulation	1
Peculiar	3
Vague	1
Arbitrary	1
Castration	1

EXPERIENCE BALANCE: 0.0/5.5

[One is immediately impressed by Helen's undifferentiated use of color. Her Experience Balance, which contains no Movement and a marked degree of gross Color, is highly unbalanced. It can be seen to what extent Helen is ruled by affect, how her emotions blurt out impulsively, and how formal aspects are arbitrarily pasted on affective judgments, so as to give a (spurious) impression of emotional integration. About one-quarter of Helen's seventeen responses contain either no form portions at all, or only highly muted ones. Such findings reinforce the impression that objective (formal) aspects of reality are of little importance to Helen, and (a finding which hardly comes as a surprise by now) that she interprets the world primarily in terms of feelings, rather than in terms of objective properties. She fails one card (the allegedly phallic one) altogether, a failure which suggests that she feels less at home with sexual matters than she tries to imply. The fact that 18-24 percent of her responses are "Populars," and thus shared by many other persons who interpret these blots, shows that Helen's perceptions are less idiosyncratic than one might predict.]

RORSCHACH PROTOCOL

Card #	React. Time	Score	Protocol	Inquiry and Observations
I	6″	WF—Ats Pec.	1. I don't know. A heart, I guess. Is that right? What are you writing it down for? (I explain why I write it down. "Do you see anything else?")	1. ("Would you describe the heart you saw?") I can't without seeing it. (I show her the card again.) Kind of the way it's spread out, because you know the way a heart is spread out. ("How do you mean?") The lines in it. You know, the way a heart has lines in it. Will you tell me what it should be? Does it mean I'm dumb because I couldn't guess it? [This is a "Peculiar" response, one that would be considered "pathological" if it appeared in the record of an adult (where it would probably be scored "Queer"). In an adolescent, the response cannot be considered so pathological because it is likely that this sort of peculiarity (fairly typical of much adolescent thinking) will disappear as the young person reaches maturity. The reasons a clinician should probably not be overconcerned when he sees such a response (in a girl so hyperemotionally organized) rest as much on empirical as on theoretical grounds.]

Card #	React. Time	Score	Protocol	Inquiry and Observations
		WF+AP	2. A bat (she laughs). An inkblot (she laughs). And . . uh . . let's see (she looks to see what I'm writing and hits me playfully). It doesn't remind me of much more. Probably it's what my mind looks like.	[Helen continues to be both playful and hyperalert. She continues to throw out self-derogatory comments for the apparent purpose of having me deny them. One cannot, however, ignore the probable underlying conviction Helen has about herself—that she is stupid and inadequate.]
II	2″	DCC′ Blood	1. Blood. That's all it reminds me of.	1. ("Would you describe the blood?") No . . . . I forgot. ("Try to remember what it looked like.") Well, bloody, with black stuff, or ink. (Lower central D.)
III	3″	DrF∓Ad	1. Your ribs (she laughs).	1. ("My ribs?") It just looked like ribs. I was kidding when I said they were yours. (Lower central Dr.)
		DC Blood	2. And blood.	2. It was just red like blood. (Upper side D's.) [The second time that this grossly modulated color response appears. Form is ignored.]
IV	8″		(She is looking at her schedule; I draw her attention back to the card.) It's nothing; just an inkblot. ("Try to see something.")	
		DF+ Ad(P)	1. Okay, feet.	1. ("Tell me about the feet.") Uh-uh, I can't. ("Tell me what you remember.") A bear's feet, I guess . . I don't know.
		WF− geol.	2. Gosh . . I don't know . . . . It could be an ice fossil, too. Or a stalactite that comes down in a cavern.	2. ("How about the ice fossil?") It was the same place as the feet. The whole thing . . like in the Carlsbad Caverns. It just seemed to kind of hang there.
		WF−pl Vague	3. Or it could be a leaf. This is real dumb, but	3. ("How about the leaf?") Hm . . I was just guessing. I was just saying something so that you wouldn't think I'm dumb. I don't think I'm dumb,

Card #	React. Time Score	Protocol	Inquiry and Observations

Inquiry and Observations

but mother sure does. (She continues to tell about her mother's poor opinion of her.) She'll think it's all an optical illusion . . . Are you married? Is that very nosy? . . Is Dr. Adams (the psychiatrist)? . . Is that lady social worker? I bet she thinks I'm just horrible. [Helen has obvious difficulty making sense out of what seems to appear to her as a vague perceptual blob. With the exception of the Popular "bat" on Card I, and the "feet" on this card, her responses so far have been arbitrary and often formless. It is quite likely that she feels she has to say "something," rather than appear "dumb." All in all, although she "sees" more on the Rorschach than did Joan, Helen's performance is not very different from Joan's even though the latter saw almost nothing at all on the ten Rorschach cards. Helen probably actually perceives little more than does Joan, but Helen feels she *ought* to report some kind of response because the examiner's opinion of her carries so much weight with her.

[One can see that Helen needs to transform the testing relationship into a much more personal one. Whether or not the members of the examining team are married appears to be of infinitely greater moment than does Card IV. Interestingly, Helen's former derogation of the social worker has changed into a concern about what the social worker thinks of Helen. Undoubtedly, a similar mechanism lies at the bottom of Helen's tendency to disparage her mother.]

Card #	React. Time	Score	Protocol	Inquiry and Observations
V	17″		Do we have to do these? Oh, I hate 'em. Do you blame me? I like all the tests except these.	[Partly because what *has not been* successfully repressed is probably stirred up and therefore threatens to achieve consciousness, and partly because what *has been* successfully repressed probably transforms the inkblot into an undifferentiated mass, the Rorschach tends to be an unpleasant experience for persons who defensively depend on repression to the degree that Helen does.]
		WF+AP	1. I'll say it looks like a bat .. so we'll hurry and get through.	
VI	3′	Failure	Nothing. An inkblot. (She starts to put the card away.) ("Look at it a little longer.") Do you blame me? I like all of these, except this. I hate it. Shall I just say anything? ("Look at it and see if it doesn't remind you of something.") It doesn't remind me of anything .. honest! .... Can I put it away? (She does.)	[The phalluslike figure often seems to make this card particularly threatening to persons who need to shy away from awareness of serious sexual thought. Failure on this "father" card is rather often seen among persons who depend to a high degree on the mechanism of repression.]
VII	6″	DrF±Ad	Nothing, really. Oh! 1. It could be two donkeys.	1. ("What did the donkeys look like?") (She starts to pick up the turned-over card.) ("Try to tell me from memory.") Oh, I can't! ("Give it a try.") They just look that way. They had long ears and a long face, just like a donkey. What do you do with these answers? Read them and see how dumb I am? (She describes how the small outer Dr could be a hoof; the small connection between the two top D's, upside down, could be the body; and the donkey might be "kicking up.") Am I the dumbest student you ever had? [Apart from the fact that this last comment is an obvious request for my support of her, Helen

Card #	React. Time	Score	Protocol	Inquiry and Observations

Inquiry and Observations

again demonstrates naïveté by trying to transform the testing situation into a pupil-teacher relationship. She can somewhat meet testing ("reality") expectations, once she is not permitted to manipulate them —even though she protests her helpless inability to do things in the required way.]

VIII 3″ Comb. { SF+At 1. A body.
             DrC blood
                body
          Pec.
          Arb.

1. ("Tell me about the body.") I can't. You know how a body has ribs. Please let me show you on the card. It looks like the inside of a body because the blood is blue at first. Is that right? Please let me show you on the card. (I show her the card. The entire middle portion of the blot is involved; the middle and lower D's are the "body," the upper middle space is the rib cage, and the central line going through the upper D is the "backbone.") [This response represents a highly arbitrary, not to say "inaccurate," organization. Not only does Helen's reaction reflect her inability to organize formal characteristics successfully; it again makes one aware of her overpreoccupation with the (her) body. It shows how she reacts immediately, impulsively, without waiting for an adequate, formal organizing function or principle to take over. Although the response is scored Peculiar and Arbitrary, Helen's poor organization probably comes about because of her lack of thoughtful restraint, and not because of any intrusive "psychotic" process.]

DF+AP   2. And these, right
Cast.   here . . Wait . . they
             could be some kind

[While this response is scored Popular, it misses being truly "popular" by a hair's breadth

Card #	React. Time	Score	Protocol	Inquiry and Observations
			of animal . . a wolf. No, not a wolf. I don't know what kind because they don't have a tail.	because of Helen's accentuated concern with her animal's missing tail. In this connection, of course, one suspects that Helen's seductiveness contains meanings which involve envy (and hence derogation) of the male (cf. her drawing of a man).]
IX	26″		Gee, we're almost through! You're not timing me because you don't look at the clock.	
		Color Denomination	A bunch of colors. A beautiful design . . the end. Are you mad that I don't like these? ("Try to find something on the card.") Okay . . a bunch of colors.	[Helen has given up trying to impose intellectual-perceptual organization in a situation which arouses so many inchoate affective responses. At first, she cannot deal with this multicolored card at all, except to describe it as "a bunch of colors." Naturally, she does not "like these" and looks forward to being through with them. A little later, she is able to recover somewhat.]
		WC/F painting Fab.	1. It could be a water painting . . or a finger painting. (She looks to check what I'm writing.) ("Anything else?") Uh-uh . . no.	1. ("What would be the difference between a finger painting and a water painting?") Because with finger paintings there's a lot of spots. You know how you paint with your spots. And it could be a water painting because the colors are very light . . . . Okay. I didn't say very much, so you shouldn't write so much. Oh, it takes so long. Are you going to miss me? [Helen's tolerance for the tension the Rorschach creates in her has obviously about reached its limits. She can barely wait to be through with a task which requires so much introspection of her. Her comment, "Oh, it takes so long,"

Card #	React. Time	Score	Protocol	Inquiry and Observations

indicates the extent to which she experiences waiting as an obnoxious constraint. Since she is asked to give some sort of response, she eventually gives one which requires almost no organization, so that the final result is barely better than no response at all. Her reaction further underlines inferences that have already been made about her functioning.

[The open "Are you going to miss me?" represents almost a parody of what she conceives to be the behavior of the tantalizing temptress; and yet, the question may well reflect Helen's sincere wish to be of importance to others, and her doubts whether others genuinely care for her.]

Card #	React. Time	Score	Protocol	Inquiry and Observations
X	20″	WC/F painting Fab.	⋁ 1. This'll be another beautiful finger painting . . a very gorgeous one. ("Do you see anything else?") That's all. ("See if you can't see something else.") Okay. (She reads the back of the Rorschach card.) Oh, it looks like it might have been printed in Switzerland. (She reads the rest of the publisher's information and then turns the card and looks at it some more.)	[Helen's use of hyperbole is typical of the histrionic aspects of strongly repressive personality organizations.]
		DF+A	2. Okay, these are sea horses right here.	2. (Bottom green D's, upside down.)
		DF−A	3. And these yellow things are fish.	3. ("What made them seem like fish?") I don't know. It was just something to say.

Card #	React. Time	Score	Protocol	Inquiry and Observations
		DF±A	4. And the blue things are lobsters. They should be red .. No, they should be blue until they're cooked.	[Although it would have been useful to inquire, it seems likely that in Helen's undifferentiated world view "crabs" and "lobsters" are equivalent. But even uncooked lobsters never had such a vivid shade of blue.]

[Although Helen responds more actively to the Rorschach than Joan does, Helen's greater *number* of Rorschach responses alone can be misleading. One can see that Helen is incapable of concrete specificity, that she is impotent to delimit perceptual areas in detail, that she finds it nearly impossible to respond to more than superficialities, and that she becomes chaotically organized in the presence of color. Her greater responsiveness (higher R), in other words, reflects much more an apparent than a real difference from Joan. Although Helen talks much more than Joan, she is not any more oriented toward reflective thought.]

THEMATIC APPERCEPTION TEST

Card 1 (A young boy is contemplating a violin which rests on a table in front of him.)

Once upon a time there was this little boy, and he didn't want a violin. I *guess* that's what it is, and ... Are you pressing it down? (She points to a lever which allows the dictaphone to record.) ("Yes I am.") He didn't want to take violin, and his mother made him, so he was sitting there, looking at it and had some music under it, and deciding why he had to take it, and that at the end he is a great violinist. ("And how is he feeling right there?") I don't know. I guess he's feeling okay. [The story is typical of Helen's approach in a number of ways: the phrase, "Are you pressing it down?," reflects her need to control and her tendency to feel that others (particularly men?) cannot be trusted to do a job right. Considering Helen's disparaging attitude toward her mother, it is not surprising that the story hero's mother *makes* him study the violin, while he passively resists her by simply sitting and looking at the instrument. Without concerning herself about any intermediate steps, Helen suddenly has her hero become a "great violinist"; she makes no attempt to explain the gap between the boy's just looking at the disliked violin with which he does not practice, and his ending up as a violin virtuoso. Such types of "fairy tale" endings, which are arbitrarily pasted onto unpleasant situations, and which appear without preparation, without any sort of expectable precursor, are typical of the action-oriented, nonreflective, nonfuture-directed person.]

Card 2 (Country scene: in the foreground is a young woman with books in her hand; in the background a man is working in the fields and an older woman is looking on.)

You got that (i.e., the dictaphone lever) on now, don't you? . . Yeah, okay . . . Well, this little girl, I guess she was about eighteen, and she lived on this farm, and they have these hired hands, and anyway her brother was running this horse, you know, plowing the field, and her mother was standing there watching, and I guess she was coming home from school, and she was mad for some reason. Anyway, it turned out that . . And they had a whole bunch of wheat, and I guess that's all. ("Why was the girl mad?") Because she had to go away to school. ("What's the mother thinking?") I don't know. It looks like she got her eyes closed, and it looks like she's trying to get her head, her face, suntanned. [Motives of others do not run deeply, so far as Helen is concerned. Her tying together elements of her story with the conjunction "and" is reminiscent of the arbitrary juxtaposition of ideas of the much younger child. It is striking to see how Helen avoids attributing serious reflection to others—even though they may look lost in thought, the appearance is misleading (e.g., "She's trying to get . . . . her face suntanned"). Her again making sure she is being recorded seems to involve more than merely a wish to control. She wants her words (and, of course, herself) to be taken seriously, to transcend the moment, to achieve some measure of durability.]

Card 3 GF (A young woman is standing with downcast head, her face covered with her right hand. Her left arm is stretched forward against a wooden door.)

Well, see, this little girl had come up to this clinic because they said it would help her. So, anyway, they were staying out at this tourist court, and they told them she would have to go away to this hospital and stay, so she was crying. She went there and the results were horrible. ("What were the results?") You mean after she got out of the hospital? Oh, she had to go, and no one understood or anything, and it was real dumb. ("Why did they make her go?") Don't ask me. [This is the first of several conscious self-references whose purpose is to demonstrate the adults' (parents', examiners') unfairness and lack of wisdom, and to force them to change their minds about what she is convinced will be their decision. Her conviction about "their" thoughts may well be a projection of her own.]

Card 4 (A woman is clutching the shoulders of a man whose face and body are averted as if he were trying to pull away from her.)

It just looks like a television program . . . . ("What's the program about?") Oh, I can't say, or you'll think I have bad thoughts, evil you know . . . . Oh, I don't know. See, it could be . . . . . Oh, it's just about this man and this woman . . . . ("What's happening?") Well, I don't know. ("Make up something.") No, I know. I *could* say something, but then you'd think, "Oh, she's insane." [Helen's sexual fantasies are probably aroused by this card. She seems to feel that revealing such thoughts would insure the examiner's thinking she is "insane" and in need of hospitalization.]

Card 5 (A middle-aged woman is standing on the threshold of a half-opened door looking into a room.)

A girl is looking in. She just got to bed, and she went to see what was on television, and the television was off. [Helen has a tendency to transform young or middle-aged women into "girls," a tendency which may be related to her wish to view herself as little in most respects. Once she omits mention of her preoccupation with hospitalization (i.e., with present, concrete reality), she is almost unable to use her imagination. Whatever story she does finally tell is extremely brief and lacking in imaginative development. She seems unable imaginatively to elaborate beyond a description of fragments of personal experience and preoccupation.]

Card 6 GF (A young woman sitting on the edge of a sofa looks back over her shoulder at an older man with a pipe in his mouth, who seems to be addressing her.)

Oh, a girl sitting down, and her father came up and talked to her, and she was real mad because she didn't want to go away to school, to a hospital. And she went, and anyway, when she got back it just ruined her, her life and everything. ("How did it ruin her life?") Oh, she . . You don't even have the button (of the dictaphone) pressed down . . There was nothing wrong with her or anything. They just made her go. ("What happened when she came back?') She was just ruined. She had an old phoney that talked to her, and he just ruined her. ("How did he ruin her?") Oh, he made her think that . . Oh, he was just . . I don't know how, he just did. ("What was her life like when she came back?") It was horrible. She ended up in the penitentiary about a month later. [Helen makes no bones about conveying what she thinks both about hospitals and psychotherapy for herself. Far from helping, such measures would "ruin" her life. It is obvious again that Helen strategically uses the TAT to help her wage various battles: to be left alone, to prevent adults from getting to know her, and to keep people from restricting her mobility.]

Card 7 GF (An older woman is sitting on a sofa close beside a girl, speaking or reading to her. The girl, who holds a doll in her lap, is looking away.)

Well, there is this mother, and the girl is holding her doll, and the mother is trying to talk to the little girl, and she's real mad because she just got back from . . . . uh . . What's the name of this place? ("Menninger's.") Menninger's. It just ruined her, but she doesn't take it out on Dr. Hirsch. I don't take it out on you; I blame it on my parents. ("Why did they take this little girl to Menninger's?") Oh, I don't know. She didn't know either. She never did find out. All she ever knew was that they made her go to this hospital, and . . . Oh, it was real boring, and there was nothing to do, and . . . Oh . . . . uh . . . . She was just ruined when she came back. ("Why would parents just take a little girl and bring her to Menninger's, do you suppose?") Oh, I don't know, just for the heck of it, just for kicks. [Here is more polemic. It is obvious that Helen cannot see any need for help; all blame for difficulty is projected. She tries to create dissension, both between her parents and the clinic and (as is apparent elsewhere) between the various members of the clinical team. She presents her parents as being callous, as lacking in understanding of her, and as persons who bring her to a clinic for their own perverse pleasure. It is not clear whether Helen actually believes the situation to be the way she describes it, but she certainly paints it vividly.]

Card 10 (A young woman's head against a man's shoulder.)

I don't know. There are two people asleep . . . . ("Two people asleep?") I'm not going to say anything that might incriminate me. [To have this couple "asleep" is an unusual interpretation. Helen's unwillingness to "incriminate" herself suggests that she is trying hard to avoid letting the examiner know that this card may have sexual implications for her; yet, while she apparently tries to keep this information from him, she also makes sure he has some knowledge about what is going through her mind.]

Card 12 F (The portrait of a young woman. A weird old woman with a shawl over her head is grimacing in the background.)

I don't know. There *is* no story. ("Try to make up a story.") I can't. I'll incriminate myself, and I don't want to any more . . . . . There's this lady and this other lady and, anyway, this girl was beautiful and, until she had to go away to this hospital, and when she came back, this (the old woman) is what she looked like. ("What did they do to make this girl look like this woman?") Oh, they just, oh, you just get to be an old hag and square and don't have any fun or . . . it's just terrible. ("What's going on right now?") That's her mother standing in front, and she's thinking, "Ah, I'm prettier than she is at last." ("And what's the girl thinking?") "Boy, I wish I were dead." [It is becoming more and more evident that Helen thinks that being sent to a hospital represents some sort of dreadful end for her. Horrible things will happen once she gets sent away. Again, one cannot be certain to what extent Helen believes these things will actually happen and to what extent she is presenting the possibilities to make her point as dramatic as possible.]

Card 12 M (A young man is lying on a couch with his eyes closed. Leaning over him is a gaunt form of an elderly man, his hand stretched out above the face of the reclining figure.)

And

Card 13 MF (A young man is standing with downcast head buried in his arm. Behind him is the figure of a woman lying in bed.)

(Helen immediately turns these cards over and says she doesn't know any story. She again says she doesn't want to "incriminate" herself.) ["Incriminate" is obviously the equivalent of "reveal."

Helen wants to avoid letting the examiner know the types of impulses and thoughts she is trying to deal with.]

Card 15 (A gaunt man with clenched hands is standing among gravestones.)

How horrible! . . . . Now I know what this is. This is my father, and they sent me to the school. He's standing there, praying that he wishes they hadn't, because I killed myself before I went. [Helen no longer even pretends to make her stories about someone else.]

Card 18 GF (A woman has her hands squeezed around the throat of another woman whom she appears to be pushing backwards across the banister of a stairway.)

I don't know. ("Try to tell a story.") (Helen explains that if she said something I would think this is what she was about to do, and I would put her in the "insane hospital.") I'll say it in Spanish. Okay? I don't know. I know, but I can't say it. [Considering the preceding material, it would not be surprising to find that Helen's reluctance to tell a story to this card springs from aggression she feels toward, or fears from, her mother.]

Card 16 (Blank card.)

Once upon a time there was this girl and her parents, and they came up to Menninger's. And, anyway, she went to see the psychiatrist. She went to see Dr. Hess or Hirsch or, anyway, and he was real nice, and she went to see Dr. Adams, and he was okay. And this old bag (the social worker) saw her parents. The reason the old bag was so bad was she got her parents to thinking that she should be sent to this hospital, and they made her go. And when she went to the hospital, she was ruined when she got back. And she didn't want to go, so she decided she would rather be dead, so she cut her wrists with the razor blades instead of going to this place where she . . . to this hospital and . . . because if she had went to the hospital it would have just ruined her. [Helen is continuing her campaign to avoid hospitalization. The fact that after more than four hours she still does not know either the name of her psychologist ("Dr. Hess or Hirsch") or the name of the clinic at which she is being examined reflects her lack of involvement in the people or things she emotionally disowns (even when she tries to convey an impression of intense involvement).]

Sentence Completion Test II

She hoped that when she grew up she could leave home. [Looking forward to leaving home is very much part of the "adolescent rebellion," but, as will become apparent later on, Helen does not think that leaving home will be easy for her.]

Her parents are awful . . sometimes. Mother mostly. [The development of an extremely angry attitude toward parents represents a typical effort to resolve the intimate early bonds of childhood. Often adolescents are unable to establish independence except by angrily disowning their parents.]

When she saw what the other kids were doing she wished her mother would let her go out and do it too.

When she compared herself to her friends she found they were quite the same. [It is important to Helen to be like "the others," to be part of her group of peers.]

She was sad whenever she thought of having to . . go away . . to school. I hate it. ("Why do you hate the thought?") I hate to leave my friends. [Although Helen says the reason she hates to go away from home is that she does not want to leave her friends, her angry relationship to her parents suggests such strong interdependence that it seems likely that her basic reluctance to go away involves leaving her parents, more than, or at least as much as, her friends.]

When she was asked about her aches and pains she didn't have any . . except in the head. I have headaches . . except there's nothing wrong with me. [Helen's wish to reveal, immediately followed by a denial of the revelation, is particularly clear in this response.]

The person she admired most was her father. [And yet, her parents "are awful."]

Her brother is a good kid (she laughs).

When the boy kissed her she . . . . I don't know (she laughs).

When her father came into the room they went outside and played tennis. No, change it . . He changes clothes and went out to play tennis. I love to play with Daddy. [This is a far cry from the punitive father who appears later on.]

When she was with her sister they got along fine.

At school she had a ball. ("In what way?") Just messing around . . goofing off.

When she looked at the work the other students were doing . . she didn't.

She was very happy when she was swimming, riding horseback, not fighting with her parents.

The thing she found hardest to do was get along with her parents . . her mother.

Whenever certain things really bothered her she had a fit. ("What would she do?") What wouldn't she do?

Her dreams were to own a farm . . with a lot of horses . . and a swimming pool.

When she saw that the man had left the money behind . . What man? ("Any man.") She said "Oh!" ("What did she do?") Nothing. I don't know what I mean.

She thought that her mother hated her . . at times . . and at other times liked her. [Helen probably projects her own ambivalence.]

Whenever she and her family disagreed she wished she were dead or run away. Did you hear about that? ("What's that?") I went to Lawrence (a college town thirty miles from Topeka). I never had so much fun in my life.

When she was very little she and her daddy were good pals. ("What about now?") They still are . . except . . I think Daddy likes Mother better than he does me. [One suspects that much of Helen's anger with her parents is related to her increasing awareness that her relationship with her father is not as exclusive as she would like.]

Her best friend I've got hundreds of them. ("How would you finish the phrase?") Put friends. Her best friends are Becky, Louise, Sharon and Mary Lou. [Helen has many "friends," perhaps because in that way she can avoid making a serious psychological investment in any one person.]

She was unhappy with her father when he'd hit me . . hit her. [Helen finds it exceedingly difficult to maintain the appearance of talking about the mythical test-third-person "she."]

When her mother asked about her boy friend she didn't get told anything. ("And what would happen then?") Her mother would knock her through the wall.

She never thought she would be able to . . hm . . have a car.

She always hoped that she could have a car.

What she liked best about herself . . . . was having friends.

[Helen apparently finds she has not many things to choose from as far as liking herself is concerned. Eventually she chooses an "other-directed" value: i.e., the ability to have friends.]

Her mother was more likely than her father to get her in trouble. ("In what way?") By always finding something wrong.

Her sister was a nice girl.

When she had nothing else to do she went horseback riding or talked on the phone.

She thought that her intelligence was . . well . . *she* thought that it was good, but her mother thought that she was a dope. [Helen consistently needs to judge her mother as degrading Helen. Her mother seems to serve as a focus for Helen's exceedingly low self-esteem.]

What she liked about school was recess . . noon hour. [This response is given by many adolescents who experience problems with authority or with studies.]

When she couldn't see a way out of her problem . . What problem? ("Any problem you want to make it.") I don't have any that I haven't been able to see my way out of . . except this. I don't even know why I'm here.

She saw the cockroach on the wall and killed it (she laughs).

Her teacher was real sweet. [Not good, or knowledgeable, but "sweet."]

Whenever she got angry she had a fit. ("What was that like?") Oh, what wouldn't I do? Golly! Throw knives and everything else. Because they won't leave me alone. If they'd let me go to my room, I'd calm down. [Once again Helen blames "them'" for her disorganized behavior. The switch from "she" to "I" is made immediately, without hesitation.]

She remembered that when she was little she always wanted a car. [To the action-oriented adolescent, the car represents the way through which intractable problems will become resolved.]

When the kids invited her to go with them to the hiding place, she thought . . To the hiding place; what's that? ("Any kind of hiding place.") She thought (she laughs) . . . . it would be real neat.

After school she usually came . . home because her mother wouldn't let her go downtown or anything. [The ubiquitous forbidding mother.]

She admired her father when he . . was in a good mood.

When the boy invited her to his party the Old Boy wouldn't let her go. ("Why was that?") Because we had to come here.

When she and her sister were together they got along good.

She thought that her body was too fat (she laughs). [Another self-depreciation.]

When she had a lot of homework to do she never did do it (she laughs).

What she disliked about school was . . hm . . work.

Whenever she spoke about her problems to someone . . she never did. ("Why was that?") It wasn't anyone else's business. [One extrapolates into psychotherapy.]

When she entered the haunted house . . it was a lot of fun. ("Why was that?") Oh, I love excitement. ("Would it be scary?") Uh-uh. Nothing scares me . . rides or anything. Only a belt. ("Why a belt?") My father uses it. [This response suggests Helen's use of counter-phobic mechanisms.]

When the other girl offered her a cigarette she didn't take it. ("Why was that?") I never smoke.

She didn't like her mother to . . to be . . I don't know.

When the baby arrived . . Whose baby? (She laughs.) . . . It was a boy (she laughs). [Helen uses an arch, two-step avoidance with this stem.]

Whenever she didn't do what she was told . . "You're grounded!"

What would make her angriest when she couldn't . . when she wouldn't be able to have *anything* her own way. Not *everything* but *anything*. When you can't have *anything* your own way! I never get angry except with my parents. [Even if Helen's parents are not unusually restrictive (and they may not be), it is probable that Helen considers any restriction, even the most objectively appropriate, as insufferable. The search for freedom (from parental restraints) is the most frequent—and in some ways (i.e., when not carried to extremes) a highly desirable—manifestation of adolescent rebellion. In this way, adult independence is achieved. Helen, of course, is unreasonable in her protest.]

In her spare time she goofed off with the car, when she could steal it. (She expresses concern that this portion of the test might be shown to her parents.) ("Why did she steal it?") Because her parents wouldn't let her have it. Do you have a car? Would you let me drive it? [Here again we see Helen's effort to create a schism between a member of the examining team and her parents.]

When she was alone in her room at night she listened to the radio.

What scared her most . . the belt.

She struck the match and . . blew it out. I love to light 'em.

She disliked her father when he spanked her . . he beat her. Honest, he does. ("Does he beat you often?") Uh-huh. Whenever my mother tells him something.

She thought that her looks were horrible. ("What was horrible?") Everything. [To Helen, "looks" are of utmost importance. So far, she has been unable to mention a single characteristic about herself (except her ability to have "friends") about which she expresses pride.]

The thing she could do best were sports.

She had no respect at all for herself. That's something mother tells me, but I think I do. [So far, there is little evidence that she does.]

She always enjoyed messing and goofing off with the kids.

She had a very uncomfortable feeling when . . hm . . Let's see . . Well, if my parents see this paper . . . No, they won't; I believe you. But that lady (the social worker) might tell them.

She found it easiest to talk to you.

[The Sentence Completion Test, although it does not bring out any new aspects of Helen's personality, further emphasizes already known features. Helen was also given a Word Association Test, but it did not demonstrate anything significantly different from what has been presented.]

THE PSYCHOLOGIST'S REPORT

Helen shuns thoughtful introspection and is ever impelled to action because of peremptory impulses over which she can exercise only a minimum of control. She lives in the moment, so that the future, particularly, has little significance. Her active way of handling situations is partially revealed by her performance on the Wechsler-Bellevue, where the Performance Quotient (97-98) is approximately ten points higher than the Verbal (86-90). Her thinking is subjective and personalized, and knowledge for its own sake has little value for her. She does not consider persons and objects to have an existence which is objective and separate from herself; rather, things exist primarily in terms of some relationship to her—she tends neither to know nor to be concerned about people, things, or ideas which she cannot use or from which she cannot gain some gratification. On the Wechsler Information subtest, for example, she locates London in France; she estimates there are six pints in a quart and twelve weeks in a year; she knows no cities in Italy or Japan; and she locates Egypt in the "north continent." Understandably, her reluctance or inability to view things objectively interferes with judgment and concept formation. Still, she apparently has some awareness of the difficulties she might get into with her impulsivity. On the Comprehension subtest, for example, she is able to distinguish between what she *would* and what she *should* do in case of a fire in a theater: she *should* call the fire department but thinks she probably *would* sit there and yell, "Fire! Fire!"

Since she does not value intellectual activity, Helen's thinking tends to be inexact. She is satisfied with approximation instead of precision and almost never pauses long enough to consider the true nature of either herself or her surroundings. She ignores what does not fit into her system of wishes, and "actuality" is what she wants it to be. While her tendency to ignore what is "true" occasionally reaches rather serious proportions, Helen never totally disregards or denies the real. She may shrug it off when it does not suit her; she may embroider it rather vividly, but she does not misrecognize or misread it.

The way Helen's needs and wishes modify and at times distort, the way exclusively affectively organized thoughts fill Helen's consciousness, so that little room is left for ideas that are not immediate sources of personal preoccupation, can be seen in her way of dealing with the Thematic Apperception material. Helen had been told that the possibility of her being hospitalized somewhere was being considered, and she became intensely angry and fearful about this. When she found out about the plan, she organized many of her TAT stories around the theme of a girl who was sent to a mental hospital and who thereupon suffered dreadful consequences: either she committed suicide, or became an ugly old crone, or got into immense trouble. Helen brought in such themes even on occasions when, at first glance at least, the pictures did not seem suitable for the purpose. To the "Graveyard" card, for example, she told the story of a father mourning over the grave of his daughter—she had committed suicide by slashing her wrists when she was told she would be sent to a hospital.

Helen's Rorschach performance further reflects the characteristics described. Impulsivity and tension intolerance find expression in her inability to integrate form and color smoothly, so that her perceptions of "blood" and "gorgeous finger paintings," for instance, contain almost no formal aspects. Color has such an affective impact that it disorganizes her; she is never able to integrate color with form to give it a more objective character. Many of her Rorschach responses are vague and at times quite peculiar. For example, she sees Card I as "a heart." She finds it difficult to explain how or why she sees the blot this way and says, "Kind of the way it's spread out, because, you know, the way a heart is spread out. ('How do you mean?') The lines in it. You know, the way a heart has lines in it." Helen rarely attempts a description of one of her percepts from memory and usually insists that she be permitted to look at the card again to refresh her memory. Her difficulties in relying purely on her own resources and her distrust of what she alone can offer find expression in her wish to find out what a percept "really" is (i.e., how "the others" see it).

Helen tries to get by through short-cutting serious work and replacing it with a flirtatious, seductive kittenishness. She hopes that people, particularly men, will excuse her lack of application and instead attend to the flattery with which she tries to take their minds off whatever needs to be done at the moment.

Helen's dependent and helpless attitude, although it seems unreal on the surface, is probably more genuine than it appears. The deeper one goes, the more one discovers her to have an uncertain foundation of basic mistrust, and fear about how others may wish to harm her. Her tendency to exaggerate and indulge in many other histrionic expressions can easily mislead an observer, who may dismiss Helen's dramatic expressions as no more than insincere requests for compliments. Actually, it seems that Helen suffers from a profoundly low evaluation of herself and needs genuine reassurance. Thus, for example, she makes use of each opportunity to announce how "dumb" she is. At the beginning, these declarations seem little more than thinly disguised requests for flattery. After a while, however, it becomes apparent that Helen is painfully concerned about her intelligence. She needs genuine and constant reassurance that she is not really "dumb," although her obtained Verbal I.Q. of 86-90 does not make the self-evaluation of her intelligence entirely unrealistic.

Helen's persistent plea for help is probably based on her suspicion, verging on conviction, that others tend to "double-cross" her, as she puts it. Adults, particularly, are banded together to frustrate her and to deny her what is rightly hers. Helen's view of the "depriving grownup" is particularly striking as one observes her attitudes toward her parents. Helen interprets the entire psychiatric examination as having been arranged by them for their benefit, and she perceives the Menninger Clinic as conspiring with her parents against herself. She says, for example, how disappointed she is in me; she had considered me a friend, but I have joined the enemy because I also recommend that she be hospitalized.

Helen's expressed feelings toward her parents are predominantly negative. Her mother, particularly, emerges as an unreasonable, restrictive, nagging and punitive ogress who does not and will not understand Helen at all. For example, she says that if her mother discovered she were "dumb," she would "kill" and "ground" Helen. A strong competitive threat binds mother and daughter together. To the Thematic Apperception Test picture which shows an old, ugly, witchlike woman standing behind a young and pretty one, Helen says the pretty one is her mother, while the witch is Helen after she has left "the hospital." The mother is thinking, "Now I'm finally prettier than she is."

The major role the family romance still plays at this time is suggested by Helen's remembered delight as she tells of the wonderful times she and her father formerly had, together and alone, when they played tennis or went swimming. On Sentence Completion, Helen says, *When she was very little* "she and her daddy were good pals. ('How about now?') They still are . . except . . I think Daddy likes Mother better than he does me." Helen now generalizes the overtly predominantly negative (maternal) and overtly predominantly positive (paternal) attitudes to adults in general. Thus, she sees the female social worker whom she has barely met as a horrible old hag who hates her and who thinks she is terrible. Her wish to re-establish a (possibly mythical) closeness to her father emerges in her general friendliness toward all adult males. Her tendency to try to divide her mother and father is similarly generalized. It emerges in her attempts to set the members of the examining team both against one another and against the parents, by her judicious use of flattery and disparagement.

While Helen's feelings toward her parents are marked by great intensity (the negative feelings no more so than the positive), her relationships with peers seem of quite a different order. The many people she describes as her "friends" ("nice" and "good kids") actually seem to be little more than acquaintances. One has the feeling that these "friends" come and go easily and that Helen is more concerned with their number than with the quality of the friendship. On Sentence Completion, for example, she says, *Her best friend* "I've got hundreds of them."

Helen's impulsivity, her vulnerability to the demands of the moment, her distrust of the motives of others and her marked tendency to act rather than think all suggest that outpatient treatment would probably meet with failure. Further, although Helen's suicidal threats are embellished by a strong histrionic component, the likelihood certainly exists that she might impulsively make a suicidal or homicidal attempt. For these reasons, it is suggested that a closed treatment setting be recommended for her treatment.

DISCUSSION

In what she conceives of as an "adult fashion," Helen is living out a parody. She is acting the role of the flirtatious, winsome, adult temptress whom she has seen in the movies and on TV. In this way, she is skipping the adolescent process—the proces of evaluating and coming to grips with the changes that are taking place within her; she is not facing how these changes refer to the past, to the future, or even to the present. Because she fears facing changes within herself, she is trying to solve the "adolescent problem" by acting as if it did not exist. She prematurely throws herself into adulthood (or her conception of it) without taking the time to deal internally with conflictual aspects. The period of adolescent uncertainty looks so painful that she attempts to ignore it altogether, jumping from childhood into pseudo adulthood.

The adulthood she chooses for herself is far from real, however. Helen assumes roles, rather than being the way she truly feels. She has adopted an adult "persona," and she uses it without genuinely involving herself in the exertion of growing up. She finds "real" adulthood difficult, if not impossible, to assume in a genuine fashion, and the adult shell she has adopted is extremely thin. Neither has she been able to deal adequately with the earlier problems of childhood. She does not seem to have given up intimate fantasies about her father in favor of establishing significant and genuine peer relationships. She is immersed in a struggle between her mother, her father and herself, and the struggle has no natural ending in sight. Only reluctantly can she admit that her father seems to prefer her mother, a situation different from what she remembers in the "good old times." Although Helen says that the problem of leaving home involves primarily having to say goodbye to her "friends," the real difficulty probably stems from her inability to leave her parents and consequently making the inevitable discovery that they can create a full life for themselves without her. Instead of experimenting with a gradual growth into adulthood, Helen sees her only solution to growing up as leaving home (at the same time that she finds herself unable to take this step).

In other words, Helen thinks her salvation lies in leaving an impossible home situation, but she finds herself unable to do so. In the meantime, she fights ghosts.

CONCLUSION

Joan and Helen share the characteristic of finding serious, reflective thought difficult to carry out. Although their personality organizations look very different on the surface, they are, at least in this important respect, quite similar. In both cases, action takes the place of reflection: Joan's action involves primarily avoidance and withdrawal; Helen's, outbursts of temper and "delinquent" behavior.

Both Joan and Helen are seriously disabled by having available such an insufficient supply of the powerful tool of thought. Thought would permit them to rehearse action internally first, so that the action could then be more modulated, and hence more appropriate.

Neither Joan nor Helen deals directly with her adolescence. Appropriately handling *any* major life stage requires reflection. When reflection is in some way short-circuited during chronological adolescence, leaving only action available, it is usual for the pubertal person to embrace the "solution" of either remaining in childhood or skipping adolescence altogether and entering a premature adulthood.

The next chapter contains test protocols of adolescents who are usually called "delinquents," either because they have already come in conflict with the law or because someone fears they soon may.

7

The "Delinquent" Adolescent

It has often been observed that the term "delinquency" has legal rather than psychological meaning. In this chapter we hope to show that young people accused of "delinquent" (i.e., illegal) behavior share only phenotypical characteristics, which may express vastly different genotypical organizations and meanings.

In order to avoid making the problem even more complex than it is, only *male* adolescents who have gotten into trouble with the law will be described here. It will become apparent that these young men have arrived at their legal difficulties via quite different psychological routes.

Most people, when they think of a "delinquent," have in mind a stereotype which never describes a three-dimensional person. Too often, those portions of the personality that do not fit the conventional and legal mold are squeezed, tugged, or ignored, so that the end product will conform to a quasi-sociological preconception.

Three young men are presented in this chapter. One is a tense, obsessive, sensitive young man, with a mild encephalopathy, quite different from the black-leather-jacketed model which the word "delinquent" usually calls to mind. The second young man's thinking is occasionally disorganized, and his conception of the world is frequently gross and degraded. Only the third young man begins to approximate the nonreflection and action orientation usually associated in popular thought with the "delinquent." But even he deals with life situations in his very own ways.

One may argue that young men who come to the Menninger Clinic for a psychiatric examination can hardly be typical "delinquents" because of the social and economic status their families occupy. True, these young men come primarily from upper middle-class homes and therefore occupy a status which lends their "delinquency" a particular quality. They are not what is sometimes thought of as "social" or "adjusted" delinquents, who intermingle with an antisocial neighborhood subgroup. On the contrary, these young men who are brought to the Menninger Clinic with an anti- and schools. For assorted conscious and unconscious reasons, they seek out persons of socioeconomic groups lower than their own. Consciously, they find their own groups boring, "square," not "cool," or whatever the momentary term of derogation happens to be. The young men who are brought to the Menninger Clinic with an anti- social history are proud of their associations with peers who (being sought out for that reason) often come from impoverished neigh- borhoods. But the new associates rarely offer more than exploitative toleration. The "outsider" who joins the well-established neighbor- hood group never seems truly to become a part of it, although he is grateful to belong even as little as he does.

Sometimes a young man who is brought to the Menninger Clinic because of his conflict with the law has a history of having rejected every sort of companionship; he commits his antisocial acts either in isolation or with a small group which exists primarily to carry out these types of activities.

These sorts of "delinquency" seem based largely on needs which involve anger, self-derogation and occasionally the wish for a certain kind of companionship. This last wish is obviously different from that of the young man who goes just outside of his own door to be "one of the boys." The young men who appear in this chapter either do not strive to be one of the boys at all, or they travel far in order to avoid their own groups and become one of "those" boys.

CLINICAL SUMMARY: Don

Don, aged sixteen, is the oldest son, the third of five children. His parents brought him for psychiatric examination because of their concern about his sullen, antagonistic attitude, his association with a delinquent boy, and because of a recent episode of minor stealing and alcoholic intoxication.

Don's father himself started drinking heavily as a teen-ager, and the father's repeated episodes of misuse of alcohol and drugs have required a number of hospitalizations for him. After several years of treatment, the father managed to control his addiction for longer periods of time, and though he still has been hospitalized off and on, his stays have been briefer. Most recently, after arranging for Don's examination, the father again resorted to excessive drinking and hospitalized himself just before coming with Don. Don's parents consider only one of Don's four siblings to be a "normal child."

Except for nausea during the first trimester, Don's mother was in good health during her pregnancy. Delivery was easy and spontaneous. Don seemed to develop normally. He accomplished bowel control before he was one year old. Bladder training, however, has never been established, as Don still wets at night. He was able to speak in sentences by the age of eighteen months. He showed no special behavior problems, except that he reacted to frustration and punishment with fear and timidity.

At the age of two and a half years, Don caught his arm in a washing-machine wringer; he suffered severe soft tissue injury to the right arm and was hospitalized for one week. A skin graft completed the repair of this injury when he was eight years old. After the age of six years, he suffered from recurrent bouts of allergic rhinitis, asthma, bronchitis and sinus trouble each winter. He still suffers frequently from the rhinitis. At the age of ten, he had bronchial pneumonia for one week, but recovered easily. At the age of fourteen, he was hospitalized because of pallor, low-grade fever and weakness. A diagnosis of nephritis, complicating an upper respiratory infection and sinusitis, was made.

Don began school at the age of six and made average or better grades. He could never adequately draw or write, however, in spite of efforts to coach him. No special problems were reported by his teachers until the sixth grade, when he started disobeying some of them.

Both parents have considered Don a troubled child since his early years. At the age of three he was already a silent, sullen boy who would not talk to people. Starting at that time, he spent hours playing by himself, telling himself stories and twirling a variety of objects. On several occasions, he walked away from home in the middle of the night. Most of his care was entrusted to an older sister and to women who were hired for that purpose. He was always resentful of direction and frightened of discipline. He generally associated with older boys, but had almost no intimate friends. When he was about seven, he began associating with a boy known in the community as a "delinquent." This association has persisted until the present.

Since the age of seven, Don has been in legal trouble, first because he broke a number of windows, later because he stole cigarettes from a filling station and, in the school locker room, money from the pockets of seventh-grade football players. About two months ago he came home drunk twice within one week. He was brought home by a sheriff who had caught him and his friends stealing liquor and billfolds from the cars of students who were at a graduation dance. Don has apparently had no significant relationships with girls.

Physical and Neurological Data: Physical and neurological examinations revealed an asymmetrical skull, convergence paralysis of the eyes, 20/100 vision of the right eye, a deviation of the nasal septum and hyperactive reflexes on the left side. These findings reflect a congenital, mild, nonspecific encephalopathy.

Laboratory, X-Ray and EEG Findings: The EEG showed consistent minor irregularities of the left temporal region, where medium voltage negative spike discharges occur in waking, sleep and hyperventilation. The impression was one of an abnormal EEG, suggesting disturbance in the left temporal region. Other laboratory findings were within normal limits.

THE PSYCHOLOGIST'S DESCRIPTION

Don manifested his great initial tension in restless fidgeting, a tremor of his hands, a persistent tugging at his shoes, a constant scratching of parts of his body, a frequent grimacing, nail biting and in an uncertain quaver of his voice. He readily admitted feeling "nervous," but gradually he relaxed, smiled, and made humorous little comments. Yet he never became really at ease, and some of the test procedures rearoused almost his initial degree of tension.

He responded appreciatively to friendliness. For example, after I gave him one of my cigarettes, he offered me one of his each time he smoked. Very early, he developed somewhat dependent feelings toward me, and he often sought my advice, help, and approbation of what he was doing. He seemed to become frightened whenever he thought I was not physically available. For example, I once suggested a break in a two-hour testing session. We both went downstairs, but when Don returned to my office I was not yet back. I had returned by the time he came again, and with anxious relief he said, "I was afraid I was going to lose you." The following day, he knocked on my closed door before his scheduled appointment and explained that he had been uncertain whether I had expected him to come on his own (I ordinarily picked him up in the waiting room).

Although he found many of the tests distasteful because they were difficult and tension producing (he experienced them as "boring"), he ordinarily showed an unusually thoughtful and cooperative attitude and put forth a strong effort to do what was expected. He never attempted to avoid doing a problem, even when he found it exceptionally difficult.

It was necessary to see Don for eight hours in order to finish the normal battery, which usually can be completed in six or seven. It took longer because Don was obsessively uncertain, a characteristic which was reflected in everything he did. His sentences were filled with qualifiers and modifiers, with words such as "perhaps" and "maybe," and with phrases such as "could be" and "I suppose." He frequently corrected himself, modifying a word to make it just a little more accurate. His entire approach, both to the world and to his own thoughts, was tentative, as though he could trust neither. He had difficulty daring to make a verbal commitment and seemed convinced that what he said would probably be wrong. At times it seemed as if he almost had to hear his thoughts aloud before he could know whether they were correct.

THE WECHSLER-BELLEVUE SCALE

[Striking in Don's Scattergram (p. 524) is the difference of more than thirty points between his Verbal and Performance quotients. A discrepancy of such magnitude leads one to think immediately of the expression of some sort of encephalopathy, particularly since it is so much more usual for persons who come in trouble with the law to be action oriented, and therefore to do better on Performance than Verbal tasks. Not only is Don's thirty-point Verbal-Performance differential striking; it is almost equally amazing to see how well he does on Verbal tasks, achieving a Bright Normal→Superior level. Again, it is not usual to find persons who come in chronic conflict with the law to be as verbally articulate as Don appears to be.

[A number of characteristics suggest the interfering effects of a rather marked degree of anxiety. The outstanding "sign" of this is the very low Digit Span performance, which is about eight points below Don's average. Another suggestion that anxiety interferes with efficient performance is Don's tendency to achieve alternate scores (on five of the subtests). The difference between actually achieved and alternate scores usually indicates the degree to which anxiety or some other intrusive agent prevents the person from performing at his optimal level.

[Although Don has more than the average number of facts at his disposal, the inverted Comprehension-Information subtest relationship suggests that he depends more on already prepared (e.g., social) standards to organize his thinking about situations than on thinking situations through for himself.]

Name: Don   Age: 16-3

	RS	WTS	0 1 2 3 4 5 6 7 8 9 10 11 12 13 14 15 16 17 18 19 20
COMPR.	15-16	13-14	x
INFOR.	16-17	11-12	x
DIG.	8-9	4-6	x
ARITH.	8-10	10-13	x
SIMIL.	17	14	
VOCAB.	29	13	
P. A.	9	8	
P. C.	13-14	13-14	x
B. D.	17	8	
O. A.	12	5	
D. S.	34	8	

TOT. VERB.	61-66
TOT. PERF.	42-43
TOT. SCALE	103-109

VERBAL I.Q.:   119-126   LEVEL: Bright Normal→Superior

PERFORMANCE I.Q.:   87-89   LEVEL: Dull Normal

TOTAL I.Q.:   105-110   LEVEL: Average

INFORMATION

(He is obviously tense, and his hands are shaking, but his manner is very pleasant.)

No.	Question	Response and Comments	Score
1.	Who is the President of the United States?	Eisenhower. ("And who was president before that?") Truman. ("And before that?") Uh . . Roosevelt.	+

No.	Question	Response and Comments	Score
2.	What is a thermometer?	It's uh .. an instrument for measuring .. uh .. Thermometer .. for measuring temperature. [His hesitant tendency is already evident.]	+
3.	What does rubber come from?	That's a good question .. Well, the only thing I can think of is "tree." [The phrase, "That's a good question," gives Don additional time to prepare his thoughts.]	+
4.	Where is London?	England.	+
5.	How many pints make a quart?	Two.	+
6.	How many weeks are there in a year?	Three hundred and sixty-five and one-fourth. ("Is that how many weeks there are?") Weeks .. oh .. fifty-two. [The minor inefficiency which causes him to distort "weeks" into "days" suggests that Don's perception is somewhat imprecise, probably because of anxiety.]	+
7.	What is the capital of Italy?	Uh .. Well .. I'll say Genoa, but I don't think that's right. ("Can you think of any other city?") Oh .. let's see .. Rome (he laughs). ("Which of the two cities would you choose?") Oh, I'll say Rome .. I don't know. [The effort to reduce uncertainty by presenting alternatives reflects Don's feelings of unsureness.]	−
8.	What is the capital of Japan?	Uh ...... Tokyo.	+
9.	How tall is the average American woman?	Uh .. five feet five inches. [Don finds it hard to make this unequivocal statement (even though he apparently "knows" the correct answer), without preceding it with an exclamation which denotes his hesitancy.]	+
10.	Who invented the airplane?	Uh .. Wright brothers. [Again.]	+
11.	Where is Brazil?	South America.	+
12.	How far is it from Paris to New York?	(He sighs.) .. Oh .. 4,000 miles.	−
13.	What does the heart do?	That .. circulates the blood .. It pumps blood.	+
14.	Who wrote Hamlet?	Shakespeare.	+
15.	What is the population of the United States?	.. One hundred and sixty million.	+

No.	Question	Response and Comments	Score
16.	*When is Washington's birthday?*	February 22.	+
17.	*Who discovered the North Pole?*	Should I just guess at these if I don't know? ("Yes, that's all right.") Byrd.	—
18.	*Where is Egypt?*	That'd be, what *continent?* ("Yes, that would be okay.") Uh .. uh .. Asia.	—
19.	*Who wrote Huckleberry Finn?*	Uh .. Mark Twain.	+
20.	*What is the Vatican?*	That's where the Pope lives.	+
21.	*What is the Koran?*	I'll pass it up. I never heard of that.	—
22.	*Who wrote Faust?*	I don't know that one either (he smiles).	—
23.	*What is an Habeas Corpus?*	Uh .. that's .. Let's see .. That's your proof that a person's dead, I guess. [Many so-called delinquents know the meaning of this phrase because of familiarity with legal terms.]	—
24.	*What is ethnology?*	E-t-h? ("That's right.") I don't know.	—
25.	*What is the Apocrypha?*	I don't know.	—

RAW SCORE: 16-17

WEIGHTED SCORE: 11-12

COMPREHENSION

(Don is able to deal well with this subtest, and there are only occasional and minor indications of doubting and other uncertainty. On the "theater" question, for example, he answers as follows: "Oh .. oh .. Tell the manager, I guess. If he's there." Although this answer is correct, Don is uncertain.)

RAW SCORE: 15-16

WEIGHTED SCORE: 13-14

SIMILARITIES

(Don's responses are clearly and precisely stated at the beginning. As the concepts to be discovered become more abstract, however, he occasionally misses dead center, becoming somewhat fuzzy.)

No.	Items	Response and Comments	Score
1-6	——	(He achieves full credit on these items.)	12

No.	Items	Response and Comments	Score

7. *Wood-alcohol*

They're compounds. ("In what sense do you mean?") Well, they're made of the same substances. They both have the same, or some of the same. ("Could you put it any other way?") No. [This is an example of Don's tendency to hit things just a bit off the mark—not to the extent of being wrong, but to the extent of not being correct enough. This sort of tendency toward vagueness is not great enough to indicate severe disturbance; the vagueness constitutes a diagnostic "soft" sign.]   1

9. *Egg-seed*

I can't think of a word ... They produce objects .. living things. [Words and ideas tend not always to be readily available to Don, and he occasionally labors mightily to produce quite an ordinary idea. This poor availability of words and concepts suggests the presence of an intrusive, interfering phenomenon of some sort.]   1

10. *Poem-statue*

.... I thought of something funny. ("About poem and statue?") That wasn't it. Can I come back to it? Like on those quiz shows. ("Would you like to come back to it later?") (He laughs.) I don't want to come back to it very bad. Well, I'll say .. they're symbols of .. uh .... Well, they could be symbols of people. ("How do you mean?") Well, like famous people, or something. [Don's reasoning is becoming difficult to follow, both for the examiner and for himself.]   1

11. *Praise-punishment*

They .. they help people .. Yes, people. ("In what way?") What way! Well................. They .. It teaches them not to do certain things. It helps them to be sure of themselves. [In addition to the recurring vagueness, Don's comment, "It helps them be sure of themselves," probably has a special meaning for him. One of Don's major felt problems seems to refer to his feelings of uncertainty. Offhand, praise and punishment have little to do with helping a person become "sure of himself." Don appears to drag this "explanation" in because he feels his own unsureness so overwhelmingly.]   1

RAW SCORE: 17

WEIGHTED SCORE: 14

PICTURE COMPLETION

(Don does well on this subtest. He fails to find only the missing portion on Item 14 and obtains alternate credit on Item 3, as follows:)

No. Item	Time	Missing	Response and Comments	Score
3. *Profile*		ear	Oh .... missing (15″) (he sighs). Gosh I can't see anything missing .. unless it's hair (20″). Oh, the ear! The ear! The ear! (32″) Gosh. [The missing ear is an "easy" item. The fact that Don requires 32″ to discover it missing underscores the spottiness of his capacity to attend and concentrate.]	0-1

RAW SCORE: 13-14

WEIGHTED SCORE: 13-14

PICTURE ARRANGEMENT

[Once again it becomes evident that Don is able to work effectively for a period of time, but eventually comes up with some statement or interpretation which, although not extraordinarily peculiar, is nevertheless unusual enough to make one question the solidity of his mental organization.]

No. Item	Correct Order	Time	Arranged Order	Story and Comments	Score
4. *Flirt*	JANET	16″	AJNET	This woman was walking down the street and this guy came along in his car. He saw her, stopped and got out, and then he put on her hat. He took her hat from her and put it on. [Apart from missing the humor of the sequence, Don mistakes the woman's laundry bag for her "hat."]	2
5. *Fish*	EFGHIJ	40″	EGFHJI	The man was fishing and .. caught a fish, and then he caught another one, and then his butler came up. The butler came up, and he was holding the fish, and that was the way he was catching the fish. [Don misses credit on this item, not because he misunderstands the point, but because he overlooks aspects which would indicate the correct sequence. Don's ignoring of these details is particularly striking because of his higher-than-average ability on Picture Completion, a test	0

No. Item	Correct Order	Time	Arranged Order	Story and Comments	Score
				which requires him to attend to and interpret perceptual detail.]	

RAW SCORE: 9

WEIGHTED SCORE: 8

BLOCK DESIGN

(Don obtains scores on only the first five designs. Although he obtains extra time credits on Design 2 and 5, even on these he gives evidence of confusion and occasional impotence. With considerable help from me, he can do the last two designs, but he requires twice as much time as the test's time limits permit for credit. He works slowly, but even so his efforts frequently look extremely unlike the model. Often Don's error is not that he simply rotates some blocks, but that his construction has little to do with the entire gestalt. Sometimes, for example, he tries to copy the given design by stringing blocks together at their corners in single file.)

RAW SCORE: 17

WEIGHTED SCORE: 8

[To give a more precise idea of the confusion which Don experiences with this type of motor-sensory task, his Object Assembly performance is presented in detail.]

OBJECT ASSEMBLY

Item	Time	Accur.	Description of Behavior and Comments	Score
Manikin	24″	Yes	(He hesitates occasionally, but experiences no real difficulty on this item.)	6
Profile	2′ 16″	Yes	(He first places the ear upside down.) It looks backwards to me. (He does not change it at this point, however. He puts the nose piece upside down in the eye area and then removes it. Then he corrects the upside-down ear.) That works better. (He first is unable to make the nose piece fit, even though he has it in the right area; but then he fits it correctly. Both the mouth and backhead pieces are in the right place, but upside down. He takes the backhead piece from the back and tries it in front; suddenly he sees how it should go and places it correctly. Eventually, by 2′ 16″, he fits the backhead piece and places the other pieces in their correct spaces.)	6
Hand	4′ 5″	No	And away we go! It'll take a while, I'm afraid. (He puts the thumb piece upside down	0

Item	Time	Accur.	Description of Behavior and Comments	Score

and tries to fit the fingers into the cavity made by it in this position. At 2', he is still contour fitting.) I'm thinking something should fit in there. (He bites his fingernails and looks at the pieces in a puzzled fashion. At 2' 30", he has gotten no further.) It must fit in here some way. (He takes the upside-down thumb piece away and tries to fit the wrist piece in its place. He turns the unfinished hand over to look at the other side and tries more contour fitting.) This is something I'll never get .... Whoops! There! (He fits the thumb piece correctly at 3' 30".) I should have gotten that a half an hour ago. (By 4' 5", he has fitted all the fingers correctly.) ("When did you realize what it was?") I thought it was a hand all along, but I just couldn't get it to fit together. [Goalless contour fitting, which occurs even when the person knows what the item should make, is typical of the sensory-motor helplessness of people who suffer some sort of organic brain dysfunction. Although Don's responses in general are occasionally somewhat peculiar, the reasons for this seem to involve desperation and frustration that nothing works, rather than a preference for or tendency to indulge in a peculiar style. One may well wonder to what extent Don's "antisocial" behavior reflects, at least in part, an effort to show himself capable, potent and of at least a little account in some area. The behavior may also express his anger about being disabled (even though he does not know the nature of this disability).]

RAW SCORE: 12

WEIGHTED SCORE: 5

VOCABULARY

No.	Word	Response and Comments	Score
1.	*Apple*	Fruit. You want just a word? ("Just tell me what it means.") A definition? [Here again is an indication of Don's uncertainty, of his need to have the situation minutely spelled out.]	1
2.	*Donkey*	Animal . . uh . . ("Were you going to add something else?") It's a . . uh . . beast of burden. [One can almost feel Don's being torn in two directions at once: to let go and not let go.]	1

No.	Word	Response and Comments	Score
3.	*Join*	That's to . . uh . . pss . . take up a membership with some party or group of people. [Don's definitions are well rounded, and they cover the area more than sufficiently. He apparently spends considerable time in thoughtful activities.]	1
4.	*Diamond*	It's . . uh . . uh . . compressed . . uh . . what is it? Carbon. Highly compressed.	1
5.	*Nuisance*	Uh . . that's something that bothers other animals or people.	1
6.	*Fur*	That's hair . . . that you take off . . . that you can get from certain animals. Outside covering.	1
7.	*Cushion*	(He sighs.) . . Uh . . I'm sitting on one here. That's something that's soft . . soft object that . . uh . . let's see . . Well . . I can't think . . . That you can put things on. ("Could you tell me a little more precisely?") (He covers his eyes.) Let's see. ("Tell me as best you can.") All I can think of . . cushion is something like I'm sitting on. ("And what is that?") Well, an object to sit on. [After a series of very good definitions, Don suddenly cannot adequately define a very simple word. One has the feeling that every once in a while Don's capacities are much less available, and at times almost absent. Such an unaccountable ebb and flow of availability and unavailability is typical of the functioning of persons who suffer from a brain dysfunction.]	1
8.	*Shilling*	That's an English measurement of money.	1
9.	*Gamble*	Well . . that's to . . uh risk.	1
10.	*Bacon*	That's part . . part of a pig . . of a pig. [At times Don seems relieved to have caught hold of a word or concept which just previously had not been available, and so he repeats it.]	1
11.	*Nail*	Let's see . . could . . A long . . uh . . It would be a . . thin, long piece of iron, iron. Do you want what it's used for? ("Tell me as much as you think will tell the meaning.") It's used for holding things down or putting them together with.	1
12.	*Cedar*	That's a tree . . a tree.	1
13.	*Tint*	That's . . shading.	1
14.	*Armory*	I'm darned if I know what that is, but I'd say . . I don't really know, but I'll guess. It's uh . . uh . . well . . cripes! For military purposes is all I know. ("Can you tell me any more about it?") (He smiles.) No, I can't. Well, maybe for storing. ("Storing	½

No.	Word	Response and Comments	Score
		what?") Weapons. [Euphemisms, such as "cripes" and "darned," do not reflect the devil-may-care toughness one usually associates with the "delinquent."]	
15.	Fable	That's a story.	1
16.	Brim	It could be the top. ("How do you mean?") Like the top of a hat. No! Wait a minute. The top of a hat would be the crown. Well, leave it that way anyway. ("What do you think the brim of a hat would be?") It would be the side. [Don obviously cares enough about intellectual adequacy to correct himself when he thinks he is wrong. Were he less involved in doing well in this test, he would not bother to correct a mistake.]	½
17.	Guillotine	That's a .. machine used for .. uh .. for .. uh .. beheading people.	1
18.	Plural	More than one.	1
19.	Seclude	It means to .. st .. be .. uh .. be by .. uh .. alone .. be alone, I guess. [Might the increased speech disturbance reflect Don's own struggle with feelings of aloneness?]	1
20.	Nitroglycerin	.. Explosive .. explosive substance.	1
21.	Stanza	Like a verse of a poem.	1
22.	Microscope	It's a .. machine for studying microorganisms. ("What does it do?") It magnifies.	1
23.	Vesper	Yeah. (He smiles.) That's about it. Pass that one up.	0
24.	Belfry	That would be the place where .. well .. for bells, I guess.	1
25.	Recede	That's to .. recede .. Well, that's to hold back, or pull back. ("Which do you think?") Well, pull back.	½
26.	Affliction	It'd be a disease.	½
27.	Pewter	Well .. a substance that .. somewhat like cement, I think. ("What is it used for?") It's used for making jars, I guess .. containers.	0
28.	Ballast	That's weight .. extra weight.	1
29.	Catacomb	Isn't that a .. be a sort of a cave, I guess.	½
30.	Spangle	Be .. uh .. decorations. ("Could you tell me more?") Well .. uh .. well, like a play, maybe.	½
21.	Espionage	(He sighs.) That's .. uh .. well, spying I guess.	1

No.	Word	Response and Comments	Score
32.	*Imminent*	That's something like something that's bound to happen . . will soon happen.	1
33.	*Mantis*	It's a bug.	1
34.	*Hara-kiri*	Suicide, I think. ("Any special kind?") Well . . you mean example? ("Where does the word come from?") Well, doesn't that come from the Japanese?	1

(He does not know the meaning of the remaining words.)

RAW SCORE: ___29___

WEIGHTED SCORE: ___13___

The BRL Sorting Test

[Only a portion of this test is shown to suggest the flavor of Don's performance. It can be seen how difficult he finds smooth conceptualization.]

PART I

Stimulus	Patient's Sorting	Response and Comments	Score
1. Don's choice: *Toy hammer*	(I give instructions.) You mean that would have something to do with it? Well, let's see . . . . (He studies the items and adds: nails, wooden block with nail.)	I'm just trying to figure something out that I'm not sure about. I'm just thinking, if everything in that line of work goes with it, you'd have a whole bunch more. But it's up to me, I suppose. What is this thing? (He points to the pliers.) ("What do you think?") It looks like a pair of pliers. (He adds all the remaining tools.) The block of wood and the nails use the hammer to work with. The rest of these are just tools around the house, so I've decided they should go with it. [Although Don's sorting is not peculiar, it reflects his conceptual, abstraction difficulties.]	Loose Concrete→ Conceptual Def. Syncretistic
2. *Fork*	(Sink stopper; spoon.) (He holds the toy spoon but does not place it right away.) Let's see here (adds sugar). These	Let's see. I think that's about the size of it there. ("Why do they all belong together?") Well, these are all eating utensils, and they're used for food, and	Loose (Symbolic) Concrete— Conceptual Def.

Stimulus	Patient's Sorting	Response and Comments	Score
	are supposedly sugar, aren't they? (He puts back the toy spoon.) Oh! (He adds the knife. Eventually he adds all the silverware.)	that's what the sugar is supposed to represent, I imagine. ("How does the sink stopper fit?") That's kind of silly, but I'd say that goes for washing them. (After he completes the next item, he adds the file card to the present sorting and says:) I should think this would go with it. ("How would it go?") Because you might use it (the file card) for putting a menu on, or a recipe, I mean.	

[The remainder of Don's Part I sortings are more or less the same as these. The lack of sharpness and clarity of his concepts, their murkiness and looseness, are vivid.]

PART II

Examiner's Sorting	Explanation and Comments	Score
1. Red objects	Oh .. (he smiles) .... This (matches) is included, too? .... Whew!.............. Hm! It would take me a million years to figure out that one, but they could all be used in school, maybe. [This response reflects Don's conceptual difficulties, although the pathological effect is softened somewhat by the fact that many persons find it difficult to make the transfer from Part I to Part II.]	Syncretistic
2. Metal	(He studies the sorting.) .... I can only think of one answer. I can think maybe that they're all machines. ("Machines?") Well, they all perform some sort of work. [Don's inability to find the rather simple conceptual realm that ties the metal objects together is striking. Throughout this test one is again impressed by the fact that Don's responses are not odd—instead, they usually reflect his helplessness. By now, it is quite clear that Don suffers from an impairment which affects both his sensory-motor and conceptualizing abilities.]	Syncretistic
4. Tools	That should be an easy one. (But he studies the grouping at length.) You just want to know why they're alike? ("That's right.")	Conceptual Def. Peculiar

Examiner's Sorting	Explanation and Comments	Score
	Because they are all simple machines. ("How do you mean?") Well, they . . uh . . . . . They only have about one certain job to perform. ("Could you put it another way?") Well, how would this be? That they all have their one certain job . . their one main job. [Does Don invoke the sophisticated concept of "machines" because he is unable to think of the much simpler and more economical "tools"? Persons with conceptual interference occasionally formulate complex ideas to hide the fact that they do not have a simpler idea available.]	
12. *Square*	(I omit the eraser to make the conceptualizing task somewhat easier.) (He bites his nails.) That couldn't be. ("It might. What were you thinking?") It might, if that nail wasn't there (the nail in the block of wood). ("How would they belong then?") They'd all be a product of plants. ("Can you think of any other way?") . . . . Well, they all change their shapes and forms when they're burned. [Don obviously understands the test's requirement, to form a general concept that will cover all items, but he goes far afield before he can think of one. This concept-finding difficulty is frequent in persons suffering organic brain dysfunction.]	Syncretistic Peculiar

The Bender Gestalt Test

PART A AND PART B (PLATES 49 AND 50)

[Although Don's Bender Gestalt reproductions are fairly accurate, in the sense that he maintains the basic configurations of the designs, both on the 5″ Exposure and the Copy, several features give away Don's graphomotor difficulties. Both times, for example, he rotates Design 3 (the "arrow") 180°. On Part A, he has considerable difficulty with Design 6; its wavy lines become jagged and irregular, and look like edgy points rather than smooth waves. Here he also has difficulties in making lines meet smoothly, and his entire drawing effort seems forced, constricted and irregular. Although his drawings are of "borderline" accuracy, they are nevertheless sufficiently distorted to suggest difficulties in the graphomotor area.

[He is extremely aware of his drawing problems, so that on almost every design he makes such a comment as, "I can't even make a circle." The effeminacy of his expressions is striking. He frequently says, "Dear me," or "Oh dear," expressions which are hardly in keeping with the stereotyped image of the "cool" delinquent.]

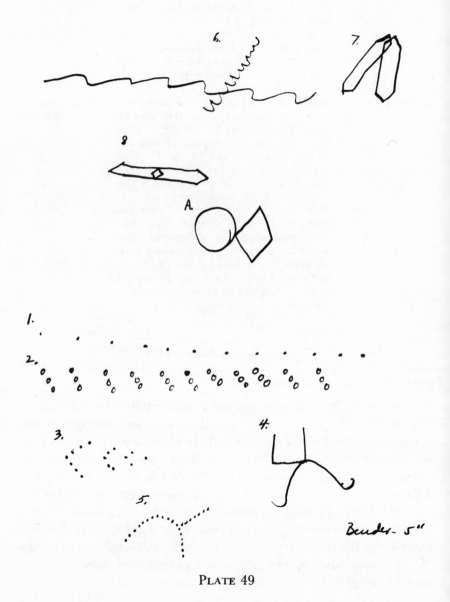

PLATE 49

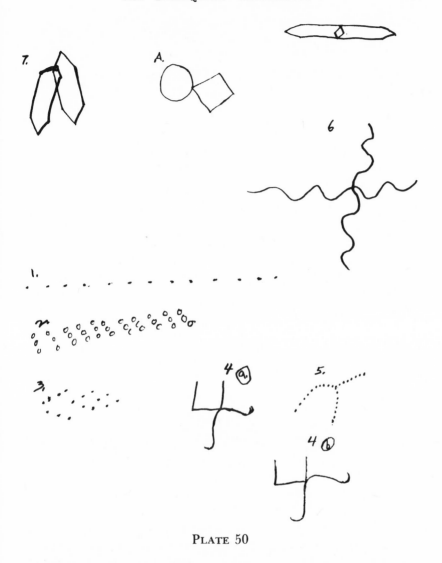

PLATE 50

THE DRAW A PERSON TEST

PART I (PLATE 51)

(As he is drawing his "man," he says:) One monstertype person
coming up. Oh dear! Of course, you know that I'm not very good
at this. Oh boy! . . . . . You want me to do the whole thing? . . . . .
(As he continues to draw:) One thing I always hated is this . . . . .
Let's see . . where am I here? . . . . I hope you're not expecting too

much. (He draws tentatively and does not appear at all sure of himself. As he slowly proceeds, his lines become mixed up. For example, he draws shoes so that their backs come out too far behind the legs he has previously drawn. While he is drawing, he is softly whistling—in the dark?——to himself. He says:) I hope you never have to bump into one of these.

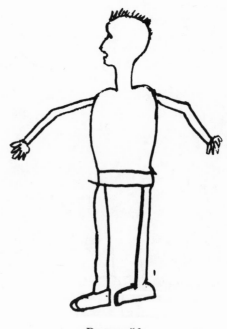

PLATE 51

PART II (PLATE 52)

(He does much erasing around the head.) Wow! That's terrible .... (He smiles.) I hate to do this to anybody. (Again, he is softly whistling to himself.) .... I'll give her some hair .. just for the heck of it .... (After he is finished) It looks more like .. I don't know *what* it looks like.

[Not only the immature execution of Don's drawings, but his awareness of the drawings' inadequacy, are significant. But in spite of his awareness, he is unable to make these poor drawings any better. Although many aspects of verbal functioning seem little affected, some behavioral areas do not function at all well (as a result, presumably, of Don's organic impairment). It is important to note that, while the "organicity" is relatively unobtrusive on neurological examination, its effect on some areas of Don's psychological functioning is considerable. Again, one wonders to what extent Don's antisocial behavior represents a reaction to an impairment of which, on some level, he may be aware.]

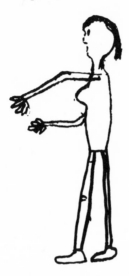

PLATE 52

RORSCHACH TEST

[Don's Rorschach Psychogram (p. 540) suggests that his disorganization is greater than had hitherto been thought. It is impossible, however, to know just how Don's "organic" features complicate this disorganization. In any case, a number of the Psychogram features present a disquieting picture.

[Although his uncertainty and doubt-riddenness were apparent earlier, one does not expect such a high percentage of his responses to have so strong a Dr (i.e., more or less arbitrary) quality. The qualitative features of Don's responses are arresting, particularly the number of fabulized components. Another significant aspect of the Psychogram is the Experience Balance, which shows that Don does not muster a single "true" M response. This lack of evidence to suggest productive thought activity is unexpected in a person who has appeared to have a relatively rich inner life. None of Don's Color responses are of acceptable Form quality; two out of four are of the unmodulated CF variety. His high responsiveness to color,

RORSCHACH SCORING SHEET

Number of Responses: 26

Manner of Approach (Location)

WS	3
W	4
D	10
Dd	0
Do	1
Dr	8
De	0
Total	26

Location Percentages

W%	27
D%	38
DR%	35
De%	0

Form, Movement, Color and Shading Determinants

F+	6		
F−	4		
F±	3		
F∓	5		
FM±	1		
FC∓	1	FC−	2
CF	2	(FC̄)	(1)
F(C)+	1	F(C)−	1
Total	26		

Groups of Contents

A	8
Ad	1
H	0
Hd	1
Monster	1
Scarecrow	1
Obj.	3
At.	1
Ats.	2
Pl.	5
Cloud	1
Geol.	1
Spots	1
Total	26

Determinant and Content Percentages

F%	69/92	Obj.%	12
F+%	50/46	At.%	12
A%	35	P%	4
H%	4		

Qualitative Material

Popular	VIII
Combination	III IV VIII IX X
Fabulation	15
Fabulized Combination	1
Peculiar	2
Identity Confusion	1
Castration	2
Masturbatory	1
Oral Aggression	2

EXPERIENCE BALANCE: <u>0.5/3.5</u>

together with his poor integration of it, suggest Don's emotional lability—his tendency not to look before reacting. One is surprised that Don constructs so few adequately formed percepts, and that so many of the ones he does construct contain an unimaginative animal content.

[Don gives more than the average number of responses, and it is obvious that he does not participate in the Rorschach task lightly or superficially. At the risk of underscoring the point too heavily, one must say again that his approach is quite different in various respects from that of the "usual delinquent."]

RORSCHACH PROTOCOL

Card #	React. Time	Score	Protocol	Inquiry and Observations
			Oh dear . . . . . Am I just supposed to tell you whatever pops into my mind?	
I	25″	WsF+Obj. Fab.	1. It looks like a jack-o-lantern with ears . . . . ("Anything else?") Hm? ("Does any part remind you of anything else?") Let's see	1. ("Tell me about the jack-o-lantern you saw.") Well, the four slits in it look something like they have in a jack-o-lantern. ("Anything else about it?") Well, those two odd-shaped pieces sticking out on top. ("What about them?") They look like something might be on a . . uh . . just for . . decorations.
		WF−Cl	2. It might be a cloud formation. (He offers this response somewhat disparagingly.)	2. ("What did the clouds look like?") What did it look like? (He laughs.) . . . . I really don't know. It looked like just . . uh . . an odd-shaped cloud. ("What made it seem like a cloud?") Well, because clouds often make funny-looking pictures. ("Was it any particular kind of cloud?") You mean, like cumulus or . . ? ("That's right.") Well, no, I guess not. I can't think of anything. [Don begins this test rather effectively, with a well-conceived, if mildly noncritically fabulized, response. Response 2, however, is much less sharply conceived. It is an "easy" percept which requires little effort to articulate. Perhaps Don offers "clouds" because he feels he ought to say something in response

Card #	React. Time	Score	Protocol	Inquiry and Observations
				to the examiner's question, even when he has no "good" response available.]
II			(He studies the card intently.) Can I turn it around? (After 20".) ("Whatever you like.") ∨ ∧ (He laughs.) . . . . . (He sighs.)	
	1' 15"	DCF Spots Pec. Fab.	1. All I can think of . . is . . it looks to me like an optical illusion . . . That's all I can think of.	1. ("Tell me about the optical illusion.") Well, I just . . . . . thinking of something *I've* seen before. Like, sometimes I look into a light and then look away, and then I see different-looking lights and different spots when you look away. Of course, *I guess* I'm supposed to have glasses. ("Do things ever look funny in other ways, too?") Sometimes things far away are somewhat blurred. Dad thinks I'm nearsighted. ("Do you get headaches?") Yes. If I wake up with one, it stays all day. ("How often do you get them?") Maybe one a month; maybe less. ("Where in the card were the spots you saw?") All the red spots. [This seemed to offer a good opportunity to inquire about various visual difficulties which might be related to Don's possible "brain damage," but except for the occasional fairly severe headaches, Don's experiences are not unusual. The "spots" appear to be afterimages. Don becomes uncreative as soon as he comes face to face with color—e.g., he is incapable of making spots into anything but "spots."]

Card #	React. Time	Score	Protocol	Inquiry and Observations
		DF±A (FC̄)	2. If it didn't have that red in it, you might say it looked like two . . what do you call 'em? . . rhinoceros. Rhinos, anyway. It's probably impossible, but	2. ("What about the rhinos?") I was thinking of the . . the . . top of the picture there . . if you want to call it the top. Something that . . to me . . looks something like a horn. Also, something that looks like a head . . a couple of heads. ("Why did it seem impossible?") It's impossible for them to stand up like that. I mean, the way I look at it, they would have been standing on their hind legs. (The entire nonred area of the blot. He differentiates the horns, which are the upper central Dd, the ears at the side and the legs at the bottom.) [After he first becomes mildly disorganized by the color on the previous response, Don makes a good recovery and describes the present response in a fairly differentiated fashion. It should be noted, however, that color is sufficiently disturbing so that it must be specifically rejected.]
			If I can't think of anything more, what am I supposed to do? ("Tell me.") (He smiles.) Well, I'm finished. (He offers me a cigarette and shows me a membership card he received from a local miniature golf course.) I'm getting to be a golfer.	
III			Let's see . . I'm not going to say anything about these red spots.	[The first thing he is aware of again, but can not integrate effectively, is color (affect).]

React. Card # Time Score	Protocol	Inquiry and Observations
45″ DoF+Ad Comb.	1. But these two on top here look sorta like chicken heads.	1. ("Tell me about the chicken heads.") The top part reminded me of, like the comb on the rooster; and they both had parts stuck out there that reminded me of a beak.
DrF+Hd Fab. comb. Ident. confus.	2. And the rest on down reminds me of a person. Let's see.	2. ("What kind of a person did it seem to be?") Well . . . . uh . . . . (He shakes his head.) Nope. ("Nope what?") Nope, I don't really know what it was . . . . ("Was it a man or a woman?") A woman. ("What made it look like that?") Well, it looked like they had the figure. ("Do the head you saw and the body belong together?") Well, what do you mean, belong together? ("I mean, are they part of the same thing?") Well, I thought they were in one piece. ("Like a human body with a chicken head?") (He smiles.) Yeah. ("The rest of the person" is the central black Dr, above the "legs" and below the "head.") [The examiner was perhaps too insistent in his inquiry here; Don's perception was probably less integrated than finally turned out. Nevertheless, it seems likely that the response reflects the kind of identity confusion so frequently found in adolescence.]
DF−Ats DF∓Ats	3. and 4. Those red spots, they might be some of the . . Well, let's see . . . . . . They might be some of the . . They might be organs . . like the inside of a person, I mean.	3. and 4. ("Tell me about the organs.") Well, I really don't know, but maybe it could have been . . uh . . large intestines, and maybe the lungs, although I don't really know what they look like for sure. That's just

React.				
Card #	Time	Score	Protocol	Inquiry and Observations

what they make me think of. (What about them made them look that way?") Well, I've seen some pictures . . of that sort of shape. (The side red D's are the "intestines," the center red D's are the "lungs.") [Although Don first announces that he will say nothing about the "red spots," he is drawn to them nevertheless. But as soon as he deals with these colored areas, his form level becomes poorer, his content loses "distance," and his responses become cruder. Is Don's rather gross, poorly differentiated use of color another reflection of his "organicity," in the sense that it suggests a poorly controlled impulse expression? To what extent, for example, does Don get in trouble with the law because of impulsive acts which he may later regret?]

		DF±At	4. And this thing right here might be part of a skeleton . . . . Oh dear (said softly), I still haven't got it all yet, have I? (He smiles.) . . . . That's about all I can get, I guess.	4. ("What kind of skeleton was it?") What do you mean? ("Was it human or animal, for instance?") Human, I guess. ("How much of a skeleton did you see?") How much? Well, I think it was just part of the chest. Yes. (Lower central D.)
IV	65"		∨ ∧	
		DF∓pl (anal?; phallic?)	1. Well, I'm not going to say I know exactly. I'm going to take a wild guess. It doesn't look like anything to me exactly. I'll say this middle part right here looks sort of like the stubble (he means stump) of a tree.	1. ("Tell me about the stubble.") I meant the stump. ("Could you tell me about that?") Well (he sighs), well, it was short and fairly thick through the middle (bottom D).

React.		
Card #	*Time Score*	*Protocol*

Inquiry and Observations

WF±Monst. Cast.

2. And the rest of this looks sort of like a headless monster.

2. ("Would you describe the monster.") Well, this is . . I'm just thinking of some shows I've seen, where they have something like that . . similar to that . . something with not much shape to it. [The headless monster without "much shape" to it might well be Don's self-representation. As with the chicken head with a human body, the "headless monster" appears to reflect Don's poorly differentiated self-image. The nonhuman aspect of both these responses is often met in adolescent uncertainty about who and what one is and what forms one may take. Is the "headless monster" related to the anal or phallic "stubble" of response 1? How?]

WFM± Scarecrow Cast. Comb.

3. Or it could be a scarecrow . . maybe. These (side D's) are feet, I guess. These things here (upper side D's) I suppose are arms. This place here is where there should be or where there is . . a head. And dot's it.

3. ("What made it seem like a scarecrow?") Because if that was a stump there and hanging on a scarecrow . . hanging on a stump, it might be out in somebody's field. ("Did it seem to have a head or not?") I couldn't tell for sure, but it looked like maybe there wasn't any. It looked like the place where there should be one. [Not only can this "scarecrow" be interpreted as another aspect of Don's enfeebled self-image, the response also reflects his tendency to become mildly confused—e.g., the stump hanging on the scarecrow, rather than the other way around. The "stump," the "headless monster," and the "scarecrow" without a head

React.			
Card #	Time	Score	Protocol	Inquiry and Observations

Inquiry and Observations

probably also represent Don's commentary apropos of his masculine potency.]

V   Oho! Well.

12″ WF+A   1. This looks sort of   1. ("What made it seem
     Pec.   . . this part here re-   like that?") It was because
     Fab. Comb. minds me sort of a   of the head and tail. ("How
     Tend.   butterfly . . with bat's   do you mean?") Well, I
     Mast.   wings. There isn't   seem to think that a butter-
              much else to say for   fly tail would be something
              it, except for these   like that. And the head
              here sticking out . .   would be bigger if it were
              maybe where his   a bat, it would seem. Be-
              wings are torn . . or   cause a bat is more like a
              else maybe for guid-   mouse, so I've heard. [This
              ing purposes.   response again reflects
              Don's confusion about what
              things *really* are. Is what he
              sees a "bat," a "butterfly,"
              or a bit of both? This sort
              of uncertainty about the
              true nature of things has
              been apparent in a number
              of Don's responses. The
              vague boundaries which he
              perceives living objects to
              have reflects the nature of
              his own uncertain bound-
              aries. More uncertainty fol-
              lows: Are the butterfly-bat's
              wings torn (i.e., damaged),
              or is the damage actually
              a "positive" characteristic
              (i.e., to help "guide")? It
              is most interesting to see
              how a blot which is usually
              so easily and quickly inter-
              preted as "a bat" can be-
              come the expression of an
              identity-diffused adoles-
              cence.]

              That's all . . for that
              bird.

(There is a brief interlude here, during which Don goes downstairs. He returns to my office before I am ready, so that my door is closed. When he returns
again and finds my door open he says:) I was afraid I was going to lose you.

Card #	React. Time	Score	Protocol	Inquiry and Observations
VI			("Here we go.") Here we go, he says . . . . Boy, this is a dilly. $\lor$	
	35″	WF∓A Fab.	1. Well, that might be some sort of a sea animal . . and . .uh . . these here would be some sort of . . I can't think of the name . . things that fly over the water. I can't think of it. And this might be the tail. I don't know what this is. This might be the head, up here, and these might be used to guide it. And *that* is all. (He smiles.)	1. ("Why did it seem to be a sea animal?") Well . . uh . . those sort of wing-shaped things, out along the side . . it reminded me of what's called . . . I think a manta ray. It's a big fish, I guess. I guess it's got a long tail. It's the only thing it reminds me of at all. (Upside down, the side sections are the "wings," and the outer side Dr's are the "guides." The "tail" is the long central protuberance, minus the jagged edges, and the "head" is the tiny lighter Dr section at the top center, as Don holds the card.) [Although fish of one sort or another are fairly frequently interpreted on the Rorschach, one nevertheless often gains the uneasy feeling of clammy sliminess from a "fish" percept. Alone, such a percept may not mean much, but in the context of Don's other responses (of headless giants, headless scarecrows, bat-butterflies, chicken-men, lungs and intestines) the vaguely seen manta-ray percept underlines Don's unstable identity. This is the second time Don has specified "guides" that would help an animal with its direction. One is inclined to feel Don would like similar guides to help him reach various goals.]
VII			Oh boy! Another dilly. $\lor$ It's such a non-descript thing, if you ask me.	

Card #	React. Time	Score	Protocol	Inquiry and Observations
	35″	WSF∓pl Fab. Oral−agg.	1. Well, we'll just take a wild shot at this one, and we'll say it's some sort of plant . . a flower, maybe. I'd say it's probably one of those types of flowers that gets insects, and this part closes up . . traps them. This would probably be the place where the nectar is, right here, and the stem would come right down this way. (He looks at me and smiles.) Enough.	[Card VII has been described as "feminine" and as the "mother" card. Whether Don is speaking primarily about his mother or about women generally (or, indeed, about the world), one is impressed by the way he juxtaposes aggressive, voracious aspects with sweet nectar. [It is probable that Don's long reaction times throughout are the result both of (a) his need to oppose what is implicitly desired of him (note his tendency immediately to turn each card upside down) and (b) his general uncertainty and confused perception, which prevent a percept from emerging clearly within the briefer time usually required.]
VIII			> ∧	
	32″	DF+AP	1. Well, these two things here might be mice.	[The popular "animals" are very rarely interpreted as "mice."]
		DrF(C)+A	2. And . . uh . . these two might be . . uh . . uh . . uh frogs.	2. (Top Dr portion of bottom "butterfly." I neglected to ask about a possible color determinant.)
Comb.		DrF+pl Fab.	3. This part right here might be a small tree . . just a seedling . . or a small part of a tree.	3. ("What did the tree look like?") You mean, what sort of a tree was it? ("What did the tree look like to you?") Well . . What did it look like? . . . . It just looked like a small tree with a little foilage (sic) on top and on the sides (combination of top and middle D).
		DrFC∓geol Fab.	4. And these might be colored rocks down here, that the tree is growing up through . . . . . . And that's the size of it.	4. (Bottom lower portion of lower central "butterfly.") [Although Don often does not make his color impressions explicit, he rarely misses the opportunity to

React.			
Card #	Time	Score	Protocol	Inquiry and Observations

react to color in some way.
[Growing things force their way through obstacles.]

IX

∨ ∧
Well now . . what do you know? (45″) The silliest things I'm coming up with here.

Comb.

DF(C)—obj.

1. This bottom part here reminds me of an ash tray.

1. ("What made it look like an ash tray?") Well, I thought the shape of it. It sort of looks like it had some grooves in it. (The [C] sections constitute the grooves.)

DrF—pl
Fab.

2. This part might be a stem . . wooden stem.

2. ("Did that stem belong to something?") No, that was a wooden stem . . probably a branch from a tree.

DrCFpl
Fab.

3. And these parts (side green sections) might be some artificial leaves.
And that's all there's to it.

3. ("Why 'artificial' leaves?") Well . . what *made* them . . well, because *real* leaves would probably wilt before too long . . They'd get all wilted up. ("Do the leaves belong to the branch?") Well, they were supposedly connected to the stem. ("Why would it matter if they wilted?") Well, it would spoil the looks . . Supposedly it's a fancy ash tray. ("Are the stem and the leaves part of the ash tray?") Yes. [This is a "forced" response, in the sense that it rather arbitrarily gathers elements that are tied together primarily by their juxtaposition. The arrangement creates an unusual combination which appears to have essentially private meanings.]

X

Well, let's see what we can make out of

React.				
Card #	Time Score		Protocol	Inquiry and Observations

this thing. On (he smiles) . . I'll tell you one thing. It's a mess. ∨

50″ | DrF+Obj. Fab.

1. Well you can always start off with this thing (top central D). It looks like some sort of iron or woodened (*sic*) post . . or rod.

Inkblots, huh? (He smiles.) (He sighs.) > ∧ (He sighs again.) ∨

1. ("What kind of post or rod?") Either wood or iron. ("What purpose does it have?") Oh . . well . . . . . . no particular purpose, I guess. [This preoccupation with purposeless phallic protuberances again suggests that Don has rather marked feelings of masculine inadequacy.]

DF—A

2. Well, these (large pink D's) might be . . this . . all this part here . . might be some sort of small organism in the ocean . . and . . uh . .

2. ("What reminded you of an ocean organism?") Well, because of the funny shape. ("How do you mean?") They're usually . . . . Well, it could have been an organism in the body . . but, as I say, I think . . they have no definite shape. ("Could you see the body?") Well, what sort of organism? ("What sort did you see?") Well, a cell. ["Some sort of small organism" is about as vague a formulation as it is possible to make. So far, Don has been able to see a post, which he has been unable to describe further, and some sort of cellular organism which might be in the sea or in the water. One would probably be correct to suspect that the vivid colors in this blot adversely affect Don's cognitive capacities. It will be important to see whether Don can recover more effective perceptual organization.]

Comb.

DFC—A Fab. Oral agg.

3. And all of these . . this . . this one . . these two yellow ones, are probably feeding

3. ("What would the yellow be?") Well, that was another of a different species, probably. [Probably a

Card #	React. Time Score	Protocol	Inquiry and Observations
		from it. Yeah ‥ this thing here, this main part here, might be separating, dividing. (The various small D areas that surround the larger pink D area.)	parasite that "feeds off" others? And is it also partly that of one who will be devoured while (because?) he grows?]
	DFC—A Fab.	4. They might be part of the same kind, but a different color, that haven't grown up yet. (Outer bottom D areas.) I give up on the rest of that thing. Is that the last one of these things? ("Yes, it is.") Whew!	4. [The wooden or iron post, poor as it was, is the most differentiated percept Don has been able to distinguish on this card. Significantly, the "post" area is gray, rather than colored.]

Thematic Apperception Test

[Only a few of Don's stories are presented, primarily to illustrate his fear of making self-involving commitments. Before he is willing to make up any stories, he needs to know the precise conditions under which they should be told. Although he uses many words when he tells his stories, he actually says little. He leaves it up to the examiner to ask salient questions, and only rarely volunteers elaborations.]

Card 1 (A young boy is contemplating a violin which rests on a table in front of him.)

Let's see. Do you want me to start from the beginning? I don't mean exactly the beginning, but where you think they will be? ("Start wherever you think will make a good story.") You mean, in story form, or just explain? ("In story form.") I'll make this up as I go along . . . . I guess there was a boy whose mother decided that he ought to take music lessons, and she probably liked this instrument . . the violin. So she bought him one, and he probably liked it pretty well the first day he got it, before he went to see his instructor. He's all caught up now. Probably after the first or second lesson he had, he began to wonder whether it was a very good idea. And right as he's sitting now, he's probably wondering how he can get out of this . . mess . . . . He'll probably continue taking his lessons for a few more days, and then his mother will probably have a pretty rough time to get him to practice . . . . uh . . Let's see . . . . uh . . Let's see . . Can I bring this to a . . Does it have to be a prolonged story? Can I end? ("Whenever you like.") Where was I? (I tell him where he stopped.) And finally he'll either quit or be forced to continue with his lessons . . and . . . . . . (he returns the card). ("Which of those two will it be?") (He smiles and studies the card.) . . . . Well, that depends on how . . uh . . uh . . I guess you'd say how persistent his mother is . . or father. ("Why do they want him to study the violin?") Well, she probably figures that he should have some musical experience. ("Why does he want to stop?") He probably doesn't enjoy it very much. ("What about it doesn't he enjoy?") Well . . . . (he looks at the card again . . Maybe it would be too hard for him. [This story illustrates Don's need to keep things open, to present alternatives, to evade final decisions. In all his stories, he depends very much on the word "probably"; using this word, he is able to carry the story along without ever closing a possibility. The story illustrates how short-lived Don's enthusiasms tend to be.]

Card 2 (Country scene: in the foreground is a young woman with books in her hand; in the background a man is working in the fields, and an older woman is looking on.)

You want a story, huh? (He smiles.) Hm . . (he studies the card). Well, I have to have a beginning, I'm afraid . . . . (He sighs) . . . . Let's see . . . . Well, I was thinking that this could be a . . uh . . . . . . Well . . . . . . I don't know how to say it right at the moment here . . . . . . I know what I think this is, but I don't know how to put it in story form. Shall I just tell you my idea? ("Yes, go ahead.") Well, I think this boy here, or man, whatever he is, working in the field, doesn't enjoy it too much and would rather be in school, and this girl would probably rather stay home and do housework than go to school . . and . . . . . . I can't think of anything for her (the older woman) except she could be the mother and just overseeing to make sure that the boy did his work and the girl went to school. ("How does it come out?") How does it come out? I'd say probably after the boy finished his work, he'd go to school, and the girl would continue to go to school . . . . . . ("Why don't they do what they want to do?") Well, they .. probably they figure that the girl should go to school and that the boy should help his father with the farm work and *then* go to school. ("Who are 'they'?") Well, the parents. [Apparent is Don's difficulty in committing himself, as well as the theme of being dissatisfied, wanting what another person has, but finding that the other person is also dissatisfied with what he has. A major theme, then, is: "Nothing anyone does for me can satisfy me."]

Card 8 BM (An adolescent boy looks straight out of the picture. The barrel of a rifle is visible at one side, and in the background is the dim scene of a surgical operation, like a reverie-image.)

(He looks at the card and laughs.) Ho-ho! . . . .
. . . . Oh .. this guy looks like he's on an operating table there. He's probably been shot in an accident . . . . And this other boy here, probably is the one that .. that .. uh .. shot him, I guess . . . . . I really can't tell from the looks of him whether he's sorry or not . . . . (He sighs) . . . . . But this other boy will probably come out of it all right . . . . . ("How does the other boy feel?") Uh . . . . . He probably feels pretty mad at him, or maybe he hates him, or something. Unless he figures it was just an accident, and that this other guy was sorry for it, he could probably not feel that way . . . . . ("What are they to one another?") Probably just friends. [This story again epitomizes Don's tentativeness and the difficulty he has in committing himself to a fact, or an emotion, or a point of view.]

Card 15 (A gaunt man with clenched hands is standing among gravestones.)

Where'd you dig up this character? (He smiles.) . . . .
. . . . It doesn't matter how long these are, because I can't think of very much for this. Well, this fellow, maybe his wife has died, and he's coming out to her grave. And he looks kind of like it might have been his fault she died, more or less . . . I can't think of anything more. ("How might it have been his fault?") Oh, he might have been mean, or .. or .. or .. Let's see . . . . That's all I can think of. ("How does he feel now?") He's probably sorry now. [Is Don afraid that his "meanness" might cause the death of someone close to him?]

Card 16 (Blank card.)

You mean I should tell you what's in it? ("Make up a story about it.") . . . . (He sighs.) . . . . (He bites his nails.)

. . . . Well, there might be some man in here, looking sort of unhappy. He was feeling pretty bad about some of the things he'd done . . like . . uh . . well . . . . (He sighs.) Let's see . . (he grimaces), well . . Can I just say the first thing that pops into my mind? ("Sure, go ahead.") . . . . . Maybe he was a politician that had gotten into office by unfair means . . . . . Maybe he was thinking that maybe he ought to make some correction for all the mistakes he made. (He hands the card back.) ("What happens to him?") Well . .hm . . . Maybe he reforms himself and goes straight. ("As a politician?") Well, maybe if he sets himself straight and does the best job he can, he'll go farther in politics, maybe. [Behind Don's indecisiveness appears to be the wish to undo what he considers have been his mistakes and to start again with a clean slate.]

SENTENCE COMPLETION TEST II

[This test is included to demonstrate how Don consciously wishes to present himself. Often the Sentence Completion Test permits the expression of feelings, attitudes and philosophies of life which are present in awareness. But in spite of the fact that the Sentence Completions are often more within conscious control, so that the individual can manipulate them to point in the direction he wishes, the endings frequently reflect layers of organization which are a good deal less conscious. If one studied only Don's Sentence Completions, one might feel more convinced that he approximates the stereotype of the "delinquent." He sometimes wishes to present himself as a fairly rough and devil-may-care character, and he is much more able to do so on a test such as Sentence Completion, where attitudes to be conveyed are apparently so much more consciously controlled. The discrepancy between Don's performance on Sentence Completion and on other tests emphasizes again the importance of using an entire test battery for each person; that way the full variety of the person's psychological organization, with all its apparent contradictions and its peaks and valleys, can emerge.]

He hoped that when he grew up he would be a man . . or . . excuse me . . an aviator. [This completion touches both on Don's conflict related to growing into a masculine adulthood and on his wish to play the dashing, masculine role. Although it has been evident that Don is afraid that he may not be or ever want to become an adult "man," he tries to disguise his anxiety by presenting himself as someone who wishes to become a romantic, action-oriented, highly masculine figure, an aviator.]

When he saw what the other kids were doing he wanted to do the same thing. [Not, "he did the same thing," but "he wanted to."]

When he compared himself to his friends . . . . uh . . he found that he was different. ("How was that?") Well, he didn't like the same things. [Don stresses his sense of alienation.]

He was sad whenever he thought of . . uh . . Let's see . . hm . . . . . . whenever he thought of what he had to . . do. ("Like what?") Oh, let's see . . Well, it could be . . in connection with some kind of work. ["Settling down" is saddening.]

When he was asked about his aches and pains he said that . . he said that he had fallen off a bridge. It takes me back to a movie I was watching last night.

The person he admired most was his father.

His brother was two years older than *he* was . . than he. [Don is not about to reveal significant feelings about his brother. Instead, he focuses on his own—grammatical—image.]

When his father came into the room he was very angry. ("Why was his father angry?") Because his son had not come home at the right time.

When he was with his sister . . a large jet flew over his house. [Don's ending concerning his relationship with his sister is as distant as was the comment concerning his brother.]

At school he had trouble with his algebra.

When he looked at the work the others were doing . . when he looked at the *work?* ("That's right.") Let's see . . he thought that he'd better study more.

He was very happy when he discovered that he had *not* failed his alphabet.

The thing he found hardest to do . . . . . uh . . Let's see . . . . hm . . . . . was to study his science. [Don's school difficulty is emerging.]

Whenever certain things really bothered him . . . . (He repeats the stem.) . . . . . . (He fidgets.) . . . . . uh . . . . . he . . went for a walk by himself.

His dreams . . . . . well . . let's see . . . . . His dreams were very mixed up. ("How was that?") Well . . well, let's see . . They were always about different and unusual things. [Don describes himself as different from others. It is not clear whether he sees this difference as putting him at a disadvantage or, possibly defensively, at an advantage.]

He liked to ride his motorcycle. [This fits the stereotype of the "delinquent."]

When he saw that the man had left the money behind he took it to him . . back to the man, I mean.

He thought that his mother had gone to a neighbor's house. [As in the cases of the brother and sister, Don does not commit himself to an evaluation of his mother.]

Whenever he and his family disagreed there was always a big argument. ("Who would win?") Eh? Oh . . father, I guess.

When he was very little he got his arm caught in a wringer . . right here (he shows the scar).

His best friend had gone away for a long trip.

He was unhappy when his father decided that he would have to work for him that summer. ("Why did that make him unhappy?") Because he had other plans for working. [The irritable interaction between parent and child is, of course, typical not only of the "delinquent" but of other adolescents as well. Once again "work" is the source of bad feeling.]

He never thought he would be able to . . Should I say the first thing that pops into my mind? ("That's right.") Would you repeat that one? (I repeat the stem.) Beat his brother in the half-mile race. [To support the masculine, action-oriented self-image which Don tries to construct, he imagines competition with a brother toward whom he apparently feels inferior, even though the brother is younger than Don.]

He always hoped that . . . . . well, someday he would own a car. [More activity—the adolescent's ubiquitous car.]

His parents did not approve of him owning one.

What he liked best about himself about himself? ("That's right.") Was that he was a fairly good rifle shot. [More activity.]

His mother was more likely than his father to . . hear out his problems.

When he had nothing else to do he rode his motorcycle. [Still more activity.]

He thought that his intelligence was below normal. [Many young people who try to solve their problems through activity have a low opinion of their "intellectual" capabilities.]

What he liked best about school .. uh .. were .. uh .. were the study periods.

When he couldn't see a way out couldn't see what? (I repeat.) Way out? (I explain.) He would move to a different position.

He saw the cockroach on the wall and . . . . . . hit it with a fly swatter.

His teacher was a very old woman.

Whenever he got angry .. It seems like I've heard that one before. (He smiles.) He'd go out and take a walk by himself.

He remembered that when he was little he had fallen on his head. ("Did that happen to you?") My sister was holding me, and I fell on my head on the floor. [Although one cannot, of course, ascribe the etiology of Don's "organicity" to this incident, it is significant that the incident has apparently become part of Don's, if not his family's, "growing-up mythology." One wonders to what extent Don thinks of himself as a damaged person who, because he is damaged, cannot think as well as others.]

When the kids invited him to the hiding place (he repeats the stem) he said he would be right there.

After school he usually went downtown to get the groceries for his mother. [Once again, the juxtaposition of the "obedient boy" and the action-oriented youth.]

He admired his father when . . . . (he repeats the stem) .. when he got the new job.

He and his brother were good friends. [Not lately, apparently.]

He thought his body (he repeats the stem questioningly) . . . . was very small. [And "unmanly"?]

When he had a lot of homework he would have his mother help him. [Don's relationship with his mother is obviously a close one. One frequently finds a hypernurturant (forgiving) mother, together with a father who tends to be seen as punitive, in the family background of boys with Don's antisocial proclivities.]

What he disliked about school was his English teacher. ("Why was that?") Oh .. Maybe she was too strict for him.

Whenever he spoke about his problems to someone they did not listen to him. [Don's conception of "his problems" are perhaps not taken seriously because he expresses them as projections or displacements.]

When he entered the haunted house he was .. a little bit shaky.

He didn't like his mother to .. to, how do you spell that to? ("T-o.") To think that he never studied while he was in school.

When the baby arrived he was very much relieved. ("About what?") (He shrugs his shoulders.) ...... Well .... because he thought something might be wrong with him. [This is an unusual completion. Although Don is probably not aware of the source of his concern, destructive wishes toward the baby may justifiably be inferred from his worry about there possibly being something wrong with it.]

Whenever he didn't do what he was told he was punished. ("Punished how?") By having some of his privileges taken away.

What would make him angriest ..... uh ..... uh ..... was when his mother would not let him see his friend. [Mother is seen not only as indulgent, but also as a depriving disciplinarian.]

In his spare time he worked on his car.

What troubled him most was what he was going to do when he finished school. [A concern about the more distant future is atypically expressed by the action-oriented adolescent, who lives almost exclusively in the moment.]

When he was alone in his room he got very bored. [Does "bored" equal "tense"?]

What scared him most .... Let's see ..... was when he almost ran into the back end of another car. [Don leaves open whose fault this near accident might be.]

He disliked his father when he would not let him use the car.

He thought that his looks .... were not very good. [And that his body was "very small."]

The thing he could do best was his science work. [Not some more gross muscular activity, such as "rifle shooting" or "working on his car"? "Science work" certainly does not conform to the stereotyped model.]

When he saw the girl he thought that she was very good-looking.

He had no respect at all for other people's property. [This appears to represent a kind of identification with law and order, possibly real, possibly manipulative, probably temporary and situational.]

He always enjoyed eating sweet foods.

He had a very uncomfortable feeling when .... when he came in at very late hours.

He found it easiest to .... easiest to do his homework his own way.

As far as girl friends were concerned . . . . he was disinterested. [This item was specially added because heterosexuality apparently involves a number of difficulties for Don. Both this stem and other material suggest that Don deals with heterosexuality primarily with avoidance.]

THE PSYCHOLOGIST'S REPORT[1]

It is in the context of Don's reluctance to make verbal or emotional commitments that one can understand some meanings underlying his explanation of how praise and punishment are alike. He says, in part, "Praise and punishment . . . . help us be sure of ourselves." It requires only a slight inferential step to make one feel fairly certain that Don requires external support before he can be sure about the "rightness" of his thoughts and actions. His obsessive organization is not at all typical of the "usual," action-oriented, nonreflective, antisocial adolescent "delinquent," and Don relies much less heavily and self-consciously on the (often counterphobic) mechanisms that are seen so frequently in such young persons. Nor does he need to swear or otherwise to "talk tough" to demonstrate his masculinity; on the contrary, he uses such effeminate terms as "Oh dear" when he discovers some task to be more difficult than he had bargained for. While Don consciously needs to present himself as a "delinquent" when he feels he has control over the creation of this "image," the image is neither stable nor solid. He is never quite able to overcome his doubts, hesitations, uncertainties, his needs to be proper, to be "good," and he seems always just on the verge of being aware of several of his conflicts. Thus, although he tries to assume the trappings of his "delinquent" peers, he usually does not quite make it. While he may speak about his interest in such typical activities of the delinquent as riding motorcycles and repairing cars, and while he tells about his school failures and his fights with his parents, he displays introspectiveness, mildness—even effeminacy—and vulnerability. He has not developed the hard shell which so often characterizes the antisocial character.

The activities which have gotten Don into trouble with the law seem associated with an impairment of various ego functions which

[1] Since more than a usual amount of Don's test material has not been included in this chapter, the report makes rather frequent reference to material with which the reader is not familiar.

involve the control, integration and clarity of perception and the efficiency of intellectual production. His gross use of color on the Rorschach reflects the difficulty he has when he tries to deal with the integrated enunciation of affective impulses. He is unable to express feeling in an appropriate, differentiated, modulated fashion. Affect tends to emerge explosively, grossly and unproductively. The large discrepancy (thirty-two I.Q. points) between Don's Verbal and Performance scores on the Wechsler-Bellevue, as well as the extreme scatter of his subtests (ranging from a weighted score of 4 to one of 14), further reflect rather severe inefficiencies. His abilities allow him to achieve a Verbal Intelligence Quotient of 119-126 (Bright Normal —Superior range), but his Performance Quotient is only 87-89 (Dull Normal range). His ability to perform tasks which require perceptual-motor organization is both qualitatively and quantitatively impaired. On the Block Design subtest, for example, as the designs become increasingly complex, he is no longer sure whether what he has made is identical with the model. On the Object Assembly subtest he is reduced to random trial-and-error contour fitting. He requires more than 6' to complete the *Hand* item, even though he knows from the beginning what he is trying to put together. His drawings of persons are primitively done. Don tends to deal with all his performance difficulties by quite literally whistling in the dark and mumbling encouragements to himself. The quality of this performance strongly suggests the debilitating effects of some sort of "brain damage." It is likely that, in addition to causing an impairment of cognitive abilities, Don's presumed brain damage results in too impulsive and otherwise poorly controlled behavior which occasionally lands him in legal hot water. It may also be, of course, that he reacts to the difficulties with which his brain damage constantly confronts him by acting through channels that are antisocial but that permit him some success and some minimum of admiration.

It is to be noted that Don's brain dysfunction seems to affect primarily perceptual-motor cognitive areas. So long as he is able to work with exclusively verbal symbols, he usually shows a higher than average ability. His vocabulary is excellent, his fund of information considerably higher than one would expect of a person his age, and his memory functioning seems altogether adequate.

It is difficult to judge to what extent evidence for "peculiar" thinking can be separated from the "organicity" referred to previously. But what one sees appears to reflect more than simply a deficit.

On the BRL Sorting Test, for example, Don's thinking is often loose, vague, fabulized and overgeneralized. These characteristics seem to be a reflection of an underlying confusion (possibly separate from "organicity"). When, on Part II of the BRL, he is asked how the *Tools* fit together, for example, he says, "That should be an easy one (but he studies the items for a considerable time). You just want to know why they're alike? ('That's right.') Because they're simple machines. ('How do you mean, "simple machines"?') Well, they . . uh . . they only have about one certain job to perform. ('Could you say the same thing more simply?') Well, how would this be? That they all have their one certain job . . their main job?" The *Tools* item is usually conceptualized immediately by most persons, and it is particularly surprising that Don is unable to make the "passive" conceptualization, since he "actively" sorted "tools" previously, on Part I.

This type of conceptual performance can still be interpreted as a kind of "gap" in functioning, a gap fairly typical of the "organic." Still, the concept of "gap" does less well in explaining Don's Rorschach performance. He perceives Card II as an "optical illusion." He sees the red portions as "spots," the same kind that he experiences whenever he looks at a strong light. He sees Card IX as a "fancy ash tray," with a stem going up through the center, and artificial leaves on either side. Of his twenty-six responses, only one is a Popular one, a finding which further underscores the unusual ways in which Don perceives. Fewer than half his responses are of an acceptable form quality, and more than half contain fabulized elaborations and ideational embroideries. Both the absence of adequate form quality and the too frequent appearance of fabulized responses suggest that Don has an active fantasy life which he uses to modify his world in terms of internally determined wishes. On the Word Association Test, in addition to mildly "distant" associations, Don occasionally blocks for as long as 17″ and fails to recall 25 percent of his first associations. What all this means is difficult to say. Perhaps the most parsimonious explanation is that the "organic" dysfunction is basic and that other disturbances are secondary to it.

Don experiences significant conflict about his wish to be both passive and active. The danger he sees in passivity can be inferred from his response to Card VII of the Rorschach, which he interprets as: "One of those types of flowers that gets insects, and this part closes up . . traps them . . . . This would probably be the place where the nectar is." The danger he sees in passivity is also suggested by his story to the TAT "Hypnosis" card, in which the hypnotist finds himself unable to wake his subject.

Anxiety about growing up and being more on his own is suggested both by a Rorschach percept of a small seedling that has to force its way through a barrier of rocks, and of a microorganism which is being devoured by parasites as it is undergoing mitotic division. Growing up faces Don with uncertainties about his eventual manhood. On the Sentence Completion Test he says, *He hoped that when he grew up* "he would be a man . . or . . Excuse me, I mean an aviator." His Rorschach percepts of a person with the head of a chicken, a butterfly with the wings of a bat, a headless monster, a headless scarecrow, an animal with "torn wings," all suggest the degree of Don's identity diffusion. That this diffusion is also partly represented by quite possibly conscious homosexual feelings is suggested by his response of "men" to the word *love* on the Word Association Test. This association is immediately followed by an embarrassed "correction." On the Sentence Completion Test he disclaims any interest in girls. He is a lonely, isolated boy who consciously feels, if not inferior to, at least different from others.

Don's Thematic Apperception Test themes reflect a rather strong superego struggle. His stories, although tentatively and often equivocally phrased, tend to deal with crime and atonement, and particularly with guilts and with wishes to make restitution for past wrongdoing. Certain of the themes suggest that the wrongdoers were not really in the wrong—were all the circumstances known, people would be less quick to accuse. Don seems to suffer rather intense guilts, not only about his antisocial acts, but also about resentful and aggressive feelings that he experiences toward members of his immediate family. Although he tries to convince himself and others that he is really not particularly guilty, he is not very successful in his efforts.

In summary, Don is an intelligent and sensitive person whose obsessive thinking reflects his uncertainties and doubts. Gaps in smooth cognitive integration, spontaneity and availability, and disturbances, particularly in areas involving perceptual-motor integration, as well as such things as a major difference between Verbal and Performance quotients, suggest the activity of either an endogenous or an acquired "brain damage." At times Don's thinking becomes somewhat vague, diffuse, peculiar, somewhat arbitrary and poorly organized, but it is difficult to know to what extent these features are secondary to a more basic encephalopathy. In other words, do the apparently nonorganic peculiarities of thinking seem determined primarily by the effort to cope with organic encroachments of one sort or another? Don's over-all psychological organization is not typical of the stereotype of the aggressive, nonreflective, counter-phobic adolescent character disorder. He seems to be experiencing a particularly difficult identity crisis. Not only does he have acute questions about who and what he is and who and what he will become, but this identity questioning is strongly interlarded with feelings of guilt and fears of retribution. In a number of ways he seems to be avoiding "manliness," and there is a strong possibility that he experiences conscious homosexual feelings.

DISCUSSION

Don's test material exemplifies the complexity which the term "delinquent" tends to ignore. Although Don tries to approximate the cultural ideal of "the delinquent," he does so rather badly. It is difficult to say exactly what lies behind his stealing. The stealing has gotten Don in trouble with the law, and in that sense he is a "delinquent." When one tries to make sense out of Don's behavior, a number of possibilities present themselves. One wonders, for example, to what extent Don's antisocial behavior represents his anger about feeling himself so much outside of things, to what extent the stealing represents an area of competence while he feels so frustrated elsewhere, and to what extent the stealing has more specific resentful meanings that are related to his feeling unable to keep up with his more heterosexually oriented peers (e.g., stealing from participants at school dances).

In any case, Don's antisocial behavior is a complexly determined phenomenon. The behavior must be evaluated from various vantage points—the organic dysfunction, the identity diffusion, and other, possibly "functionally" determined, confusion. But whatever the specific cause or causes, it seems clear that Don feels lonely, frightened, confused and puzzled, and that his antisocial behavior is somewhat associated with his distressful feelings about these states.

Chuck has also gotten into difficulty with the law. He has shown his disturbance since the age of four, possibly concomitant with his sister's adoption. His antisocial behavior is part of a more generalized and more basic and severe disturbance. He has been able to maintain a façade of appropriateness, and this façade has kept him from being hospitalized previously.

CLINICAL SUMMARY: Chuck

Chuck, aged fifteen, is the oldest of three adopted children. His parents are concerned about his long-standing difficulty in school and at home, specifically about his rebellious behavior, his incivility to adults, his fights with other children, his generally poor self-control and his tantrums. He has recently been getting into serious legal trouble, which has brought him into contact with the courts.

A marked change took place in Chuck at the age of four, at the time his parents made plans for adopting a girl. Whereas Chuck had been affectionate and loving, he became distant, independent, dissatisfied and unhappy. He was extremely resentful toward the baby, and on several occasions tried to hurt her seriously. In nursery school, he was a severe disciplinary problem. Although he did better in kindergarten, one of Chuck's teachers spoke to the parents even then about Chuck's possible need for psychiatric help. Chuck's difficulties continued in the first grade: he refused to do the school work, was resentful, talked back to the teacher and threw books and other objects. From the sixth grade on, he had increasing difficulties, and as a result he was moved from one school to another. At thirteen, he was expelled from a military academy because of "stealing, fighting, bullying and obnoxious behavior." Only the father's political influence has prevented Chuck from being expelled totally from the public schools.

Chuck was also very difficult to control at home: he threw tantrums, lied, defied the parents' authority, attacked his sister, and made himself socially disagreeable in many ways. In the past two years, he has begun to associate with a group of "delinquent" boys and has avoided people that his parents considered to be in his own social and economic group. Recently, Chuck has been getting into more trouble with the law, primarily as a result of speeding, running away from home and vandalism. A month ago, he and nine other boys broke into a neighbor's home, did $2,000 worth of damage and stole, among other things, a revolver and two wrist watches.

Chuck's parents first sought psychiatric help for him when he was eight years old. Since things seemed only to get worse during his treatment, the parents discontinued it. He was again seen in therapy a few years later, but once again he showed no improvement and the parents discontinued treatment. After he returned from military school, Chuck was seen in psychotherapy a third time, for a period of a year and a half. This treatment was also considered to be unsuccessful by the parents.

The parents received Chuck from a children's home when he was two weeks old. The only information they had about his background was that his mother was a young girl from a poor family who had had the child out of wedlock, and that there was no insanity, epilepsy or diabetes in the family history.

During the first three months of life, Chuck had considerable difficulty with eating. When he was four weeks old, he got what was diagnosed as whooping cough with fever, frequently coughing and vomiting. After the first three months, he was described as a sweet, lovable, good and happy baby, who, however, always had to have someone with him and who could not play by himself. Development, including sitting, walking, eating, speaking, bowel and bladder control, all developed normally. During his first three or four years, Chuck was overindulged, with his parents attempting to meet his every whim. Whenever his demands were not immediately met, he would throw severe tantrums, and these have continued through the years. Chuck has been in excellent physical health throughout his life.

Physical and Laboratory Findings: The results of physical, neurological and laboratory examinations were all within normal limits.

THE PSYCHOLOGIST'S DESCRIPTION

Chuck came to all testing appointments looking resentful and sullen. Because of this initial impression, it was surprising to see how well he cooperated in the various testing procedures. Frequently, he spent considerable time thinking about his answers, and only rarely did he seem to give up too readily. Even in the latter instances, however, he quickly resumed trying to solve test problems when he was encouraged. Throughout, his face showed little change of expression, and only rarely did he allow himself a brief, shy smile. One initially felt that Chuck was chronically angry, but eventually it seemed that the apparent resentment and sullenness one saw were actually expressions of Chuck's hopelessness and depression.

His apparently considerable tension was expressed primarily as frequent yawning, sighing and stomach gurgling. At the beginning of our testing sessions, he constantly addressed me as "sir," but in a way which did not seem to reflect much respect. This apparent remnant of military school discipline disappeared quickly, however.

THE WECHSLER-BELLEVUE SCALE

Name: Chuck   Age: 15-2

	RS	WTS	0 1 2 3 4 5 6 7 8 9 10 11 12 13 14 15 16 17 18 19 20
COMPR.	11-12	10-11	
INFOR.	14	10	
DIG.	9	6	
ARITH.	2-3	1-3	
SIMIL.	12	10	
VOCAB.	18½	8	
P. A.	8	7	
P. C.	14	14	
B. D.	18-24	9-11	
O. A.	20	12	
D. S.	44	10	

TOT. VERB.	39-42
TOT. PERF.	52-54
TOT. SCALE	91-96

VERBAL I.Q.:   91-95   LEVEL: Average

PERFORMANCE I.Q.:   104-107   LEVEL: Average

TOTAL I.Q.:   97-101   LEVEL: Average

[Chuck's Verbal-Performance relationship is what one would expect. This sort of interconnection, which reflects action orientation, is frequently found among persons in trouble with the law. Such young people feel much more at ease *doing* things, rather than reflecting about them. Chuck's extremely wide scatter (1-14) suggests a rather profound disorganization. Still, a number of his subtest scores are located fairly close together (ranging from about 8-10), a homogeneity which suggests that a fairly tight intellectual organization is also maintained. The fact that Chuck does so poorly on Arithmetic suggests both that his present concentration is impaired and also that it has been impaired in the past, specifically at school, where he should have been able to concentrate and learn basic addition, subtraction, and so on. The question of motivation probably also enters—learning arithmetic requires a kind of patient application which Chuck was probably neither ready nor willing to give to it. Chuck's poor performance on Digit Span also does not come as a surprise. It is difficult for a presumably action-oriented young man to attend well enough to carry out this task effectively. Chuck's best performance is on the Picture Completion subtest. One wonders to what extent his ability to find the missing items successfully reflects his alertness to small inconsistencies in his environment. Of his Performance tests, he does most poorly on Picture Arrangement. This is somewhat surprising, since persons with antisocial character organizations tend to do well on such a task, which depends on a sensitivity to social events and interpersonal interactions. Judging by his below-average performance on Picture Arrangement, one suspects that Chuck has poorly developed social skills and awarenesses; perhaps rather than (more or less subtly) "conning" persons into the positions where he wants them, Chuck tends to shove them there. If that is so, Chuck's interpersonal maneuvers are probably less precise, and therefore perhaps less successful, than those of his peers.]

INFORMATION

No.	Question	Response and Comments	Score
1.	Who is the President of the United States?	Eisenhower. ("Who was president before that?") Truman. ("And before that?") .... I don't know. [Chuck's waiting a moment before saying he does not know what president preceded Truman shows that he is willing to reflect somewhat, at least. He is not so action oriented, in other words, that he cannot bear any tension at all to develop. Even though Chuck was very young at the time of President Roosevelt's death, it is surprising, considering Roosevelt's fame, that Chuck does not know that he preceded Truman as president. Is Chuck so immersed in the present that the past has extremely little meaning for him?]	+
2.	What is a thermometer?	Tells the temperature.	+
3.	What does rubber come from?	Tree.	+

No.	Question	Response and Comments	Score
4.	*Where is London?*	England.	+
5.	*How many pints make a quart?*	.... Two. [Chuck answers briefly, economically, without elaboration.]	+
6.	*How many weeks are there in a year?*	.... Sixty-two. [Even though his answer is incorrect, he does not simply blurt it out, but thinks about it a while. Again, the evidence suggests Chuck's ability to bind at least some tension.]	–
7.	*What is the capital of Italy?*	.... Rome? [Again the brief period of thought. This time it pays off.]	+
8.	*What is the capital of Japan?*	Uh ...... I don't know. ("Does any Japanese city come to mind?") Tokyo isn't in Japan, is it? I'll say Tokyo. [Although Chuck's answers remain brief, his manner of responding reflects at least some involvement.]	+
9.	*How tall is the average American woman?*	About five foot four .. five foot five.	+
10.	*Who invented the airplane?*	Wright brothers, I guess.	+
11.	*Where is Brazil?*	In .. uh .. uh .. South America.	+
12.	*How far is it from Paris to New York?*	I don't know. ("Make a guess.") One thousand.	–
13.	*What does the heart do?*	Pumps blood.	+
14.	*Who wrote Hamlet?*	... Shakespeare? [It is surprising to find Chuck knowing this item.]	+
15.	*What is the population of the United States?*	I don't know. ("What would you guess?") (He sighs.) Ten thousand. ("Do you know the population of Kansas City?") No sir. ("What would you guess?") About a thousand. That's just a guess. I don't really know. [Chuck displays an extraordinary naïveté about numbers. His estimate is so unrealistic that one finds oneself wondering about a considerable degree of intellectual disorganization. Still, one should keep in mind that Chuck's responses have been pertinent until now.]	–
16.	*When is Washington's birthday?*	I don't know. ("Do you have an idea about what time of year it is?") No.	–
17.	*Who discovered the North Pole?*	North .. I don't know.	–

No.	Question	Response and Comments	Score
18.	*Where is Egypt?*	In .. uh ..... Africa, I think.	+
19.	*Who wrote Huckleberry Finn?*	Mark Twain. [Another literary fact available!]	+

(He does not know the remaining items.)

[With the exception of his response to the "population" question, one would estimate Chuck to be a fairly well-informed, if a somewhat inarticulate, young man who wastes no words but is willing to try even when he feels unsure. His gross underestimations of the populations of the United States and of Kansas City (his birthplace), however, cause one to wonder about possible other unexpected instabilities in his cognitive organization. Although one might suspect a lack of involvement to be the culprit in his extraordinary answer to this item, there are the signs that he does try, even when an answer is not easily and immediately available to him.]

RAW SCORE: ___14___

WEIGHTED SCORE: ___10___

COMPREHENSION

No.	Question	Response and Comments	Score
1.	*What is the thing to do if you find an envelope in the street, that is sealed, and addressed and has a new stamp?*	It didn't have any address? ("It's sealed and addressed and has a new stamp on it.") I'd probably just put it in a mailbox. [Inattention probably produces this very slight "inefficiency."]	2
2.	*What should you do if while sitting in the movies you were the first person to discover a fire (or see smoke and fire)?*	I'd run out! I'd tell .. probably tell the manager there's a fire and run out .. an usher or something. [Although this answer achieves full credit, Chuck's impulsive concern about his own safety almost overwhelms his ability to give the "appropriate" response. The suddenness and, in a sense, primitiveness of his imagined immediate reaction, point to the thinness of the appropriate response which Chuck can give once he recovers from the impact of the question.]	2
3.	*Why should we keep away from bad company?*	Uh .. you get in trouble.	1
4.	*Why should people pay taxes?*	.... Help the government, I guess. ("In what way?") To .. uh .. make things .. you know .. like planes and stuff .. and army and stuff. You know, stuff like that. Things for the forces. [The word "stuff" reflects Chuck's lack of cognitive differentiation.]	2
5.	*Why are shoes made of leather?*	Well, they wear longer than just about anything else, I guess.	1

No.	Question	Response and Comments	Score
6.	Why does land in the city cost more than land in the country?	It's harder to git (sic) and more close to everything. ("In what way is it harder to get?") Well . . uh . . uh . . well . . just more people live there, and you know, everybody wants to live in the city because it's closer to everything, and people pay more for it.	1-2
7.	If you were lost in a forest (woods) in the daytime, how would you go about finding your way out?	I'd go back the same way I came. ("And if you didn't know how you came?") I'd just start walking. [Even though Chuck was brought up in the city, this response is poorly thought through. It seems to show a not caring what he says or how well he does, and, in that sense, Chuck exhibits the sort of behavior one expected of him at the beginning but saw so surprisingly little of. The inexactness of verbal formulations in all parts of Chuck's tests is notable.]	0
8.	Why are laws necessary?	What laws? ("Any laws.") So that . . uh . . (he sighs) cause everybody'd be stealing and stuff, and killing people and stuff . . bad people would. It wouldn't be a good place to live, if there wasn't any laws.	1
9.	Why does the state require people to get a license in order to be married?	I don't know. ("Can you think of any reason?") I don't know. [Sometimes when Chuck has no answer immediately available, he makes no effort to find one. This is in contrast to the times he *does* put forth effort, even though it may mean the prolongation of unpleasant tension. One might speculate that the "marriage" question raises so much discomfort in Chuck that he cannot let himself deal with it at all.]	0
10.	Why are people who are born deaf usually unable to talk?	Cause they can't . . uh . . hear anything . . so they just don't know when they're talking. They can't hear themselves speak. They don't know what they're saying, even. [The comment, "They don't know what they're saying, even," suggests that Chuck separates action from thought. One wonders whether he fears he may say something he does not "really" mean.]	1

RAW SCORE: 11-12

WEIGHTED SCORE: 10-11

ARITHMETIC

No.	Problem	Time	Response and Comments	Score
1.	How much is four dollars and five dollars?	1"	Nine.	1

No.	Problem	Time	Response and Comments	Score
2.	If a man buys six cents worth of stamps and gives the clerk ten cents, how much change should he get back?	2″	Four cents.	1
3.	If a man buys eight cents worth of stamps and gives the clerk twenty-five cents, how much change should he get back?	20″	Uh . . uh seventeen cents?	0-1
4.	How many oranges can you you buy for thirty-six cents if one orange costs four cents?	34″	One orange costs four cents . . . . Uh . . eight. ("Are you sure?") Pretty sure. [Chuck misses the correct answer by one. Are these "misses" motivated (he also misses the next three problems by very little), or are they the result of carelessness? Although Chuck's thinking is poorly disciplined, the lengths of many of his reaction times reflect, as has been suggested, his occasional efforts to reach correct solutions. Once again, the ebb and flow of Chuck's motivation to demonstrate his capabilities is apparent.]	0
5.	How many hours will it take a man to walk twenty-four miles at the rate of three miles an hour?	32″	Uh . . about . . seven hours. [He misses by one hour.]	0
6.	If a man buys seven two cents stamps and gives the clerk a half dollar, how much change should he get back?	19″	About . . about . . thirty-two cents. [Although his answer is in the right general area, it is incorrect by four cents. The "about . . about" shows Chuck's tendency to approximate and to be satisfied with generalized guesses.]	0
7.	If seven pounds of sugar cost twenty-five cents, how many pounds can you get for a dollar?	25″	What? (At 15″.) (I repeat the problem.) Four. ("How did you get four?") Well, if seven pounds cost twenty-five cents, you'd get four for a dollar . . four times twenty-five is a dollar . . or a hundred. [Although Chuck shows he has made the effort to use	0

No. Problem	Time	Response and Comments	Score

some kind of arithmetical manipulation to solve this problem, he is not aware of any inconsistency when he says that twenty-five pounds would cost less than seven pounds would. He has previously shown that he does try to make a response of some sort, but it becomes increasingly apparent that his commitment to an answer which makes logical sense is not very great. One does not quite know what to make of his asking to have the problem presented again, 15″ after it was first read to him. One cannot be sure whether Chuck never heard the problem properly in the first place, or whether (more likely) he "lost" its elements as he was trying to manipulate them mentally. While the first possibility would again suggest Chuck's lack of involvement, the second would once more alert one to the possible effects of some sort of disruptive, disorganizing process.]

8. *A man bought a secondhand car for two-thirds of what it cost new. He paid $400 for it. How much did it cost new?* 1′ 33″ About . . about $1,000. [This matter is so far from correct that Chuck clearly has no idea how to approach the solution to the problem. His "$1,000" is an obvious guess.] 0

[Chuck's ways of handling these arithmetic problems show a combination of involvement and noninvolvement. Although he puts forth effort to attain an accurate answer on some problems, he guesses rather wildly on others. Does Chuck's arithmetical reasoning reflect a specific disability, or is this type of activity, which requires concentration and application, something to which Chuck has always been unwilling to commit himself? At no point does he say he has never been able to do arithmetic, and it may be that he does not care whether he does well or not. Still, if Chuck does not care, what should one make of his fairly frequent efforts to achieve correct solutions in other portions of this test?]

RAW SCORE: 2-3

WEIGHTED SCORE: 1-3

SIMILARITIES

No. Items	Response and Comments	Score
1. Orange-banana	Fruit. Is it okay if I sit over there? (He nods toward a soft chair, some distance from my desk.) ("Sure, if you like.") (He moves to the chair and sprawls in it.) [Although Chuck makes this move ostensibly to be more comfortable, one wonders to what extent he wishes to create "distance" be-	2

No.	Items	Response and Comments	Score

tween himself and the examiner. Is the examiner (i.e., an adult, or even just another person) too close for comfort? To what extent is Chuck's careless sprawl a rather complex disguise (of which he himself is only partly, if at all, aware) of his social discomfort?]

2. *Coat-dress* — Clothes. — 2

3. *Dog-lion* — Animal. — 2

4. *Wagon-bicycle* — Transportation. [Until this point Chuck has given his abstractions clearly, concisely and without unnecessary wordage. So long as problems are not too difficult, so that he can respond with a minimum of reflection, he functions efficiently.] — 2

5. *Daily paper-radio* — They tell things. [Now Chuck begins to get too vague and nonspecific to be given full credit.] — 1

6. *Air-water* — Uh . . . . . They're both things that we need. [Even though his formulation is vague, Chuck reflects about his answer.] — 1

7. *Wood-alcohol* — Rubbing alcohol? ("Just 'alcohol.' ") Uh . . . . I don't know that. ("Can you think of any way?") (He thinks some more about possible answers.) I can't. I don't know. [Again Chuck does not outrightly dismiss a question for which he is unable to find an immediate answer.] — 0

8. *Eye-ear* — They're both . . part of the human body. — 1

9. *Egg-seed* — They're both things that we eat. — 0

10. *Poem-statue* — A poem? ("That's right.") . . . . I don't know. [Chuck hardly ever feels it necessary to disguise his inability to succeed with this sort of intellectual task.] — 0

11. *Praise-punishment* — . . . . Both are something that you do. ("How do you mean?") Well, you praise somebody and you punish somebody. — 0

12. *Fly-tree* — . . . . They both die. [It is significant that Chuck picks on death as the aspect which conceptually binds two living organisms together. His choice of "death" rather than "life" may reflect his convictions about the way life is turning out for him; it might also reflect a view of life as offering little in the way of viable qualities.] — 1

RAW SCORE: 12

WEIGHTED SCORE: 10

PICTURE COMPLETION

(He fails to solve only Item 14. He tends to refer to the pictured objects or their parts as "things.")

[As was suggested earlier, Chuck's good performance on this subtest probably reflects his alertness to what goes on around him. That he is not a man of words is again shown in his vague references to objects as "things." On the *Mirror* item (11), for example, he says the following about what is missing: "The hand and arm in the thing . . the powder puff thing. ('How do you mean, "the thing"?') In the mirror." This avoidance of precision of speech is consistent with Chuck's apparently lackadaisical attitude, e.g., with the way he sprawls in his chair. It is *not* consistent, however, with the fairly intense efforts he frequently seems to exert as he tries to think of a correct answer.]

RAW SCORE: __14__

WEIGHTED SCORE: __14__

PICTURE ARRANGEMENT

(Chuck does the first three items correctly, in 5″, 8″ and 9″ respectively. He completes Items 4, 5 and 6 as follows:)

No.	Item	Correct Order	Time	Arranged Order	Story and Comments	Score
4.	*Flirt*	JANET	23″	ANJET	I don't know what that thing was on her head. I don't know the story. I guess he just wanted to carry it for her. [Here is the omnipresent "thing" again. Apparently Chuck's use of the word "thing" reflects not only his *tendency* to evaluate the world vaguely; it may well also cover his *inability* to see it in more precise terms.]	0
5.	*Taxi*	SAMUEL	38″	SALEUM	That was wrong. ("Wrong in what way?") I guess it was okay. ("What was the story?") They had that thing. He had that woman . . . . . I guess he was showing somebody he had a girl friend or something. It seemed more like a joke or something to me. ("What was it he had?") A dummy. [Chuck's vagueness often seems to be a stylistic preference—here, and possibly elsewhere, he is able to meet the demand for greater precision.]	1

No.	Item	Correct Order	Time	Arranged Order	Story and Comments	Score
6.	Fish	EFGHIJ	43″	EGFHIJ	He had that guy give him the fish. [Short and to the point, even if rather globally put.]	1

RAW SCORE: 8

WEIGHTED SCORE: 7

[Had Chuck not carelessly interchanged two cards on the *Fish* and *Flirt* sequences, he would have achieved a weighted score of 11, instead of 7. Once again, we see the paradox of careless involvement side by side with considerable application. But, in any case, Chuck's low Picture Arrangement score seems to be much more the result of carelessness than of a lack of social sensitivity. The mysterious discrepancy between the scores on Picture Completion and Picture Arrangement seems largely clarified.]

BLOCK DESIGN

(Chuck builds the designs slowly but accurately. He uses only one hand and never hurries. Even so, he achieves time credits on Designs 1, 3 and 4. On Design 5, he begins correctly but then takes three additional blocks from my pile and adds an extra line to the bottom. He sees his error and continues correctly. About halfway through Design 5, with no more errors, he says, "I can't do that one. I couldn't do it before." With encouragement, he completes the design well within the time limit. He does Designs 6 and 7 accurately, but he is so slow that he can be given only alternate credit.)

[Were Chuck to hurry himself a little, he could probably obtain a considerably higher score on this subtest than he does. The reason he approaches the task so lackadaisically, although not clear, may well represent part of his wish to create an "image" of the "cool," uninvolved person who does things in his own good time. But the slowness may also disguise Chuck's lack of certainty, which might come to more obvious expression if he seemed to be trying his best and working as quickly as possible. His readiness to give up, even though he is doing well, might also be a reflection either of uninvolvement or of a sporadic perceptual vagueness which interferes with Chuck's accurate evaluation of his perceptual performance.]

RAW SCORE: 18-24

WEIGHTED SCORE: 9-11

OBJECT ASSEMBLY

Item	Time	Accur.	Description of Behavior and Comments	Score
Manikin	40″	Yes	You mean, just so it'll fit like this? (He puts the legs in the sockets intended for the arms and otherwise demonstrates confusion, even though he begins to put together something recognizable.) Is it supposed to be a girl or a boy? (He finally puts the figure together, although with difficulty.) Oh, I see now. [Chuck's ability to achieve a full score on this item hides	6

Item	Time	Accur.	Description of Behavior and Comments	Score
			his confusion. This simple item should not require him 40″ to complete. While it might be unclear whether the pieces will make a boy or a girl, Chuck's question suggests a preoccupation with this kind of uncertainty. Placing the legs in the arm sockets suggests a sudden rupture of reality testing.]	
Profile	67″	Yes	(He completes this item accurately, although slowly and with instances of mild confusion.)	6
Hand	43″	Yes	What is it? ("Put it together as best you can.") Just put it together? (After he hesitantly fits the thumb and wrist pieces correctly, he completes the rest of the hand quickly.) ("When did you know what it would make?") When I put that on (referring to the thumb). [Chuck's "What is it?" and his "Just put it together?" reflects his unexpected perplexity. There have been enough hints by now to indicate that Chuck at times finds his environment unstable, uncertain and confusing. Although he wishes to give the impression that he has things under control, one begins to feel that this control has little substance.]	8

RAW SCORE: 20

WEIGHTED SCORE: 12

DIGIT SYMBOL

(Chuck makes several errors on this subtest. He tends to modify the   into an N and makes and spontaneously corrects this error three times. He begins to make the ∧ item into an N, but does not complete the error. He draws the symbols fairly neatly.)

RAW SCORE: 44

WEIGHTED SCORE: 10

STORY RECALL

IMMEDIATE RECALL

+1   +1   +1   +1   +1
In this little town / it flooded. / And this man / was trying to save a boy /
+1
and he cut his hand.

SCORE: 6+4 = 10

[Chuck repeats only the barest essence of the story. This Immediate Recall illustrates Chuck's tendency to make do with as few words as possible. Again, one does not know if he could do better if he "tried"; that is, whether he presents his meagerly worded paraphrase to show how he is not really involved in this sort of task.]

DELAYED RECALL

    0   +1   +1   +1

It was December 6 / in a little town / ten miles / from Albany. / I think it

  −1   0

killed sixteen people / and injured about 600, I think, / and . . no, 600 people

          −1   +1

were put out in the cold or something from the flood. / It went into the houses /

  +1   +1   +1   +1

. . and this man / cut his hands / trying to rescue / this boy.

SCORE: 8−2+4 = 10

[This Delayed Recall passage shows how ineffectively Chuck's memory is articulated. The distortions suggest that things do not get through to him clearly, particularly that he is unable to keep areas which should be separate from merging with each other (e.g., "600 people were put out in the cold or something from the flood"). This memory item, badly garbled in a context of "normal" intelligence, raises questions about the degree to which Chuck, beneath his laissez-faire attitude, is rather significantly disorganized.]

The BRL Sorting Test

[Except for his tendency to sort in a rather nonconceptual fashion on Part I, Chuck does quite well on this portion. He does even better on Part II, where most of his definitions are abstractly stated. He is able to conceptualize even such difficult items as the *Double* and the *White* categories.

[Such a relatively unimpaired capacity to conceptualize must be kept in mind as one notes future evidences of disorganization. Chuck's stable performance on this test is a major positive factor to put on the organization side of an "organization-disorganization" balance.]

The Bender Gestalt Test

PART A (PLATE 53)

(He makes the drawings very quickly, frequently modifying dots into dashes.) [Even though the Bender designs are quickly and rather carelessly drawn, they are essentially accurate. That he plans poorly is apparent when he writes the date so it collides with one of his previously drawn designs.]

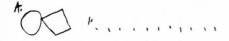

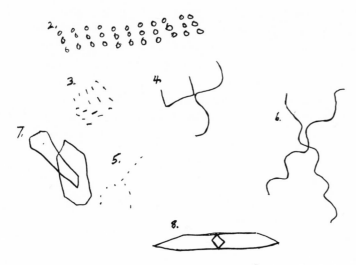

PLATE 53

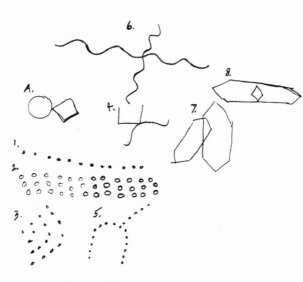

PLATE 54

PART B (PLATE 54, p. 579)

(He draws this series much more slowly and carefully. The drawings are placed essentially in the center of the page, but although Chuck's planning ability seems much improved here, the placement of his designs is still somewhat erratic, e.g., he starts in the middle of the page, rather than near the top. His eagerness to do this job well can be observed in his tendency to "correct" his first efforts, changing dashes back into dots, filling in dots and refining lines with which he is dissatisfied, either by erasing them or by drawing over them.) [Once again one is struck by the strong possibility that Chuck is "careless" in order to disguise his difficulties. At any rate, his carelessness is no longer apparent, once the difficulties are lessened. It is apparent again how much more at home with nonverbal than with verbal activities he is. It is surprising to see so much constriction in the drawings of someone who is ordinarily so alloplastic.

RORSCHACH TEST

[Chuck's Rorschach Psychogram contains a number of surprises. One would hardly expect a person whose everyday responses tend to be so casual and so apparently uninvolved to offer a total of thirty percepts and no Failure on any card. Nor would one expect such a relatively high percentage of responses with good form (76/73%). Nor, certainly, would one expect to see so many (C) responses, since they are considered to reflect a sensitivity and capacity for fine differentiations. True, the "positive" impact of these (C) responses is attenuated by the finding that the form quality of almost half (three of the seven) is poor. But still, formal qualities (the F%) predominate in every response, so that the impulsivity which is evident in other tests appears to be controllable. It is striking that Chuck never allows pure color (either C or CF) to come to expression. On the less positive side, one is impressed by Chuck's constricted Experience Balance, a constriction which suggests not only an impoverishment of his internal life but of his affective contact with the world as well. Although ways of seeing reality appear to conform to what is appropriate (as suggested by the five Popular responses), Chuck has a tendency to overdo conformity and to approach matters in too "easy," conventional a fashion (half his responses have an Animal content). That he nevertheless organizes his perceptions in somewhat

RORSCHACH SCORING SHEET

Number of Responses: 30

Manner of Approach (Location)

W	2
D	16
DS	2
Do	3
Dr	5
DrS	1
De	1
Total	30

Location Percentages

W%	7
D%	70
DR%	20
De%	3

Form, Movement, Color and Shading Determinants

F+	14		
F−	3		
F±	2		
F∓	2		
M±	1		
F(C)+	2	FC(C)−	1
F(C)±	2	F(C)C′−	1
F(C)−	1		
FC′+	1		
Total	30		

Groups of Contents

A	9
Ad	4
Ad (Horror)	2
H	1
Hd	2
Skull	1
Obj.	4
At.	1
Pl.	1
Thorns	1
Trap	1
Blood	1
Bomb	1
Sex	1
Anus	2
"Bowels"	1
Total	33

Determinant and Content Percentages

F%	70/100	Obj.%	13
F+%	76/73	At%	3
A%	50	P%	17
H%	10	Sex%	10

Qualitative Material

Popular	IV V VIII X X
Fabulation	4
Confabulation	3
Fab.-Combination	1
Vague	2
Confusion	2
Deterioration	2
Peculiar	3
Queer	2
Arbitrary	1
Castrative	1

EXPERIENCE BALANCE: 1.0/0.5

unusual ways is attested to by a fairly high DR%, a situation which may have either "positive" (in the sense of "original" and "creative") or "negative" (in the sense of "arbitrary") meaning.

[But it is when one looks at the qualitative aspects of his responses —the confabulations, the fabulized combinations, the queer, arbitrary, confused and peculiar responses, and so on—that one becomes aware of the apparent degree of Chuck's disorganization.

[Nevertheless, in spite of these qualitative aspects, one must keep in mind that the formal aspects of Chuck's thinking (as judged by the Rorschach) reflect satisfactory organization. The discrepancy in the qualities of functioning should be kept in mind as one evaluates the seriousness of Chuck's pathology.]

RORSCHACH PROTOCOL

Card #	React. Time	Score	Protocol	Inquiry and Observations
I	11″	WF±A	1. Some sort of bird or	1. ("Is it more like a bird or an insect?") In places it looks like an insect. In other places it looks like a bird. ("Would you tell me about the insect?") Do you want me to show you? ("Try to tell me without the card.") The middle of it. ("What about the middle?") It just looked sort of like an insect (total center D). ("And the bird?") Well, there were sort of wings.
		DF±A Vague	2. Insect. ("Do you see anything else?") Uh-uh.	("What kind of an insect?") Sort of like a beetle. The top part. ("Show me here on the card.") Those things up there (top center Dd), sort of tentacles, I guess you'd call them. [Although these two percepts are vaguely perceived and described, they are nevertheless "popular" enough to merit a separate and a plus-minus score. These scores, however, do not reflect very accurately Chuck's poorly differentiated ways of perceiving and describing.]
II	25″		That doesn't remind me of much of anything. It doesn't look	

React. Card # Time Score	Protocol	Inquiry and Observations

like much of anything.

Sex
DrSFC(C)—
Anus
Blood
Deterior.
Vague
Queer
Arb.
Confab.

1. It's something nasty. (He laughs. His stomach is gurgling; he picks the card up, then he puts it down and looks away.) ("What do you see?") I mean, I could tell you, but . . . . ("Try to tell me.") It's nasty, though . . . It looks like a bloody butt hole, or something, or a cock, on top. It looks more like a bloody butt hole, though.

1. ("Could you tell me about it?") (As he looks at the card, he finds it difficult to differentiate between the "butt hole" and the "cock," but he thinks the percept might be composed of the middle space and the bottom red D.) Right there, with blood coming out. ("Does it look like that?") No, I just imagined it would. It doesn't really remind me of one. You know, just something like it. [This response involves not only a highly unusual content, but also much vagueness as far as formal perceptual aspects are concerned. The penis, the anus and its bloody extrusion, seem to be combined into a kind of cloacal organ. This response is notable in several ways: (1) in that it appears at all in consciousness; (2) in that it is badly organized; and (3) in that it is said aloud. Even though such a response might occur to a person, he would ordinarily be reluctant to tell someone else about it. Actually, Chuck does display a reluctance to tell what he sees. This reluctance reflects his effort at least to try to hold back what he obviously considers inappropriate. This, by the way, is Chuck's only response to any color.
[Unusual sexual interest and possible unusual

Card #	React. Time	Score	Protocol	Inquiry and Observations
				practice is also suggested by the response.]
III	19″	DoF+Ad	1. It looks like two birds, or one.	1. (Popular "head" area.)
		DoFC'+Hd Confusion	2. Two niggers.	2. ("Tell me about the niggers.") It was the only thing that I could see that was any . . uh . . uh . . I don't know what you call it . . oh . . the only thing I could see that resembled them. The head looked something like it. The head of a colored person or something. ("Did you see just the head?") (He smiles.) I didn't see any more. It was the only thing that reminded me of it. ("Why does it seem to be Negro?") It was black. It sort of had a nose. Sort of eyes. It didn't have any mouth, so it didn't look much like one. In fact, it didn't look like *anything*, but it just reminded me of it.

[The degree of Chuck's interpersonal sensitivity is suggested by his modifying the word "niggers" to "colored person." Although the examiner was not aware of it, he must have conveyed, in a nonobvious way, his distaste for the word "nigger." While Chuck may appear gross in his attitudes in many ways, there is considerable evidence by now of his readiness to do what is expected and to abide by the explicit and implicit rules of the psychological examination.]

	React.			
Card #	Time	Score	Protocol	Inquiry and Observations
		DoF(C)+Obj.	3. And that right there looks sort of like a high-heeled shoe, you know, that a woman wears.	3. (Popular "foot" area.) [Chuck's Do tendency reflects his difficulty in smoothly integrating percepts and his need to keep together-fitting aspects of reality isolated, both from each other and, probably, from himself. The tendency to separate in this way is frequently seen among persons who use repression to a marked degree; the fact that it appears in Chuck's record suggests that he experiences difficulty in bringing together the varied aspects of his life. The tendency to focus on details in this way is also consistent with Chuck's tendency toward constriction, already evident on Part B of his Bender drawings.]
IV	21″	DF+Obj.P	1. Well, that right there looks like a shoe . . like a man's shoe.	1. (The side "shoe" D.)
		DF+AdHorror Fab.	2. And that looks like a either . . you know, either a horror creature that you see in the movies, or a caterpillar. That's about all.	2. ("What made it look like a horror creature?") It sort of had eyes, and little things kind of sticking out and everything. ("How much of it did you see?") Just the head. A little bit of the neck or whatever you call it. I don't know. ["Horrible" things of one sort or another play a rather prominent role in Chuck's fantasy life, as will be seen in future responses. While "horror" is not only "horrible," but also "funny" and "exciting" to teen-agers (so that "horror" can be thought

Card #	React. Time	Score	Protocol	Inquiry and Observations
				of as a "normal," or at least an "expectable," content for them), Chuck's apparent infatuation with horror, particularly as the infatuation is present in a person who is otherwise so lacking obvious interests, is conspicuous.]
V	25″	WF+AP	1. That looks like a butterfly . . uh . . a little bit like a bat. That's all. ∨ ∧	
VI			(He sighs at 35″.)	
	53″	DrF(C)C′—Ad Pec.	1. That right there . . those two little dot things, look like nostrils.	1. ("Would you describe the nostrils?") From above, sort of like on a horse or something . . some animal that has sort of big nostrils . . openings, and like that. (Topmost Dr point of "pole.") [This is certainly an unusual percept. Chuck has sensitively differentiated the shadings of the blot, but he presents an idiosyncratic response with poor form. The response is all the more striking in that it requires 53″ before it appears to Chuck.]
		DrF—Anus, feces Confab. Deterior. Queer	2. That right there, looks like a butt opened up . . Those look like bowels. That's about all.	2. (Bottom central Dr.) [It is rare to get anal material of this magnitude— now for the second time. Just what these anal preoccupations tell us about Chuck is difficult to know. It is not contributing much understanding to say that Chuck is "anally preoccupied" or "an anal personality." On a descriptive level, one might suggest that Chuck's fecal preoccupations are a sign of the unwholesome, de-

Card #	React. Time	Score	Protocol	Inquiry and Observations

moralized, unhealthful quality of his inner life. This time Chuck reports his percept uncritically, perhaps because his previous percept of similar content met with no disapproval. Whatever "good mental health" may be, this type of fecal preoccupation seems not to reflect it. The preceding "nostrils" appear to represent a further type of anal (i.e. aperture) preoccupation.]

VII

(After 20″.)It doesn't remind me of anything. ("Look at it a little longer.")

Does it have to be with the whole? ("Any part of it that you want.") Just little parts of it? [Chuck has, of course, reported "little parts" in the past.]

1′ 15″   DrF — Thorns

1. Those little things right there look like thorns or teeth.

1. (Tiny top Dr of "Indian's head.") [Another example of Chuck's seizing on a tiny, relatively irrelevant portion of the total percept. "Thorns" or "teeth" suggest the attacking, uncomfortable, rough quality Chuck attributes to his environment.]

DrF ∓ Trap
Confab.
Pec.

2. Well, that going right down here looks sort of like a plan to a trap, or something. Like one of those sand bugs has. Do you want me to explain how? See, like a sandbug has little things going down

2. (Central Dr portion of bottom D.) ("How did you mean, 'a plan to a trap'?") Well, I mean .. I don't know what brought it to mind. There's this boy in school, and he draws all these pictures. He draws traps and stuff like that. It doesn't really

Card #	React. Time	Score	Protocol	Inquiry and Observations
			like that. Somebody going alone would tumble down. That would be showing the hole right there.	look anything like a trap . . just . . . . . [More and more Chuck describes his unpleasant life situation. His world appears to be made up of things which are, at best, nondescript and, at worst, peculiar, dangerous, or disgusting.]
VIII			It looks like a bu . . oh . . Is it okay if I turn it? <	("What did you start to say at the very beginning?") I started to say it looked like a bunch of colors, but . . . . [Here an example of Chuck's ability, at least partially, to control nonproductive impulsivity on occasion. A "bunch of colors" would have resulted in a score of "C", and the absence of this type of gross color response has already been noted. Here one can see how the impulsive response was begun but not completed; instead, Chuck was able to spell out more differentiated percepts.]
	15″	DF+AP	1. That (he covers everything except the side "animal" with his hand) looks like an animal walking . . some sort of a pig or rodent. That's all I can think of.	
		DSF+At	2. Unless that right there looks like a spine, with the ribs coming out like that. ∨ ∧	
IX	30″	DSF(C)± Horror head Fab.	1. This is something else that looks like in a horror movie . . not much, but a little.	1. ("Something like in a horror movie?") Down at the bottom (he is picking at his lips). If I had it

React. Card # *Time Score*	*Protocol*	*Inquiry and Observations*
		turned the way you had it, you know, when you first put it there. (He has forgotten that he has returned it to its original position.) ("Could you describe what you saw?") It just looked like something you see in a horror movie. ("Why a horror movie?") It just did . . just about anything looks like something you see in a horror movie, something like that. ("How much of it did you see?") Just the head. (The center space: the bottom spaces are "eyes" and the topmost Dr's jutting out are "tentacles.") (I'm not sure whether he sees this head from the front or back.) [More horror.]
DF+bomb	2. And *this* . . just this top part, looks like just the top of a bomb. You know, just the mushroom part. ∨ (He yawns.)	2. ("Then you saw part of a bomb?") Oh . . uh . . just the top part . . You know, when it sort of comes down the bottom, then the top looks like it. (Bottom pink D.) [Chuck seems unclear about what is "top" and what "bottom"; his "explanation" makes it no clearer. A "bomb" is not at all unusual here, but it is nevertheless consistent with the general picture of horror which Chuck describes.]
DF(C)−A	3. It looks something like a crab, too, if it had legs.	3. (Bottom pink D.) [Chuck's perceptual and expressive (cognitive?) vagueness emerges strongly on this card. One is never sure whether things are up or down, back or front, or inside or outside for him. Although Chuck

Card #	*React. Time*	Score	*Protocol*	*Inquiry and Observations*
				often tries to convey that he cannot be bothered to express himself clearly, his effort at other times to convey precisely what he means suggests that the "not caring" may not be genuine but is simply an effort to throw others off the scent—the scent being that he cares a good deal but cannot function as efficiently as he would like.]
X			(He laughs.) ∨ . . . . . (He sighs at 30".) Well . . ∧ ∨	
	45"	DF+Obj. Cast.	1. That would look like . . you know . . one of those things you see on a pawnshop, with one of those things gone.	1. ("What's gone on that pawnshop thing?") You know, you see three of them (he motions). (Upper center D, "maple seed.") [Here again we see Chuck's expressive vagueness, as he refers to an object as "one of those things."]
		DF+pl.	2. Or like a leaf from a tree. I don't know what you call it.	2. (Same location as 1.) ("Like a leaf?") You know, one of those seed things that the wind brings down.
		DF+A	3. That looks like a bat.	3. ("Would you describe the bat?") Well, it looks like a bat. (Central blue D.) [A nonreflective response to inquiry.]
		DF(C)±Skull Fab. Comb.	4. Or a skull with wings. ∨ ∧	4. ("Would you tell me about the skull with wings?") It was the same thing. ("Did it remind you of something definite?") No, not unless it would be in my dreams or something. [This unusual response is presented uncritically, as though Chuck frequently came in con-

React. Card #	Time	Score	Protocol	Inquiry and Observations
				tact with a skull that had wings.]
		DF+AdP	5. That right in there looks like a rabbit . . the head of a rabbit.	5. (Popular rabbit's head.)
		DrF—Hd Pec. Fab.	6. That right there, without those things . . . it looks sort of like a bowlegged Texan, like you see in the pictures.	6. ("And the bowlegged Texan?") Just his legs. (Popular "sea horses," without heads.)
		DF+AP	7. That looks like sort of like a crab.	7. (Popular blue D.)
		DM±H	8. It looks a little bit like two men on a post, waving at somebody.	8. ("The two men on a post?") It didn't look much like it . . just sort of. ("As though they were how?") Like two men on a telephone pole. (Topmost gray D.) [Chuck's only, and not very carefully perceived, M response.]
		DF(C)+Obj.	9. That little thing right in there reminds me of a nut.	9. (Darker portion inside yellow "dog.")
			. . . . ∧	
		DF+A	10. Oh yeah. That reminds me a lot of a dog . . a collie dog.	10. (The usual yellow-area "dog.")
		DF+A	11. That reminds me of one of those things that you see in the sea . . round-looking, it has four legs.	11. ("How about that round-looking thing you see in the sea?") I don't know the name of it. I could draw you a picture. (He does.) It's real simple. I've seen it on TV. It's the real thing, though. (Side sepia D.)
			. . . . > ∨ <	
		DrF∓Ad	12. That reminds me of the head of a duck. That's about all.	12. (Back section of bottom outer D, "sleeping dog."

THEMATIC APPERCEPTION TEST (Partially Reproduced)

Card 1 (A young boy is contemplating a violin which rests on a table in front of him.)

(He smiles as he recognizes this card.) I'm supposed to tell you what he's doing? ("That's right.") Well, this little boy is supposed to play the violin, so he got a violin, and he broke it. He never did want to play one the rest of his life. ("Why was that?") Cause he broke it. So if he thought it was as fragile as that, well, he just didn't want any more. ("How did he happen to break it?") He was playing it. He was holding it up like that (he shows me), and he was so strong, it just crumbled. [Chuck seems to conceive of himself as a muscularly gross bull in a china shop, who, with his nondirected great strength and awkward clumsiness, inadvertently destroys things that are valuable, beautiful and fragile.]

Card 3 BM (On the floor against a couch is the huddled form of a boy with his head bowed on his right arm. Beside him on the floor is a revolver.)

Is that a girl? ("You can make it whatever you like.") Is that a gun? ("You can make that whatever you like, too.") It is supposed . . if it's not a gun, he's crying . . or she's crying. Since that isn't a gun, it's a soldering gun, so here she burned he or she self. And he or she cried. That's all. ("How does it come out?") Well, the burned place heals. [Although questions regarding the hero's sex are fairly common on this card, it is rare to find the question amplified into such a production. One feels fairly convinced that Chuck's need for certainty regarding the sexual identity of the TAT person reflects the unsureness he feels about his own masculinity.]

Card 4 (A woman is clutching the shoulders of a man whose face and body are averted as if he were trying to pull away from her.)

(He laughs.) That woman is trying to stop a man from beating up another man . . I guess. Trying to keep him from doing *something*. He looks like he's mad . . like he's trying to rescue him . . no, wait, that wouldn't be right, because unless his wife was an *evil* woman, she would want him to, but she doesn't look like an evil woman, so . . I guess he's trying to get somebody. ("What happens?") He beats him up. ("What is it all about?") No . . *he* gets beat up.

("How does he feel?") How does he feel about what? ("How does
he feel about getting beat up?") Cause the guy was *tougher* than he
was. His wife told him *not* to . . but . . he had to be a hero. ("How
does his wife feel?") She's glad. ("What was the fight about?") I don't
know. I'm just making it up. ("Make up something the fight might
have been about.") Let's see . . Oh! Oh! . . . .
Well, that other man . . . . raped his wife. ("Why was she glad?") I
don't know. Well, let's see . . cause she wanted to be raped. [This
extraordinary story illustrates Chuck's disposition to say things that
are startling and not "appropriate." One has the feeling, however,
that Chuck does not set out to startle—rather, his unexpected comments come as an afterthought, as a need to find and offer some sort
of explanation. For example, it is probable that Chuck impulsively
said the wife in the story felt "glad," but had no conscious idea why
he said it. Still, in response to the examiner's question, he had to
make his statement reasonable and then gave an explanation which
turns out to be startlingly unconventional. It is a question whether
Chuck enjoys and seeks unconventionality, or whether what he says
uncritically simply turns out to be outside the conventional frame-
work. Although one occasionally wonders to what extent Chuck
presents his ideas with tongue in cheek, he shows in many ways
that he tries to respond seriously and thoughtfully. What is also
striking again is Chuck's tendency to show his uncertainty about the
world by substituting the *opposite* of his original thought, e.g., "He
beats him up . . no, *he* gets beat up"; "Unless his wife was an evil
woman, but she doesn't look like an evil woman." Probably two
(superficially conflicting) response tendencies are true of Chuck: his
responses are often intended sincerely, even though at times he wants
to ridicule and degrade everyone and everything, including himself.]

*Card 6 BM (A short elderly woman stands with her back turned to a
tall young man. The latter is looking downward with a perplexed
expression.)*

Hm. (He sighs.) Well, that's that . . that man right there is this
boy's brother, and his brother was put in jail, they're both sad about
it. He came from some city to see about it. ("What happens?") (He
stares into the distance.) . . . . . Oh . . . . Let's see . . . .
Oh, he gets a lawyer, they convict him and he gets put in prison.
("Who's the woman there?") This guy's mother. ("How does she feel
about her son?") Sad. ("What did the boy do?") Oh . . he got in

trouble. ("How did he feel about jail?") They felt .. well .. they just felt bad about it .. you know. ("How come the lawyer didn't help?") Because they proved that he did it. [Despondency, hopelessness, as well as nonproductivity, are the hallmarks of this story.]

Card 7 BM (A gray-haired man is looking at a younger man who is sullenly staring into space.)

That's his father .. That's this boy's father. And this is the boy that got in trouble. And he's asking about what happened. ("What does the boy say?") He said, "I didn't do it." ("Had he done it?") Yeah. They convicted him. ("What does the father think?") The same thing as the mother and brother do. [The last two stories, filled with hopelessness and the inevitability of failure, reflect Chuck's pessimism about deriving worth-whileness out of life. Although his family is sad about what happens to the boy, they are unable to change the downward course his life is taking. Chuck makes no value statement about the boy's lying—things simply are that way.]

Card 12 M (A young man is lying on a couch with his eyes closed. Leaning over him is a gaunt form of an elderly man, his hand stretched out above the face of the reclining figure.)

.... That guy's seeing whether that guy's asleep or not. (He looks away from the card.) ("And what happens?") And he finds out that he is asleep. ("Who are these fellows?") People .. two boys. ("Why is he checking?") Cause he didn't think he was asleep. ("Why does he care?") He doesn't. He's just seeing whether he's asleep or not. [Chuck's discomfort with this card may well have to do with its homosexual implications. There is by now a good deal of evidence to suggest that Chuck has a (possibly consciously felt) homosexual tendency. Such a tendency is most usefully thought of as part of Chuck's general identity diffusion, as part of his cognitive and affective disorganization, rather than as an isolated problem.]

Card 13 MF (A young man is standing with downcast head buried in his arm. Behind him is the figure of a woman lying in bed.)

(He yawns.) That guy's wiping the sweat off his head. And he'd just gotten on all of his clothes .... And he went home. ("What was that all about?") He just got through screwing her.

("Why was he wiping the sweat off?") Cause it was hot. ("Who are these people?") Oh .. he .. he's just a man she met. ("How does this woman feel?") (He smiles.) Oh, she feels okay. She got her money and everything. ("How does he feel?") Just fine. [Most adolescents, when they speak with an adult, do not speak as openly as they do with one another. Chuck, however, takes no special care to sound "proper." His use of such words as "screw" is not appropriate in the context of being examined by an adult. Chuck's story probably has the goal of shocking, particularly in view of its obvious absence of intimate feeling between the TAT man and woman. Chuck (who after all, comes from a "good," middle-class home) expends no effort to make the intimate relationship between a man and woman complicated by gentle feelings. Instead, he stresses the couple's lack of mutual tenderness and cynically sets the stage for a business arrangement which involves a financial transaction in exchange for the man's purely physical gratification.]

Card 15 (A gaunt man with clenched hands is standing among gravestones.)

(He laughs and sighs.) That looks like a guy that has risen from his grave. (He yawns.) . . . . And he's reading what they've put on his tombstone . . . . ("And then what happens?") He goes back to his grave. ("Why did he rise from it?") He wanted to see what they wrote about him. ("What did they write?") That he was a bum. ("And what did he think of that?") Oh, from his expression it looks like he didn't like it. ("Was he a bum?") Yeah. ("In what way?") He didn't dress very nice. ("He was a bum because of the way he dressed?") Uh-huh (he smiles). [Chuck's frequent laughs, his sighs and yawns, particularly at the beginning of most of his stories, reflect his tension about the themes which the TAT cards evoke. One is taken aback again by the uncritical, matter-of-fact way in which Chuck presents his strange tale. Again, too, one wonders about the extent of tongue-in-cheekness which Chuck shows when he speaks as he does. Nevertheless, one is once more brought to the view that, were Chuck only trying to tease, the teasing alone could by no means explain the strange content which emerges so effortlessly. Chuck needs to have available raw material for any teasing he might wish to indulge in, and this material is generally of a highly unusual quality.

[Once more one comes face to face with Chuck's conviction that his life will be useless and that no one will take serious account of his departure from it.]

Card 18 BM (A man is clutched from behind by three hands. The figures of his antagonists are invisible.)

(He laughs and casts a puzzled look at the card.) (He smiles.) These hands .. uh .. This man had glued them on to his coat. He'd chopped them off another man and glued them on to his coat (he laughs) . . . . And that's all. ("Why did he do that?") Glue them on to his coat? He wanted to be funny. ("So what happened?") Everybody screamed and everything, and he got a big charge out of it. He had to attract attention some way, so he glued hands on to his coat. ("How do you mean, he chopped them off?") Oh, he dug up this grave, and cut the skin off this man, and dissected him, and cut off his arms and legs, and chopped off his head. And he carried the head around in his briefcase. And when he wanted really to scare people, he'd .. ram it on his hand like that and hold it up like that (he demonstrates). See, he'd cut away about half the skull, and left the brain showing. He'd popped out one of the eyeballs, so that it was hanging down, see, and he cut away the mouth so that the teeth were showing, real bloody, and everything. (He continues in this vein.) [Chuck obviously enjoys telling this gruesome tale—one bloodthirsty idea leads to the next, so that the whole sequence becomes amplified into a terrible description. It may well be that Chuck's usual audience reacts dramatically to his horrible stories. It must be stressed again, however, that, although such stories may be told in order to shock and tease, the fact that Chuck is able even to think of them is extraordinary. Just as the hero of Chuck's story has to "attract attention some way," so Chuck apparently uses his grisly stories to become the center of attention.]

Card 16 (Blank Card.)

Can I sit over there? (In the soft chair, away from the examiner.) I don't need that (laughing, as he returns the blank card). Well, it starts off that .. uh .. the police had found a box with .. uh .. no, let me see. It starts off with this man. He was at the docks. He saw this sort of box thing, and he got it out of the water .. and he kicked it, and .. it busted open (he smiles) .. and it was just a whole pile .. of bloody skin. And .. and .. uh .. so he was horrified. And he took it to the police, and the police started investigating. Finally, they found the murderer. And this is how the murderer tells the story, what had happened: and the police came to find out that this girl had been arrested . . this was in England. And they came to find out that this girl had been arrested on being a prostitute . . and . . and what does l-a-i-r spell? (I tell him.) What does l-i-a-r spell? (I tell him.) Well, she'd been arrested for that, too. Well, anyway, and a whole bunch of times for being arrested and stuff. This is how she tells the story. She finally settled down to making an honest living. She got a job as housekeeper. She worked for this real gripey woman, and they were always having arguments. So this one night . . it was Sunday, Sunday night in the park. She'd been drinking. She came in sort of drunk, so, one night she came in drunk. This woman was always griping . . every time she did some work, she'd run her hands over it and tell her what she'd done wrong. So she'd gotten tired of that. They had a big argument that Sunday night. They started screaming at each other. The woman she worked for, she was going off to church. When she got back, they had another big argument. They went to bed. The woman she worked for was real scared, you know, and she had people come in to spend the night. She asked this girl to leave, but she wouldn't leave. So she'd have people come in and spend the night and stay . . but at the same time, she'd always gripe at this girl, tell her to get out, but she wouldn't leave. So one night she came in drunk again and . . uh . . so they had another big argument (he smiles). They were upstairs, and so this girl pushed her off the stairs . . the top of the bannister . . and she fell. The girl got real scared, so she went downstairs . . and . . uh . . and got her and put her on the table in the kitchen, and cut off her head and started dissecting her, see . . and . . uh . . and . . uh . . so she had been cutting her up . . bloody mess . . So she went to bed . . left her on the table. The next morning she came in and started cutting her up again (he smiles) and . . uh . . ("We have only a few minutes left. Do you think you can finish your story by then?") I doubt if I can do it. You see it's a long story. Well, anyway, she went out and hung up all the clothes, as if she was working there. She put the body in this tublike thing, and it started boiling and stuff . . . . . and so finally she went out and . . that sort of . . that took away everything except the bones, and skin, and part of the body . . legs and skin . . so she put them in a great big box.

This girl was going to try and sell the house. She left for the next town with some friends. (I interrupt at this point.) [Chuck probably enjoys the thought of giving the examiner a run for his money. But while this type of "gruesomeness" may be a good deal more available to adolescents than to children or adults, Chuck seems much too much at home with it. After one subtracts possible teasing intentions, possible intentions to fool the examiner, and possible intentions to draw attention to himself, one is left with a too easily available, unusually bizarre content.]

Word Association Test

(Chuck always gives a coarse equivalent for words which concern some aspect of sexuality or of bodily function. Thus, he associates as follows: *breast*—"tit," *bowel movement*—"shit," *penis*—"dick," *vagina*—"pussy," *nipple*—"tit" and *intercourse*—"fuck."

(He shows several long delays—some as long as 15, 16 and 17″—both after "conflictual" words and in places where the pauses are not immediately comprehensible.

(By and large, his reaction times are 1″ to 4″. His recall is excellent, and he fails to remember only four of his fifty initial associations.)

[This test reflects the varied facets of Chuck's inconsistently organized and disorganized behavior. While his recall is excellent, suggesting an efficient cognitive organization, and while his initial reaction times are mostly short, they are also often long, sometimes for no apparent reason. While he reacts apparently blandly with coarse synonyms to sexual words, one infers considerable underlying disturbance when his reaction times after these sexual words are very long. One gradually suspects that Chuck tries hard to maintain the appearance of being casual and reacting off the cuff, but that he undergoes considerable turmoil as he tries to maintain this appearance.]

Sentence Completion Test II

He hoped that when he grew up that . . uh . . he would be a successful businessman.

His parents were successful people. [Success is important, even though he seems convinced that he will be a bum.]

When he saw what the other kids were doing he laughed. ("Why did he laugh?") Cause they were doing something funny. ("Did they mean it to be funny?") Something that just struck him funny. [This completion demonstrates the distance that Chuck feels exists between himself and his peers. A number of other completions show how little he considers himself to be part of his age group.]

When he compared himself to his friends he was better.

He was sad whenever he thought of his dead mother. [The "mother" prior to his sister's adoption?]

When he was asked about his aches and pains he said, "I don't have any." [Anything else would not be "cool."]

The person he admired most was Superman. [Although Chuck tries to treat this test as a lark, it is nevertheless interesting to see what shape his legpulling assumes. Throughout this test, in one way or another, he tries to demonstrate how superior he is to others.]

His brother was eighteen.

When the girl kissed him he fainted.

When his father came into the room he ran away. [Again one can see how little contact Chuck permits himself with persons who should be important to him.]

When he was with his sister . . . . . they went places.

At school . . at school! . . uh . . he worked.

When he looked at the work the other students were doing he laughed. ("Why was that?") Cause . . uh . . he had already finished. [One wonders to what extent Chuck's "gruesome" stories represent his way of laughing at people who, he may feel, take life too seriously.]

He was very happy when he got a motorcycle. [Cars and motorcycles, of course, are the trademark of the action-oriented adolescent.]

The thing he found hardest to do was take apart the shocks.

Whenever certain things really bothered him he didn't think about them. [And yet, he is more thoughtful than is consistent with the impression he tries to create.]

His dreams were almost real.

When he saw that the man had left the money behind he took it. [Although taking the money might not happen in just this way, it nevertheless has considerable shock value for him to say so.]

He thought that his mother was pregnant. [And then she would not have adopted Chuck's sister.]

Whenever he and his family disagreed . . . . he agreed with them.

When he was very little he was about five.

His best friend was gone. [Whatever the particulars of the situation, this type of completion reflects Chuck's feelings of isolation.]

He was unhappy with his father when he beat him up.

When his mother asked about his girl friend he said, "I haven't got one."

He never thought he would be able to walk again. ("Why was that?") He was crippled. He had polio. [Again, when one does not take this completion too literally, it is reminiscent of the boy who, because of his strength and clumsiness, breaks the fragile violin.]

He always hoped that he could walk again. [His clumsiness is the result of illness.]

What he liked best about himself . . uh . . was . . that he was smart. [By "smart" Chuck probably does not mean the kind of intelligence usually measured by "intelligence" tests. More likely, he means that he is "wise to the ways of the world," that he "knows what's cooking," that he is "hip." Even here, one wonders how convinced Chuck truly is of his "smartness."]

His mother was more likely than his father to be pregnant (he smiles). [Chuck is apparently demonstrating, in part, that he is not about to let himself be tricked into any self-revelation.]

His sister was more likely than his father to have a baby, too. [Again.]

When he had nothing else to do he worked on his motorcycle.

He thought that his intelligence was good.

What he liked best about school . . . . . . was Industrial Arts.

When he couldn't see a way out of his problem . . uh . . he read books.

He saw the cockroach on the wall and put it out . . side.

His teacher was Miss Brown. Can I sit over here (in the easy chair, at the other side of the room)? [Tension is rising again.]

Whenever he got angry he went to his room.

He remembered that when he was little . . (he sighs) . . that he played cowboys.

When the kids invited him to go with them to the hiding place, he thought (he laughs) . . . . he thought they had some girls there.

After school he usually . . rode around . . went over to girls' houses.

He admired his father when he . . (he sighs) . . (he yawns) leaves him alone. [The degree to which the thought of his father has an unsettling effect on Chuck is becoming increasingly evident.]

When the girl invited him to her party he went.

When he and his brother were together they played.

He thought that his body . . had syphilis. [Although this ending is intended as a real shocker, and probably a "joke," Chuck's deep concerns about his bodily and psychological integrity are most probably involved in it.]

When he had a lot of homework to do he threw it away.

What he disliked about school was the work.

Whenever he spoke about his problems to someone . . . . they listened. [Does this ending mean that Chuck has not given up at least some efforts to make contact with others? But does it also mean that he considers "listening" not to be enough to help?]

When he entered the haunted house he looked around.

When the other fellow offered him a cigarette he took it.

He didn't like his mother to . . . . . (he yawns) . . . . go out with other men. [Is a serious message concealed in this "whimsical" ending (i.e., that Chuck is jealous of his mother's attention to his father and siblings)?]

When the baby arrived he said to his daddy . . told him that his mother was more likely to have a baby than he was. [This stem appears to be disturbing and results in the resurrection of a previously offered, rather eccentric, response.]

When the fellows asked him to join them in a rough game he said "Okay."

Whenever he didn't do what he was told . . . . . he got beat up.

What would make him angriest . . . . . . for his motorcycle not to start, after he pushed it about a mile. [That ending Sentence Completion stems with psychological trivia is not always easy for Chuck is suggested by his occasionally rather lengthy reaction times. Although he would probably have denied such a possibility, the examiner might have asked Chuck if other endings had occurred to him previously.]

In his spare time he read . . hot-rod and motorcycle books.

What troubled him most was that he didn't have a motorcycle.

When he was alone in his room at night . . . . he listened to the radio.

What scared him most . . . . . the police.

He struck the match and lit his cigarette.

He disliked his father when he griped at him.

He thought that his looks he did what? (I repeat the stem.) Were real good.

The thing he could do best (he yawns) . . was work and ride a motorcycle and cars.

He had no respect at all for . . . . for punks. ("How do you mean?") Oh, that little . . you know the little guy that comes here and has short hair. ("And what about him?") I don't even know him (he smiles). He may be all right. But he seems like one . . the way he acts. ("How does he act?") Like a girl. [One can understand this rejection of feminine aspects as belonging to Chuck's (conscious or unconscious) quite possibly homosexual preoccupations.]

He always enjoyed . . . . uh . . looking at nekkid (*sic*) women. [In contrast to the "punks," Chuck shows how truly masculine he is.]

He had a very uncomfortable feeling when he did something wrong. [Here one again sees the other side of the devil-may-care portrait which Chuck tries to offer of himself.]

He found it easiest to talk to his mother. [Is his mother the only person toward whom Chuck does not feel great distance?]

THE PSYCHOLOGIST'S REPORT

Probably the most remarkable feature of Chuck's test performance is the unexpected emergence of grossly shocking material. For instance, after first saying that Card II of the Rorschach reminds him of nothing, he responds to the examiner's urging to "see something" by explaining that the blot is "something nasty." He continues, "I mean I could tell you, but . . . . . ('What do you see?') It's nasty though. ('Tell me as best you can.') It looks like a bloody butt hole or something, or a bloody cock, on top." Similarly, on Card VI, with less difficulty, he tells that it "looks like a butt, opened up, and these look like bowels." To Thematic Apperception Test Card 18, he tells the story of a person who glues a dead man's hands on his coat to be funny. The hero of the TAT story digs up a grave, peels the skin off the cadaver he finds there, then cuts off its arms and legs and chops off its head. "He'd cut away about half the skull and left the brain showing. He popped out one of the eyeballs, so it was hanging down." He tells a similar, but much longer, story to the blank card (Card 16). While these examples are the most striking, there are a number of other occasions when the listener tends to be shocked. Thus, Chuck tells of a woman who enjoys being raped, he gives the Anglo-Saxon equivalents to all sexual and sexually related words on the Word Association Test, and he completes a Sentence Completion stem: *He thought his body* . . "had syphilis."

With these and with somewhat less stark examples, it seems clear that part of Chuck's goal is to show up others and to tease them. Nevertheless, while many of these gross responses are presented apparently with tongue in cheek, it is of significance that Chuck has this content so easily available to him and that he can express it with such ease. Although Chuck himself would like to believe, and although he would like others to believe, that he has control over the availability and expression of this frequently grotesque material, it is sometimes apparent that he cannot help himself, that the material pours out whether he wills it or not.

In a number of other ways Chuck presents himself paradoxically. On the one hand, he seems eager to show himself as an uninvolved, devil-may-care person who views the world as an amused observer and who laughs at what others take seriously. On the other hand, however, he does seem to take certain things quite seriously. On occasion he tries hard and obviously wants to do well. Often he keeps trying to solve problems, even though he finds them difficult. In spite of his nonchalance, he is concerned and wishes to create a favorable impression.

Another apparent inconsistency involves the ebb and flow of the tightness of Chuck's thought organization. Sometimes his thinking runs smoothly, efficiently and without flaw. At other times, however, one comes up against sudden faults in the psychological terrain. Poorly integrated cognitive functioning is occasionally apparent on the Wechsler-Bellevue Test, where his weighted subtest scores range from 1 to 14. (He achieves a Total Intelligence Quotient of 97-101, a Verbal Quotient of 91-95, and a Performance Quotient of 104-107.) The following are some of the peculiarities which emerge even on well-structured intelligence items: he estimates the population of the United States to be 10,000; when he is asked the population of Kansas City, his birthplace, he guesses it to be 1,000. (At the same time, he knows that *Hamlet* was written by Shakespeare and *Huckleberry Finn* by Mark Twain.) Chuck's confusion is particularly evident on the Arithmetic subtest, where his answers, which he attempts to justify on the basis of some type of arithmetical logic, are often nonsensical. Even on performance tasks, where he feels much more at home, there are times when reality testing suddenly becomes highly inefficient. For example, when he is presented with the simple *Manikin* figure on Object Assembly, he fits the leg pieces into the arm sockets, saying, "You mean, put it together, just so it fits, like this?" Again it must be stressed, however, that usually Chuck is capable of functioning fairly efficiently. It seems as if occasional, rather than constant, ruptures in reality testing take place. For example, while on the Word Association Test he sometimes blocks on a word for as long as 15 to 17″, he is able to recall all but four of the words with which he initially responded.

On such tests as Thematic Apperception and Sentence Completion, Chuck manifests a pervasive underlying feeling of isolation, pointlessness and hopelessness. His preoccupation with death and decay, evident on these tests, finds its way even into more structured areas. For example, asked how a fly and tree are alike, he explains that "both die." His TAT stories are filled with themes of impotence and with themes involving giving up—trying can have no satisfactory results. His first TAT story deals with a boy who wishes to play the violin, but he is so strong (and apparently so clumsy) that he breaks the instrument. The boy feels that, if the violin is as fragile as all that, he will never want to play it again. Chuck's feeling regarding the uselessness of trying is further reflected in his story of a boy who is sent to prison, even though he tells his father he is not guilty. The boy's lawyer also cannot help. Underneath it all, Chuck confides, the boy really is guilty. His brother eventually also gets in trouble with the law. Under the superficial guise of superiority to others is Chuck's conviction of essential hopelessness about himself. Thus, he tells the TAT story of a man who rises from his grave in order to find out what people said about him on his tombstone. He discovers that he is described as a bum. On the Sentence Completion Test, he says, *He never thought he would be able to* "walk again . . . . he was crippled. He had polio." Reference to his "syphilitic" body has already been made. His reactive need to overcome his intensely low self-esteem, to be better than others, to be a kind of hero and to get attention from others, is an ever-recurring theme.

The feelings of emptiness which Chuck's stories contain are particularly marked in the sphere of personal contacts. Just as he occasionally removes himself physically from the examiner's desk (in order to sit in a softer chair at the other end of the room, ostensibly to be more "comfortable") so, too, the people he tells about on the

TAT seem to have almost no significant relationships to one another. Parents may be upset about sad events that happen to their children, but they are impotent, helpless, static people, who can do nothing to change their child's unfortunate situations. Sexual relationships involve no feelings of tenderness, but are carried out on a cash basis, an arrangement with which the persons involved seem satisfied. Chuck's relationships with his peers are distant and characterized by his contempt for them. He does not allow himself to be closely involved in their activities and reacts to comparisons with them by announcing his superiority.

Chuck tells little about his parents, either directly or indirectly. When his father appears in the tests, he does so as a carping, punitive person whom Chuck wishes to avoid. Although Chuck considers his mother to be psychologically much closer than his father, she emerges as a rather helpless and passive person. On the Sentence Completion Test, Chuck says, *He didn't like his mother to . .* "go out with other men." And, *His mother was more likely than his father to* "become pregnant." While these responses are intended, in part at least, as "jokes," it is significant that the jokes take this particular form. One wonders, for example, how much of a grudge Chuck bears his parents, particularly his mother, for not having been satisfied to keep him as their *only* child.

He makes strong efforts to assert his masculinity and to deny all suggestion of any "feminine" interest. He tells how much he dislikes "punks" (effeminate boys and men) and soon afterwards says that he likes "nekkid" girls, but it seems clear that he is fighting a chronic battle against his own feminine wishes. The extent of his masculine-feminine conflict is suggested by the almost purposeful confusion which is evident in his story to TAT Card 3 BM.

> Is that a girl? (!) Is that a gun? (!) Is it supposed to be? If it's not a gun, she's crying . . or he's crying. Since that isn't a gun, it's a soldering gun so he or she burned he or she self. And he or she cried.

This masculine-feminine self-questioning is part of a much more inclusive identity confusion. Chuck seems almost literally unsure whether outer and inner things are right side up, upside down, backside or frontside. Rather than having *no* self-qualities of any sort of which he can be certain, he assumes *negative* ones, i.e., he assumes a "negative identity."

In summary, Chuck functions grossly at an average intellectual level at this time. Although he tries to embed his "grotesqueries" in a context of teasing, the quality of his morbid, grossly sexual content, the rather frequent breakthrough of vagueness, confusion, arbitrariness, illogicality, fluidity and peculiar thinking, suggest a diagnosis which involves severe disorganization. The relative lack of disruptive, acute anxiety suggests the condition's chronic quality. Of significance is Chuck's feeling of hopelessness, as well as the hollowness and distance of his relationships with others. A significant conflict with regard to identity, and particularly masculinity, is apparent.

DISCUSSION

Superficially, Chuck seems to fit the stereotype of the antisocial, "delinquent" adolescent. He gets into trouble with the law, does poor work in school, spends much of his time zooming around on a motorcycle or in a car, talks obscenely, and is generally alloplastic. But it is apparent that the antisocial behavior is only phenotypical and that Chuck's personality organization is a much more complex, stratified structure. Although his behavior may be "bad," the reasons for the "badness" are complex. At superficial glance, Chuck looks so well integrated that one would not suspect such a degree of underlying disorganization. In his everyday dealings, he puts his worst foot forward to gather attention, to be admired and recognized, but, and apparently primarily, because he lacks sufficient organization to do anything else.

Of the three adolescents discussed in this chapter, Jack seems most nearly to fit the stereotype of what people have in mind when they think of a "delinquent": action oriented, nonreflective, too polite to adults, with a history of antisocial activities. Yet, as one studies Jack's test protocol, one again finds how complex this "delinquency" is. Even a cursory reading of his history makes one wonder about certain factors, e.g., the history of his jealousy and aggressiveness since the age of five, the resentment of his sister and, possibly, of his and her adoption. One wonders what literally destructive experiences he might have suffered during the first thirteen months of life, e.g., why he was "close to rickets" when he was first adopted. These are some factors which may have played a role in Jack's developing in the way he did, and they once again emphasize that "delinquency" is neither a simple nor a unitary phenomenon.

CLINICAL SUMMARY: Jack

Jack is fourteen years old, the oldest of three adopted children. He is at present under the jurisdiction of the juvenile court for stealing five cars and $1,000.

Jack's current legal difficulties began when he and a friend took the family's new car, without permission, and wrecked it. Neither Jack nor his friend suffered personal injuries, but the accident caused $1,900 worth of damage to the car. Two days later, following an argument with his mother, Jack, with a different friend, stole another car and drove it until it ran out of gas. Subsequently, Jack and his friend took four other cars. They were apprehended the following day for "snooping around" parked automobiles. A while later, Jack was enrolled in a military school, stayed there about three weeks, again stole a car, but was easily apprehended. Within the following week, he was enrolled in, and suspended for truancy from, two other junior high schools. A month later, he again ran away from home, taking nearly $1,000 of his parents' money. At that time, he was apprehended on a bus about fifty miles from home.

Because the mother was unable to have a child, the parents, through a nonagency source, obtained Jack when he was thirteen months old. He had been living with his biological mother, but she no longer wanted him. He "was close to rickets" when he was adopted, but he was walking and saying a few words. Jack's adoptive father feared to touch him because he did not want to drop or hurt him, and he did nothing to help with Jack's care. The adoptive mother indulged and infantilized Jack. The paternal grandmother, who lived with the family, strongly protested any correction or discipline of the boy. Jack's tantrums started early. He was an active, restless and nervous child, demanding much and seldom showing or seeking love or affection from his parents. Toilet training was difficult; bowel control was not established until Jack was six years old, and he had occasional relapses even after that. Night wetting was not controlled until he was twelve years old.

Jealousy and aggressiveness have marked Jack's relationship to his sister, who was also adopted, when Jack was five. The parents are afraid to leave the two children alone because of what they think Jack might do to his sister if he were to become angry.

At the age of eight, Jack had to be returned from camp, after he had been there two weeks against his wishes. The mother had earlier been hospitalized on at least four occasions. Each time she departed, Jack needed continual reassurance that she would return home. During his mother's absences, Jack was very difficult to manage. For example, he told his father that he hated him and that he was not his real father anyway. He never asked about his natural parents, however.

At the age of twelve, Jack was hospitalized with rheumatic fever. There were no sequelae to this illness, and he is now on no specific treatment, although he is not to indulge in vigorous exercise. At the ages of seven and eight, he had two episodes of concussion from falling off bicycles. He was unconscious about one hour each time, hospitalized overnight, but he recovered, again without sequelae.

From a very early age, Jack frequently stole money from his parents, usually to purchase treats or entertainment for himself and his friends. When he was seven years old, he began treatment with a psychiatrist because of his hatred for his sister, but when the family left the state (when Jack was ten), they did not seek further help for him.

Jack's interest in school has steadily decreased in the past year and a half, and he has failed all his subjects within the past six months. His school behavior has also been considerably more disturbed during the past six months, and he has been absent from school a great deal. During the past year and a half, he has begun to associate "with the wrong kind of boys," and he has insisted on a "duck-tail" hairdo, a motorcycle jacket and black boots.

Physical and Laboratory Findings: The physical, neurological and laboratory examinations were all within normal limits.

THE PSYCHOLOGIST'S DESCRIPTION

Jack presented himself as an extremely polite, accommodating young man who seemed always to be trying his best to comply with the test requirements. He frequently addressed me as "sir" and seemed to go out of his way to express disapproval of "delinquent" behavior. In a discussion of the TV program, "The $64,000 Question," for example, he gratuitously suggested that he would not want to have so much money, since that much could only lead to trouble. He worked hard to make an impression of propriety and occasionally corrected one of his responses when he felt I might not consider it "good."

He was particularly tense during the first several sessions—pale, restless, and breathing shallowly. He cracked his knuckles nervously, grimaced as he found questions more difficult, and asked each day whether there were any more tests. He was obviously relieved once he completed all the testing.

(The year of testing was 1956, but when I asked Jack for his birth date he said, "April 22, 1952." He spontaneously made an abortive effort to correct his error, saying that 1952 would make him only six [sic] years old.) [One cannot know yet whether Jack's temporary confusion about his birth date is referable to a high degree of tension or to the carelessness about time which one so frequently finds in persons who take a cavalier attitude toward precision of all kinds. Actually, of course, 1952 would make Jack only *four*, not *six* years old.]

THE WECHSLER-BELLEVUE SCALE (Partially Reproduced)

Name: Jack   Age: 13-11

	RS	WTS	0 1 2 3 4 5 6 7 8 9 10 11 12 13 14 15 16 17 18 19 20
COMPR.	12-13	11	
INFOR.	12	9	
DIG.	9-10	6-7	
ARITH.	7-8	9-10	
SIMIL.	12	10	
VOCAB.	17½	8	
P. A.	13	11	
P. C.	12	12	
B. D.	22-28	10-13	
O. A.	23	14	
D. S.	36	8	

TOT. VERB.	47-48
TOT. PERF.	55-58
TOT. SCALE	102-106

VERBAL I.Q.: 104-105   LEVEL: Average

PERFORMANCE I.Q.: 112-117   LEVEL: Bright Normal

TOTAL I.Q.: 109-112   Level: Average→Bright Normal

[One sees here the Verbal-Performance relationship of the action-oriented person, with the Performance quotient higher than the Verbal. Although most of Jack's Verbal subtests tend to cluster rather closely, the range of all subtests involves a considerable distance—eight scale points. The lowered Digit Span score probably reflects the higher degree of Jack's tension, which interferes with his attention. The Comprehension-Information relationship suggests Jack's tendency verbally to emphasize what is "proper" and conventional, even though he may not act accordingly. It is difficult to know what to make of the relatively high, isolated Object Assembly score, although the alternate Block Design score is only one point lower. It may well be that tension impairs Block Design somewhat; perhaps if Jack were less tense, both Block Design and Object Assembly would be equally high and so be in part another reflection of his action orientation. The low Digit Symbol score is complexly determined. The items are well drawn, although Jack pauses rather frequently to erase errors (even though he has been told not to waste his time this way). One also wonders again about the effect of tension on this performance, and one wonders, too, to what extent Jack's impulsivity (which he later tries to inhibit) penalizes his performance.]

INFORMATION

No.	Question	Response and Comments	Score
1.	Who is the President of the United States?	President Eisenhower. ("And who was president before that?") Truman. ("And before that?") Roosevelt.	+
2.	What is a thermometer?	Something to measure heat or coldness.	+
3.	What does rubber come from?	Tree.	+
4.	Where is London?	England.	+
5.	How many pints make a quart?	Oh .. uh .. four, I think ... I don't think that's right. ("What would be the other possibility?") Two? Two, I guess. ("Which answer would you choose?") Four. [Answers which require the stating of a specific number are often the first to suffer in an imprecise person who does not value exactness for its own sake.]	—

No.	Question	Response and Comments	Score
6.	*How many weeks are there in a year?*	Uh (he smiles) uh . . I can't divide here . . Can I divide if I want to? ("Sure, if you want to.") About forty-five. ("How did you get that?") Seven into 336 . . into 360. [Information which should be instantly available to Jack is obtained (incorrectly) in a roundabout fashion. The number of weeks in a year constitutes the kind of everyday knowledge which most children grow up with. Although Jack is very proper and very polite, e.g., asking if he might divide, he not only divides incorrectly but apparently does not know the correct number of days in a year. Jack seems to be trying to impress the examiner with the amount of effort he puts forth, but the effort seems to consist primarily of window dressing.]	—
7.	*What is the capital of Italy?*	Rome.	+
8.	*What is the capital of Japan?*	Tokyo.	+
9.	*How tall is the average American woman?*	About five feet six inches.	+
10.	*Who invented the airplane?*	Wright brothers.	+
11.	*Where is Brazil?*	South America.	+
12.	*How far is it from Paris to New York?*	About 3,000 miles.	+
13.	*What does the heart do?*	It . . it pumps in blood and pumps it out . . just keeps it circulating. [Jack has given the last seven answers (even the two that involve numbers) quickly and accurately, with no hesitations or unnecessary embellishments. So long as the information required is not too unusual and is therefore easily available to him, Jack is intellectually efficient and organized.]	+
14.	*Who wrote Hamlet?*	(He smiles.) I don't have no idea. ("Have you heard of it?") *Julius Caesar?* No. ("The same man wrote a play about him, too. Any idea who it might have been?") No. I don't know. [When questions no longer deal with Jack's immediate concerns, his answers become less available.]	—

No.	Question	Response and Comments	Score
15.	*What is the population of the United States?*	Fifty-five million. [Another "numbers" question.]	—
16.	*When is Washington's birthday?*	(He smiles.) .. Uh .. I don't know. ("Do you have an idea about what time of the year it is?") About a month or so after Christmas. [Another "numbers" question.]	—
17.	*Who discovered the North Pole?*	Byrd .. or what's his name? He died last night. Do you watch "The $64,000 Question"? That boy won. (He continues to tell me about the program.) That's too much money. I wouldn't know what to do with it. Money only gets you in trouble. I found that out. [It may be that Jack sincerely feels what he says at this moment. A characteristic of Jack's type of personality structure is that feelings change rapidly, although the feelings of any particular moment may be truly felt. Because such adolescents (and older persons of similar character structure) may do something which is opposite from what they just previously said, it is often (but erroneously) thought that the intentions, attitudes, or values which they present at any particular moment are insincere.]	—
18.	*Where is Egypt?*	Egypt is in .. uh .. Europe. Where all that trouble is. ["All that trouble" covers a great range of possibilities and, for Jack, constitutes a typical vagueness.]	—
19.	*Who wrote Huckleberry Finn?*	I've read that so many times. I don't pay too much attention to authors, though, Mark Twain. He wrote *Tom Sawyer*, too, didn't he? [The phrase, "I've read that so many times," may represent another way of saying, "I'm not sure about that." Although it is somewhat surprising to find Jack knowing the author of a literary work, particularly after he has failed the five preceding questions, it may be that Jack finds *Huckleberry Finn*, who in some ways is so similar to himself, an appealing figure.]	+
20.	*What is the Vatican?*	(He scratches his head.) You left me (he smiles).	—
21.	*What is the Koran?*	(He shrugs.)	—
22.	*Who wrote Faust?*	What's that?	—

No.	Question	Response and Comments	Score
23.	What is an Habeas Corpus?	A dead person, I think. A murdered person, or something like that.	—

(The last two items were not administered.)

RAW SCORE: 12

WEIGHTED SCORE: 9

COMPREHENSION

No.	Question	Response and Comments	Score
1.	What is the thing to do if you find an envelope in the street, that is sealed, and addressed and has a new stamp?	I'm sure not going to open it. That's a federal offense. I'd put it in the mailbox or give it to the police. ("Which would you give as your answer?") Mail it, probably. That's what it's for . . Wait a minute. It would depend on whether the address . . No, it wouldn't. [This response reflects Jack's sensitivity to the "legality" of his activities. The legality of acts probably often intrudes into his conception of them.]	2
2.	What should you do if while sitting in the movies you were the first person to discover a fire (or see smoke and fire)?	I'd go tell the manager. [Clear and to the point.]	2
3.	Why should we keep away from bad company?	They get you in trouble. ("How do you mean?") When you're with them . . Boys, you know boys— they just have a tendency to get in trouble. [It is not clear whether Jack identifies himself with the boys who get in trouble, with the adults who sit in judgment of them, or with both.]	1
4.	Why should people pay taxes?	Keep the government up. Without taxes, the government wouldn't be any place. They wouldn't have the federal buildings they need to stay in. [Jack exaggerates to make his point. His use of hyperbole helps further to make his answers vague and imprecise, however. Although he is able to think abstractly, he has a tendency to become involved in concrete details that may not be particularly relevant.]	2
5.	Why are shoes made of leather?	They hold up better.	1
6.	Why does land in the city cost more than land in the country?	Well, in the country . . In the city, it's harder to get, and in the country it's not. But in the city you wouldn't buy it to build a house, unless it's in the outskirts. ("Why is it harder in the city?") There's not much more of it left. ("How would you sum it all up?") It's scarcer in the city.	1

No.	Question	Response and Comments	Score

7. *If you were lost in a forest (woods) in the daytime, how would you go about finding your way out?*

If you had a compass? ("No compass.") You'd get in one place and get up in a tree and look around .. and get in a place and make something you can recognize easily and then start out in one direction, and if you didn't find anything, you'd go back to that place and start off in another direction. ("Why would you get up in a tree?") You'd look out and maybe see the edge of the forest. [This response could perhaps earn a score of 2 were it more precisely stated. Jack obviously has the scorable idea of using natural phenomena of some sort, but he gets lost in detail, and his vagueness of thinking prevents him from achieving a concise solution.]

Score: 1

8. *Why are laws necessary?*

So people won't do wrong. If they don't have laws .. people would just be shooting and killing people. There wouldn't be order. There wouldn't be a democracy. ("How do you mean?") There wouldn't be any country. It wouldn't be organized if they just had people do what they want. They'd just do what they want, and they wouldn't have to do anything anybody else wants. [The comment about "democracy" is a typical, nonthought-through reliance on cliché.]

Score: 0-1

9. *Why does the state require people to get a license in order to be married?*

Well, so they know they're married. So they have a record. Just like, if two people meet and decide to get married, and that's it. You wouldn't have to let anybody know. [Jack's first vague "they" seems to have some sort of governmental, societal referent.]

Score: 2

10. *Why are people who are born deaf usually unable to talk?*

Something's wrong with them .. with their body. ("How do you mean?") They have things .. vibrations in the throat, and they learn to read lips and all that. [Jack is bluffing. He finds it extremely difficult to say he does not know an answer; instead, he straight-facedly offers some sort of "explanation," which sometimes turns out to be no explanation at all.]

Score: 0

RAW SCORE: 12-13

WEIGHTED SCORE: 11

DIGIT SPAN

(Although Jack does poorly on this test, his performance is remarkable only in his inability to remember the age-appropriate number of digits. He remembers five to six Digits Forward and four Backward.) [Jack's poor achievement here suggests the degree to which his attention is interfered with, quite possibly by tension.]

RAW SCORE: 9-10

WEIGHTED SCORE: 6-7

ARITHMETIC

(Although Jack obtains an Arithmetic score almost appropriate for his age, the following items suggest the types of qualitative maneuvers he typically displays when items offer even mild difficulty.)

No.	Problem	Time	Response and Comments	Score
3.	If a man buys eight cents worth of stamps and gives the clerk twenty-five cents, how much change should he get back?	3″	Sixteen .. uh .. seventeen. [This is an example of Jack's quickly corrected impulsivity.]	1
4.	How many oranges can you buy for thirty-six cents if one orange costs four cents?	10″	(He asks me to repeat the problem.) You can't buy a whole orange. (It turns out he misunderstood me to say that one orange cost forty cents. I correct his misunderstanding.) Nine? [Again Jack is able to recover, but his mishearing suggests a disruption of alertness which may at times result in rather severe and nonsensical distortions of judgment.]	1
6.	If a man buys seven two cent stamps and gives the clerk a half dollar, how much change should he get back?	68″	Oh, that's a hard one. You give the clerk fifty cents? And you want fourteen .. uh .. forty-six cents. (36″) That don't seem right. ("Do you want to change your answer?") It would be .. thirty .. three .. (he counts on his fingers). It would be thirty-six cents (68″). [Apparent is not only the impulsive error, but also Jack's tendency to keep trying until a correct solution is reached.]	0-1
9.	If a train goes 150 yards in ten seconds, how many feet can it go in one fifth of a second?		Oh, that's hard .. (he whispers to himself as he does the problem mentally.) .. three times 150 .. 400 yards .. one-fifth second .. oh murder .. 400 feet in 150 yards .. (Then in his normal voice:) You got me. (He continues trying, however. He writes portions of the example in the air. Finally, after much overtime, he obtains the correct nine feet.) [Once again we see that Jack first becomes mildly disorganized but still keeps trying until he is able to achieve the correct solution.]	0
10.	Eight men can finish a job in six days. How many		Twelve .. oh .. sixteen .. oh .. a half day .. six times eight .. six days. How would you work that? Twelve times eight .. six-	0

No.	Problem	Time	Response and Comments	Score

men will be needed to finish it in a half day? — teen (35" have gone by) ninety-eight men. Is that right? (I say nothing, and he continues to work on the problem.) Twelve times eight *is* ninety-eight. ("Tell me your answer.") Ninety-eight. You kind of fooled me. [It is apparent that Jack's difficulty here involves the arithmetical mechanics of the solution, rather than the logic. The computation falls easy prey to Jack's impulsivity.]

RAW SCORE: <u>7-8</u>

WEIGHTED SCORE: <u>9-10</u>

SIMILARITIES

No.	Item	Response and Comments	Score

[Jack's performance on this subtest reflects the subtle shift from his performing adequately when the items do not require a great deal of intellectual exertion, to his giving more and more impulsive-determined responses, increasingly marked by action concepts and by impoverishment of abstract conceptualizations, as the required intellectual effort mounts.]

1. *Orange-banana* — Fruit.   2

2. *Coat-dress* — Clothing.   2

3. *Dog-lion* — Animal.   2

4. *Wagon-bicycle* — Carry somebody. [A reliance on the more "functional" action orientation begins at this point.]   1

5. *Daily paper-radio* — Give .. both give news.   1

6. *Air-water* — Both .. we need 'em both to live. [Although this answer receives a full score, the way Jack presents it reflects his functional action preference.]   2

7. *Wood-alcohol* — Don't you get some kind of alcohol off a tree? ("Can you tell me a way they're alike?") We use 'em both .. for our needs. You use wood to build houses, and alcohol .. (he gives himself an imaginary injection) to put on the cotton when you got sore muscles or joints. [Jack is preoccupied with himself here. He resorts to action (giving himself the imaginary shot in the arm) when words do not offer a sufficient avenue of expression.]   0

8. *Eye-ear* — Two senses. [A reversal of the trend—a good conceptualization.]   2

No.	Item	Response and Comments	Score
9.	Egg-seed	Egg is . . uh . . egg and seed. They're alike in one way? ("Yes, they are.") Well, an egg we eat, and a seed'll grow something we eat.	0
10.	Poem-statue	Poems about statues. ("How are they alike?") Memories or . . Quite a few poems about the Washington monument. [Jack "conceptualizes" individually.]	0
11.	Praise-punishment	Let's see. One, it gives you . . . . they're thanking you, and the other . . They're two different kinds of ways of telling you what you did . . or whether you've been good or bad.	0
12.	Fly-tree	I don't know. ("Try to think of some way.") A fly eats some of the stuff off a tree.	0

RAW SCORE: 12

WEIGHTED SCORE: 10

[As Jack begins work on the Performance subtests, one can see how much more important it is to him that he do well and that he not miss items than it was on the Verbal section. He feels obvious pride when he does well and obvious disappointment when he does not. He is more alert to what goes on. On Picture Arrangement, for example, he notes that the backs of the cards have letters which indicate the correct placement order and says, "I'm not supposed to look at the back, am I?" On the Block Design and Object Assembly subtests, he achieves weighted scores of 13 (alternate) and 14, respectively. He works effectively on both tests, and one has the strong impression that he is most efficient when he can actively manipulate inanimate objects. Although this type of work requires thinking, of course, the thinking is neither verbal nor personal. He is interested enough to want to know answers from the examiner when he cannot derive them alone. "Doing" things is obviously of a different and greater order of importance than reflecting about them.

[If Jack is truly more comfortable and more efficient with inanimate "things," one would expect that he would also do better on the Digit Symbol subtest. His low weighted score of 8 here is the combined result of (a) slow performance, (b) uncertainty about the right substitutions (at the beginning, he requires the use of his finger to help him find the correct symbol) and (c) several errors. At the end of this test, he says, "Do you ever get anybody who could finish them all? It tests your reflexes, I guess." Just what interferes here is difficult to know, but his relatively poor performance on this subtest which relies so heavily on smoothly functioning activity is inconsistent with what one has come to expect.

[On the Vocabulary subtest, Jack obtains a weighted score of 8, a below-average score by which one is not surprised. As he becomes less sure of the meaning of words, he resorts to guessing. He is not critical of himself as he casts about impetuously, trying to attribute meaning to a word by way of a clang or another illogical association. On the word *ballast,* for example, he says the following: "It's not like a ballad . . it could be a . . that's ballerina." He explains *belfry* as, "Your head. ('How do you mean?') A head." On *amanuensis,* he says: "I know that one . . analysis?"]

STORY RECALL

IMMEDIATE RECALL

$$-1 \qquad\qquad +1 \qquad -1 \qquad\qquad +1$$
Whew! March 6 / uh . . . . . There was a flood. / ninety miles / out of Albany. /
$$\qquad\qquad 0 \qquad\qquad\qquad\qquad +1$$
And . . uh . . water was coming up . . and flooded the streets / and it was running
$$+1 \qquad\quad +1 \qquad\quad -1 \qquad\qquad +1 \quad +1$$
into the houses. / A man / cut his head / trying to save / a little boy / who was
$$+1 \qquad\quad +1 \qquad\qquad 0 \qquad\qquad\qquad -1$$
caught / under a bridge. / Lots of people were cold and / six persons / died . .
$$0$$
were killed. How do you remember it?

SCORE: $9+4-4 = 9$

[Jack's memory organization is inexact. He considers that vague, imprecise approximations do as well as accurate repetitions.]

DELAYED RECALL

$$-1 \qquad\qquad +1 \qquad\qquad\qquad +1 \qquad\qquad +1$$
March 6 / there's a flood / ten side . . ten miles outside / of Albany. / And . .
$$+1$$
uh . . the water was running over . . over the streets, / covering the streets, and
$$-1 \qquad\qquad\qquad +1 \qquad\quad 0 \qquad\quad +1 \quad +1$$
. . see . . houses / . . and it was fourteen persons / killed / and 600 / caught cold /
$$0 \qquad\qquad\qquad +1 \qquad\quad -1 \qquad\qquad +1 \quad +1$$
from . . the thing / . . and . . uh . . a man / split his head open / saving / a little boy.

SCORE: $10-3 = 7$

[Not only does the repetition of the passage not help Jack achieve a better score; his score is lower than the first time. Although he is able to correct some of his first errors, he maintains others and exaggerates one—from "a man cut his head" to "a man split his head open." This test demonstrates how memorial accuracy is not one of Jack's major concerns when the thing to be remembered is not of concrete relevance to him.]

THE BRL SORTING TEST

(With the exception of a few functional sortings, some occasional loosening and split-narrowing, Jack's sortings are good, i.e., conceptually, ordered and economically organized.) [One would expect Jack to offer many more Concrete or, at least Functional, sortings and definitions. The fact that his definitions are primarily conceptual once more demonstrates how most behavior is unexpectedly multifaceted. It appears that conceptual thinking is not as unavailable to Jack as it first seemed. Not only can Jack think conceptually when the situation forces such an approach; he occasionally does so even when he has a choice, so that a conceptual attitude represents one of several possibilities.]

RORSCHACH TEST

RORSCHACH SCORING SHEET

Number of Responses: 20

Manner of Approach (Location)		*Groups of Contents*	
W	5	A	14
DW	1	Ad	4
D	12	H	1
Dd	0	Hd	1
Dr	2	Total	20
Total	20		

Location Percentages

Determinant and Content Percentages

W%	30	F%	75/100	Obj.%	0
D%	60	F+%	67/70	At%	0
DR%	10	A%	90	P%	30
		H%	10		

Form, Movement, Color and Shading Determinants

Qualitative Material

F+	9	Failure	IX
F−	3	Popular	I II III V VIII
F±	1	Combination	IV VI VIII
F∓	2	Fabulation	5
M+	1	Fabulized Combination	1
FC+	2	Peculiar	1
F(C)∓	1 F(C)±	1	Masturbation	1
		Castration	1
Total	20	Aggression	2

EXPERIENCE BALANCE: 1/1

[Jack's manner of approach to the Rorschach is consistent with what one expects by now. He focuses primarily on W and D areas, with only a few that have a Dr quality. He fails one card altogether and has a high percent of Popular (easy) responses. In a similarly "easy" way, his animals and animal details represent 90 percent of all content. His relatively void Experience Balance reflects his constriction, both ideational and emotional. Two exceptions to one's expectations are (a) that his Color responses are well modulated and (b) that he gives two (C) responses, both tendencies suggesting better control over impulse and greater sensitivity to the environment than one would have thought from studying Jack's test protocol up to this point. Jack's Form Level is fairly adequate, or at least on the safe side of borderline, and suggests that he interprets his environment fairly realistically and not particularly unusually. The relatively large number of Fabulized and Peculiar notations, however, takes away from the certainty one feels about this last statement (particularly when one also discovers a Fabulized Combination), but the meanings of these responses need to be further investigated as they occur. Knowing what one does about Jack, one would not be surprised to find the Fabulized and Peculiar responses to be primarily a reflection of a lack of precision and of a tendency impulsively to blurt out uncritically whatever comes to mind.]

(As I put out the cards, he says:) I've had this before.

RORSCHACH PROTOCOL

Card #	React. Time	Score	Protocol	Inquiry and Observations
I	13″	WF+AP	1. It looks like a . . a bat . . or a bird of some kind. That's all. ("Does it remind you of anything else?") It could be *hundreds* of things. You don't feel like writing them all. ("What else could it be?") Can I turn it? (He turns the card in various directions.) Do they make these things on purpose? . . . . (He sighs.) I still think a bird.	[One can see what happens when Jack's pronouncement of the many things he can offer is challenged. He promises much ("It could be *hundreds* of things"), but he offers nothing in addition. Similarly, Jack may often "promise" a good deal about himself, about what he can do or offer, but these promises are potentials only so long as they are not challenged.]

Card #	React. Time	Score	Protocol	Inquiry and Observations
II	5″	DF+AdP	1. Two dogs . . with their . . . . . . noses together on a little pointed object.	1. ("Would you tell me about the dogs?") I'm not too good on dogs. ("Describe them as best as you can remember them.") Let's see . . . . ("Tell me what you can remember about them.") Well, they . . look like dogs. Just . . dogs look like dogs, don't they? All I can figure out. (I show him the card.) It's half of a dog. [This response demonstrates the poverty of Jack's associative life. He can make almost nothing of the two dogs he sees. He can only say, "Dogs look like dogs, don't they?"]
		DFC+A Fab.	2. Two blu . . bu . . *butterflies.* That's it.	2. ("Would you tell me about the butterflies?") Hm . . like butterflies. They were *red.* They were over the dogs' heads. They were looking at each other, just like the dogs were. ("Does there seem to be a connection between the butterflies and dogs?") There was a real thin line coming from them down to the dogs' heads, but I didn't think it had any connection with the dogs. (He sees the butterflies in lateral view.) [Although Jack denies the connection of the butterflies to the dogs, one is nevertheless struck by the "concrete," position quality of the butterfly response. Jack seems occasionally trapped by such a "concrete" view of the world and lacks a flexibility which would free him to go beyond the boundaries of the immediately given.]

Card #	React. Time	Score	Protocol	Inquiry and Observations
III			Oh! (He turns it swiftly.)	
	11″	WM+HP Fab. mast. Pec. Comb.	1. Two men leaning over to pick up two jugs of water.	1. ("Would you tell me about the men?") Well, they . . . . . It was rough around the edges from . . . . from where the ink was . . oh . . . . And they were kind of faded. ("Faded how?") Smeared. That's about it. ("What kind of men were they?") Ink-smeared men. ("Why did they seem to be men?") Well . . just the way the body was shaped. [One constantly has the feeling that Jack's response promises greater richness than it eventually turns out to have. The expectation is that Jack is about to elaborate on the men's appearance, but the "rough around the edges," the "faded" and the "ink-smeared" coments turn out to relate only to the way the inkblot is made; they do not represent an imaginative elaboration of the "men."]
		DFC+AP	2. It looks like a butterfly in the middle. I couldn't tell you what those (upper side red D's) were . . just blobs of ink. > ∨ (He studies the card and lays it down.)	2. ("Would you tell me about the butterfly?") It was red. You could see both of the wings . . his head . . and . . that's about it.
IV	13″	WF(C)∓A	1. Say . . looking up at a cat . . . . Hm . . looking up at a *cat.*	1. ("Tell me about that.") You'd be laying on the floor and looking up, and the cat would be standing on its hind legs. ("Could you tell me about the cat?") It had a tail. The way the face was.

React.				
Card #	Time	Score	Protocol	Inquiry and Observations

| | | | | ("How was it?") The way it was shaped . . the way the mouth was shaped. ("Did it seem to be a particular kind of cat?") No, cats are cats. You can't tell on that picture, because there's no color. [This is Jack's first mildly peculiar response, but actually more unusual than peculiar. He sees the cat in a somewhat unorthodox fashion, but the unorthodoxy is not great enough to create uneasiness about the response. Jack's lack of imaginativeness is underscored again when, in lieu of elaborating his response, he can say only, "cats are cats."] |

V

			∨ ∧	
14″		WF+AP	1. Hm . . it looks like a bat.	
		DF+Ad	2. It looks like crocodile heads out there.	2. ("Would you tell me about the crocodile heads?") Hm . . oh . . well . . long . . long and thin. ("Anything else?") No [Jack elaborates only when he is pushed, and even then as little as possible.]

VI

			∨ ∧ I wonder how they make these things. (He laughs.) ∨ Is this the right way?	
42″		WF∓A Comb. Fab.	1. It looks like two birds standing on a little . . well, stick here. Here's the mouth, up here. Two legs are standing on this stick . . that's an arm on each side. This whole body.	1. ("Did you say there was an arm on each side?") Well, a wing. (He smiles.) ("Could you tell me about the bushes?") I don't know. It just looked that way. Just messed up, and the only thing I could think of to picture there. ("You said

	React.		
Card #	Time	Score	

Protocol

Inquiry and Observations

And these (side Dr extensions) could be bushes.

they were standing on a stick?") (He shrugs.) I don't know. [This response demonstrates again how unstable Jack's perception tends to be. Things have a way of appearing and disappearing, and Jack does not feel called upon either to justify his percepts or to defend them. He says aloud what appears to him at the moment, but he does not feel any requirement later on to make sense out of what he has said.]

VII

∨ . . . . ∧ I'll make it as good as I can out of it.

27″ DWF±A
Fab.
Cast. agg.

1. Two rabbits looking at each other. The middle's cut out of them or . . . . Here's the ear and mouth and eyes and head . . and paw . . some . . . . . . That's it.

1. ("The middle seemed to be cut out?") The stomach's cut out. ("Anything else about the rabbits?") They're looking back, over their shoulder. [Jack turns the card upside down automatically as soon as it is offered. While previously such activity seemed to reflect a kind of opposition to the examiner, Jack's turning the cards over may have much less of a resistant meaning here; instead, the immediate turning seems more to reflect Jack's imaginative impotence. He sees nothing when the card is first presented in the usual fashion, but he hopes that some percept may emerge when he turns the card. It seems doubtful, too, that the stomachs' being "cut out" of the rabbits represents the usual castration meanings. More likely, Jack is unable to overcome his

Card #	React. Time	Score	Protocol	Inquiry and Observations
				literalism—since a space is there, Jack thinks what was originally there must have been "cut out."]
VIII			Hm . . ∨ ∧ ∨ ∧	
	35″	DF+AP Comb.	1. Those look like wolves or dogs.	
		DrF(C)±Ad	2. Two of 'em look like two heads.	2. ("What kind of heads did they seem to be?") Oh . . turtle? (Upper part of bottom middle D.)
		DrF≠(Hd) Fab. Agg.	3. That looks like two things reaching out to grab the wolves. (He shrugs.)	3. ("What did those 'two things' look like?") I don't know . . but . . two arms . . something. (Side Dr extensions of top D.) [When Jack does finally elaborate, his elaboration is a rather disturbing, aggressively toned one. It is obvious, from a study of Jack's lengthy reaction times, that he must work hard before a percept crystallizes sufficiently in his awareness to be verbalized.]
IX	2′	Failure	∨ < ∧ M'm. (He shakes his head.) I can't see anything in this one (at 30″). (He looks at the card from an angle. He still gives no response, but only shrugs and grimaces. After 2′ I remove the card.)	
X			(He heaves a big sigh.) ∨	
	11″	DF−A Fab. Comb. Pec.	1. Well, to start out, these look like . . they look like a butterfly with two sea-horse heads on it.	1. ("Tell me about the butterfly.") The body of the butterfly was in between two wings—the sea-horse heads are on the wings. (Bottom green D.) [This is probably not so much a

	React.			
Card #	Time	Score	Protocol	Inquiry and Observations
				peculiar response as an uncritical one. Jack reports precisely what he sees, and he is not particularly concerned about whether it makes much sense.]
		DF+Ad	2. ∨ Two elephants.	2. ("How about the elephants?") It looks like the two things that came together were trunks. (Center blue D, seen upside down.)
		DF−A	3. ∧ Two rats.	3. ("What made them seem like rats?") Just the way they looked. ("How was that?") The way they . . just the way they looked. You can tell something by the way it looks, but you can't really tell what it is. (Top green D just above the blue "crab.") [Once more, Jack's inability to amplify precisely is apparent.]
		DF+A	4. Dog laying down.	4. ("Could you tell me about the dog?") It was a dog laying down with its head up in the air, looking around. (Outside bottom sepia D.)
		DF+A	5. > Uh . . . . . . a dinosaur.	5. (Outside yellow D, seen sideways.)
		DF−A	6. ∧ This is another dinosaur.	6. (Blackish D under and attached to preceding yellow D "dinosaur.")
		DF+A	7. Two dogs with awful big eyes.	7. ("What kind of dogs with big eyes did they seem to be?") Chihuahuas. ("Why?") Because of their big eyes. (Central yellow D's.)

THEMATIC APPERCEPTION TEST

[Jack's stories are brief. His people simply act, mostly destructively, and their action is not preceded by the attribution of significant awareness regarding the motivations which give rise to their action. The actions are grossly described, roughly hewn, poorly differentiated, lacking fine gradations. The examiner, though he tries rather actively to discover the causes for things happening in the stories, meets with little success. Jack is not concerned with offering reasons for the occurrence of any happening—things just do happen, without prologue or epilogue. A few of Jack's stories follow, and one quickly feels their quality of impoverishment.]

Card 4 (A woman is clutching the shoulders of a man whose face and body are averted as if he were trying to pull away from her.)

This man is . . looks like he is going after somebody, and his wife is trying to hold him back. She is just trying to hold him back. Probably been doing something, I don't know . . . . . . ("What happens then?") Well, he tells her no, and he goes on out . . . . . . ("Then what happens?") He goes out and shoots somebody . . . . . . ("Why did he want to shoot somebody?") He broke into the house. ("Is it someone he knows?") Yes. ("Who is it?") A very good friend of theirs. It is a man that they don't like. ("Why did he break into the house?") He needed some money or something, I guess he needed it. [Jack's story to Card 4 illustrates the impoverishment of his capacity to think empathically, to think in anything but a kind of shorthand in which he notes only peaks and valleys and does not recognize or describe the terrain which lies between. His stories and the motivations of his characters are obscure and his statements are confusing and often contradictory (e.g., the phrases "a very good friend" and "a man they don't like," describing the same person in succeeding sentences).]

Card 7 BM (A gray-haired man is looking at a younger man who is sullenly staring into space.)

This judge is talking with this boy about taking five cars down to St. Louis from Florida, and he is talking it over, and the boy said both of his parents are dead, and he ran away from the orphanage, and he has to stay cooped up all the time, and the judge said, "Okay," and he left him, and the boy was eighteen, wasn't a juvenile any more, and so he left him alone, and he went on out and made his living. ("Why did he take the cars?") He took the cars so he could go down . . up to St. Louis to get a job. ("Why did he take five; why not just one?") When he left the orphanage, he didn't have any money. After one car was out of gas, he just took another one. ("And how did it all finally work out?") Well, there were no charges against him, and so the judge let him go and made him report to the probation officer. ("How did the boy feel afterwards?") He didn't feel too happy, but he learned to live with it. [This is a frankly autobiographical story. Many of Jack's stories deal with delinquent activity, and very often the hero of the stories is an orphan. Jack conveys a kind of romance about the orphan who runs away, or the fatherless boy who leaves home in order to lighten his mother's burden. He talks about delinquent behavior in a matter-of-fact way. The young minor criminals he tells about act in ways that are "natural," ways that represent the "ways of the world." Jack neither condemns nor extols the illegal behavior, and one is left with the feeling that he is saying, "What's everyone making such a fuss about?"]

Card 16 (Blank card.)

This horse was wild when he was born, and he wanted to stay wild for a long time, for the rest of his life, but the ranchers caught him, and he was a real black horse with a white mane and a white tail, and they took him to a rodeo, and nobody could ride him. He is put in a stall, and they put a saddle on him, and they put a man on him and took him out there, and he bucked that man. He bucked five more off, and they put him back in, for that day it was late. The man that caught him sold him to a rodeo, and it went on for years and years, and finally he just gave up one day, and jumped over the fence, rode out into the prairie, and laid down and died. [This is an obvious metaphor. In this way Jack tells of his wish to remain free of the demands that family, school, the law and other social institutions place on him. He knows that efforts to "tame" him will continue, and he sees his only release as coming in the form of a romantic death, which will permit him freedom forever. He is able to tell a much fuller story when he speaks about himself in this minimally disguised way.]

SENTENCE COMPLETION TEST II

[A great proportion of Jack's conscious preoccupations concern themselves with cars—having them, driving them, repairing them. Engrossment with automobiles permits the diversion and focusing of a great deal of the poorly organized and disturbing impulse which appears during adolescence and which, when not channeled, causes the adolescent much distress and may well result in chaos for him and for persons and things that surround him. Jack's concern with cars has almost erotic significance—he makes it clear, for example, that his preoccupation with cars substitutes for a preoccupation with girls. If Jack grows into adulthood easily, then this diversion of interest from heterosexuality to automobiles) will be relatively temporary. Optimally, as he grows older and becomes better able to deal with impulses, his fascination with cars will give way to more future-oriented preoccupations, in addition to more heterosexually directed activities.]

He hoped that when he grew up he would . . be a mechanic.

His parents bought him a car. Is it okay if I sort of tell a story with it? ("You can end the sentences in whatever way you like.")

When he saw what the other kids were doing he too wanted a car.

When he compared himself to his friends . . . . his friends . . . . knew more. [For a moment, Jack lets us see through the car diversion to his underlying feelings of inadequacy.]

He was sad whenever he thought of . . oh . . of . . . . losing his car. ("Why did he lose it?") I don't know. Oh . . . . he was in a wreck.

When he was asked about his aches and pains he said he didn't have any. [Denial is one of Jack's prominent defense mechanisms.]

The person he admired most the person? Was his . . that's a *hard* one. (He smiles.) . . I know what you're getting at there. If it's mother, it shows I favor her, and if it's father, it shows I favor him. ("You can end it in whatever way you like.") His best friend is the person. ("Why does he admire him?") Oh, admire! It wouldn't have to be parents . . is his teacher. ("Why does he admire the teacher?") How much he knows, and what he can do. [Jack indicates that he "sees through the examiner's methods" and that he is not about to be trapped into any sort of significant, but involuntary, revelation.]

His brother had just bought him a car . . had just bought a car.

When the girl kissed him he . . uh . . . . got out of the car and started walking. That's not much in my line. I never liked girls and horses, period. [So much for girls and horses.]

When his father came into the room he got up. ("Why was that?") To show his respect. [Jack lives much of his life in accordance with external tokens which reflect little more than the thinnest forms of "appropriateness."]

When he was with his sister he felt lonely. ("Why was that?") Girls aren't much companionship. It seems like boys don't like to do what girls do, and vice versa. [Another expression of his negative feeling about girls.]

At school we had a man teacher. ("How was he?") A lot harder. [Male or female occupy an important position in Jack's life. The feeling toward males is usually more positive.]

When he looked at the work the other students were doing he decided that he would try to do as good as they are.

He was very happy when his father bought him a car.

The thing he found hardest to do .... to .. rearrange the ..... transmission.

Whenever certain things really bothered him .. uh .. he went out and talked to the boys .. that doesn't sound very good. ("How do you mean?") He should go to his father or mother. [Here is another superficial "propriety," an act Jack feels he ought to perform, such as stand when his father enters a room.]

His dreams were all about cars.

When he saw that the man had left the money behind he picked it up and ran after the man and gave it to him.

He thought that his mother was a wonderful .. mother. [The relationship between the "typical" delinquent and his mother is often intense and positive.]

Whenever he and his family disagreed ..... he'd get mad. ("What would he do?") Jump up and down and shout. [Discussion, the exchange of ideas, does not offer an effective way in which Jack can express himself.]

When he was very little .. hm .. he used to watch cars go by on streets .. to tell what kind it was. [Jack's interest in cars has probably come to serve its present psychodynamic meaning only relatively recently, however.]

His best friend .. Well .. his best friend was a school instructor .. of his auto-mechanic class. That is, his best friend in *teachers*. [It is hard to know what a "best friend" here represents. Perhaps this particular teacher has expressed some interest in what Jack is doing, and Jack has been able to talk with him.]

He was unhappy with his father when his father tried to sell his car.

When his mother asked about his girl friend he told her he didn't have any.

He never thought he would be able to tear an engine down and put it back together.

He always hoped that he . . would get a . . new car.

What he liked best about himself was . . he knew how to fix cars. [I.e., he was well defended.]

His mother was more likely than his father to understand . . why he liked cars . . so much.

His sister liked to ride in a car with him.

When he had nothing else to do he would work on his car.

He thought that his intelligence was normal.

What he liked best about school was . . mechanic class.

When he couldn't see a way out of his problem he'd go to his mother. ["Mother" serves as an effective comforter. As Jack has already said, she is more likely to "understand" than is his father.]

He saw the cockroach on the wall and took a fly swatter and (he motions swatting a fly) hit it. [Actions supplement words.]

His teacher was very nice.

Whenever he got angry he'd go out and work on his car . . to get rid of things.

He remembered that when he was little he was a . . . . . . the same way. ("What way was that?") He . . . . liked to pull things out . . and put 'em back again.

When the kids invited him to go with them to the hiding place, he thought that it'd be fun. That's the longest one [i.e., the longest stem], isn't it? [Jack's alertness is evident again here. He finds it important to know exactly what is going on "out there." Even though he may make no startling inference about the nature of the things involved, he rarely lets anything noteworthy slip by.]

After school he usually went home and worked on his car.

He admired his father when he helped him out on his car.

When the girl invited him to a party he refused.

When he and his brother were together they would have lots of fun.

He thought that his body . . His body? . . . . was getting wider.

When he had a lot of homework to do he would . . do it and go out and work on his car then, after he'd finished.

What he disliked about school was teachers. ("How was that?") Oh . . just . . they didn't seem fair to him.

Whenever he spoke about his problems to someone . . Oh . . he would put a lot of . . emotions into it. ("Why was that?") Oh . . just . . he wanted to get their attention. [Jack implies that he is not sincere, or at least does not feel sincere, when he speaks about his feelings.]

When he entered the haunted house he was scared (he laughs).

When the other fellow offered him a cigarette he took it.

He didn't like his mother to shout at him.

When the baby arrived it was . . sixteen pounds. ("It weighed that much?") When it got home.

When the fellows asked him to join them in a rough game he . . he accepted.

Whenever he didn't do what he was told his parents would get mad. ("What would they do?") They would scold him and tell him he shouldn't do that.

What would make him angriest was when . . his father wouldn't help him on the car. I'm just about sticking to the story, aren't I? [Jack wants his father's help in strengthening his own defenses. When the father is not helpful in this way, it makes Jack angriest.]

In his spare time he would work on the car. Oh, I get it. You're going over them to see if I . . remember what I put down on the others. [Jack constantly thinks he is being tricked.]

What troubled him most was when his father wouldn't help him on his car.

When he was alone in his room at night he would work on . . a model . . model car that . . he could . . He was customizing the model car to see how it looked . . and put that on his car.

What scared him most was . . when he got his report card.

He struck the match and . . hm . . lit the fire.

He disliked his father when he wouldn't help him on his car. [Jack apparently divides his parents into the one who supports his car interests (his defenses)—his mother—and the one who opposes them—his father.]

He thought that his looks were pretty good.

The thing he could do best was fix cars.

He had no respect at all for somebody who drove a car and didn't know what they were driving . . if something happened to the motor, and they couldn't fix it.

He always enjoyed working on his car.

He had a very uncomfortable feeling when the teacher was looking at him.

He found it easiest to talk to his shop teacher.

WORD ASSOCIATION TEST

(Jack's association rate usually varies from 1″ to 3″. There are, however, occasions when reaction times take as long as 4″, 11½″, 12″, 14½″ and once over 33″. Primarily, these delays occur after sexual and aggressive words (the 33″ delay comes on delayed recall to the word *fight*). Jack's recall is fairly adequate. There are occasions, particularly on the "oral" words, when he "mishears"—e.g., "mouse" for *mouth*.) [Jack's performance on Word Association shows that his calm is relatively superficial and rather easily disrupted. He appears to have specific conflicts in the area of orality and aggression, and his efficiency is rather easily disorganized in areas which relate to sex. Jack's air of bravado seems to be a rather thin veneer.]

THE PSYCHOLOGIST'S REPORT

Jack's ineffectively concealed anxiety gives rise to temporary thought disruptions and inefficiencies. For example, when I ask him his birthday, he replies , "April . . April, 1952." He spontaneously corrects himself, saying that this would make him only six years old. (Actually, it would make him four.) When, on the Wechsler-Bellevue, I ask how many weeks are in a year, he tries to solve the problem by dividing seven into 336, a number he later corrects to 360. Recent and remote memory seem particularly vulnerable to anxiety. He recalls only half the memorial elements of a paragraph I read to him and on Delayed Recall loses some credits he previously achieved because of fairly serious memory distortions. For example, instead of repeating the phrase, "A man cut his hands," Jack says, "The man split his head open."

But while anxiety undoubtedly has a disorganizing effect, it is difficult to separate it from Jack's basic noninvolvement in the solution of problems that require a verbal response. Thus, one is never sure to what extent Jack does not remember because of disruptive anxiety and to what extent he does not remember because he does not find the area involved particularly important to his life. He does not prize thinking, particularly thought which involves factual elements unrelated to his present interests; and his doing poorly in tasks which require reflection may well be a symptom of this lack of involvement.

On the Wechsler-Bellevue, he functions in the Average to Bright Normal range. His Verbal Quotient is 104-105; his Performance Quotient is 112-117; and his Total Intelligence Quotient is 109-112. His capacity for abstract thought is surprisingly well developed for a person who seems to value conceptualization so little.

On this same test, Jack's action orientation is suggested by the discrepancy which exists between his Verbal and Performance Quotients. His penchant for activity is further expressed in his tendency to express ideas through descriptive gestures and through explosive, onomatopoetic sounds (instead of, or in addition to, words). Jack often seems to find it easier to act than to resort to the introspection required for reflective thinking. His difficulty in looking inward is also manifest on the Rorschach, where eighteen of his twenty responses have an "easy," uncreative Animal content. He finds it almost impossible to respond thoughtfully to inquiry on this test. The following is a typical example of this inability: he sees two dogs, and when I ask him to describe them, he says, "I'm not good on dogs. Let's see . . Well, they look like dogs . . dogs look like dogs, don't they? That's all I can figure out." On Card I, after seeing the popular "bat," he says, "It could be *hundreds* of things," yet he is unable to give a single additional response. Jack's lack of careful, disciplined thinking results at times in a carelessness and occasionally in a certain arbitrariness. On Card X of the Rorschach, for example, he sees a butterfly with two sea-horse heads attached to its wings. Although such a response might at first glance suggest a schizophrenia-like disorder of thinking, the response is much more probably the result of Jack's somewhat cavalier and stimulus-bound attitude toward reality.

Jack's lack of involvement (or is it his anxiety about having to deal with the uncertain?) is particularly striking when a task is poorly structured, so that he does not know what is "right" or "wrong." When he *is* fairly sure, he is eager to proceed and to be correct. Nevertheless, one feels that Jack's tendency to wish to do well reflects almost exclusively his desire to make a favorable impression.

Jack is exceptionally alert to his environment. Once, for example, when I had misplaced my cigarettes, he casually pointed over his shoulder to where he had briefly seen them when he entered the room. He uses his alertness to discover what possibilities he can exploit as potential shortcuts and "gimmicks." On the Picture Arrangement subtest, for example, he correctly guesses the meaning of the letters on the back of each card and says, "I'm not supposed to look at the back, am I?" He often projects this somewhat wiley tendency, so that he will see others' motives as insincere and "tricky." Thus, for example, he may say what he thinks my "real" intention might be when I (ingenuously) ask a particular question.

Jack's suspiciousness largely operates in a world which to him seems composed of cops and robbers. Thus, he tends to view even relatively innocuous situations in terms of their "legality." When, for example, he is asked the Wechsler-Bellevue question about what he would do were he to find a sealed, addressed envelope on the street, he answers, "I'm sure not going to open it. That's a federal offense." Literally three-quarters of his Thematic Apperception Test stories involve delinquent or criminal themes, including: staying out late, running away from home, narcotic addiction, car theft, burglary, armed robbery and murder. Possibly because he wishes to present himself as reformed, and possibly because he feels so plagued by guilt that he performs delinquent acts in order to be caught, the criminals about whom he tells stories are all caught and punished.

Jack seems to see himself as the victim of a malevolent fate. He has little conception of his own responsibility in getting into his difficulties and experiences himself as propelled by some force over which he has no power. He seems to express his philosophy as, "Well, that's the way things are. Boys will be boys." On the Thematic Apperception Test, his heroes have to make the best of their unpleasant situation, and there is nothing they or anyone else can do about it. He consciously sees delinquent and criminal acts as realistic events, neither "good" nor "bad."

That the "delinquent" behavior may nevertheless represent a wish to be punished is suggested by one Thematic Apperception Test story in which a boy, troubled by insomnia, goes to a psychiatrist. The psychiatrist finds the boy's sleeplessness to be the result of guilt caused by a past crime he has committed. The boy is able to sleep peacefully again after he has confessed to the police and been put in jail.

Jack expresses little direct aggression. Only once does he permit himself an even mildly caustic comment: I misunderstood him, and he smiled sarcastically and said, "We all make mistakes." The conflict he experiences around expressing direct aggression is suggested by his blocking 33" to the word *fight* on the Word Association Test. It may be that Jack's antisocial activities and fantasies represent a less direct outlet for the aggression which he finds so difficult to express face to face, at least toward adults.

Jack feels very close to his mother. In his Thematic Apperception Test stories, he tends in some fashion to eliminate his father, usually by means of an accident or illness which results in the father's death. On the Sentence Completion Test, Jack states, *He thought that his mother* "was .. a wonderful .. mother." At the same time it is important to note that, once Jack eliminates his father and finds himself alone with his mother, his stories concern the boy's running away from home.

This intimate feeling for his mother is probably related to Jack's delayed interest in girls. Jack's present attitude toward girls is much more typical of a boy eleven or twelve years old. On the Sentence Completion Test, he says, *When the girl kissed him he* "got out of the car and started walking. That's not much in my line. I never liked girls." Jack feels that girls are no fun, offer no companionship and don't like to do the things that boys like. Several times on the Thematic Apperception Test, Jack wonders about the sexual identity of different persons, even though one of them is wearing a necktie. Such doubts suggest the degree to which Jack had not yet resolved his identification struggle.

Possibly because he finds erotic impulses too psychologically disorganizing, Jack is intensely preoccupied with cars. Literally half his Sentence Completions refer to riding in, working on, and being given cars, or having them taken from him. At least superficially, his preoccupation with cars colors all his relations—to peers, parents, siblings, teachers and even to strangers. He is happy with his father when his father gives him a car and angry with him when he takes it away. He says his mother is more understanding than his father because she can accept his interest in cars. The person "he admires the most" is his automotive-mechanics teacher. He has "no respect at all" for people who simply drive cars but have no understanding of the cars' inner workings. When he is bored or angry, he finds relief by working on his car.

Jack's view of himself, of his freedom to operate the way he wishes, and of the involvement of adults in his present situation, is poignantly captured in the following story he tells to the blank Thematic Apperception Test card:

> This horse was wild when he was born, and he wanted to stay wild for a long time, for the rest of his life, but the ranchers caught him, and he was a real black horse with a white mane and a white tail, and they took him to a rodeo, and nobody could ride him. He is put in a stall, and they put a saddle on him, and they put a man on him and took him out there, and he bucked that man. He bucked five more off, and they put him back in, for that day it was late. The man that caught him sold him to a rodeo, and it went on for years and years, and finally he just gave up one day, and jumped over the fence, rode out into the prairie, and laid down and died.

Jack seems poorly motivated to undertake any treatment that would depend primarily on talking, such as psychotherapy. He seems unable and unwilling to involve himself in an introspective investigation of himself. Introspection gives rise to so much anxiety in Jack that he could probably not long remain in outpatient psychotherapy without needing to run away. It is recommended, therefore, that his fascination with cars be somehow exploited in his treatment. Work with cars seems literally to be the only constructive activity in which Jack is interested, and the persons associated with such work seem to be the only adults toward whom Jack feels respect and admiration. For these reasons, automotive mechanics seems suited as a treatment entry.

DISCUSSION

In many ways, with some pulling, tugging and other adjustments of edges which do not fit the stereotype precisely, Jack, of the three adolescents discussed in this chapter, seems most nearly to constitute what one thinks of as a "delinquent." He fits the stereotype in terms of his nonreflectiveness, his action orientation and his apparent unconcern regarding "right" ways of behaving. But he does not fit the stereotype as soon as one looks at his so very easily aroused anxiety, which causes him to block, to become confused and otherwise to behave in a number of tense ways.

Is there such a thing as "the" delinquent? Jack is a real person, three-dimensional and combining both strengths and weaknesses within his personality structure. One is able to consider him as a "delinquent" only if one disregards the "concrete" Jack in favor of the theoretical one.

CONCLUSION

The three young men whose test protocols are presented in detail in this chapter argue much more effectively than can the author for a critical look at a diagnostic concept that has been robbed of its individuality. Once more it needs to be said that the term "delinquency" is an abstraction which fits real people only as well (and as poorly) as any abstraction can. All diagnoses, of course, are abstractions. There is no such thing as "the" schizophrenic, or "the" hysteric, just as there is no such thing as "the" delinquent. People tend to be grouped as equivalent once they hold the same diagnosis, even though the individuals in the grouping may be exceedingly different from one another, similar only in an abstraction which has been taken out of the concrete context of the personality organization of which their diagnosis is a part. Just as there is no "schizophrenic," "obsessive compulsive," "hysteric," "organic," or "mental retardate," if one means that all persons in such a group are identical in all important respects, so there is no such thing as "the" delinquent. It cannot be said often enough that when one thinks in individualistic terms, one cannot deal with diagnostic abstractions because such abstractions eliminate the very thing which gives clinical practice its special quality. One thinks diagnostically primarily for epidemiological reasons—for the institution of large programs which will meet some needs of many. But since no large program can be individually tailored, such a program can never meet the totality or the unique configuration of a particular person's needs.

8

Final Thoughts

This brief, final chapter will serve primarily as a way of drawing a few threads together. One thread is a kind of caution—namely, to watch out for the confusing effects of the brief diagnostic *label*, which may hide more than it reveals. Even a superficial glance at the cases in each of the preceding chapters will show how different each individual is from others, even though he may have the same or a very similar diagnostic designation. This is not at all to say that diagnostic categorization is either invalid or useless. Diagnostic categories are usually gross and may therefore describe inexactly, but efforts have been and are being made to eliminate or circumvent traditional simplistic groupings and to substitute more complex and useful ways of ordering. A good diagnostic category is a shorthand communication, intended to help in the exchange of clinical information. When one says, for example, that a patient is "schizophrenic," one finds that a group of behaviors is mentally evoked and a section of discourse blocked out. Unfortunately, the "help" may sometimes turn out to be a major hindrance because the diagnostic category sets up expectations which concrete reality does not support. "Chronic schizophrenia," for example, is a diagnostic category which sets up expectations that probably have not too much to do with the kind of person that Chuck (Chapter 7) turns out to be. In Chuck's case, were one to take the diagnostic nomenclature completely seriously, one would discover a relatively poor fit, since, in a variety of ways, Chuck does not fulfill one's expectations of "the" chronic schizophrenic. And yet, what label would more effectively capture the kind of person Chuck is? What (nowadays) would describe the pathological-clinical aspect of his psychological situation more tersely, effectively and accurately? Surely such a category as "adjustment reaction of adolescence" is not an adequate alternative.

639

It is apparent that even the "mentally retarded" do not constitute as homogeneous a grouping as the nomenclature suggests. Chapter 2 contains the test protocols of three adolescents, all of whom are "mentally retarded," yet each of whom deals with his unfortunate situation in his individual way. Thus, although a diagnostic categorization may break off a relatively workable clinical segment which causes one's thoughts to travel along a certain path, such a brief categorization cannot capture the person's concrete individuality. Diagnoses are useful for quick clinical characterizations, for the setting of a clinical scene, for epidemiological studies (and for organizing this type of book), but they tend to muddy a person's individuality and thus to minimize the particularity on which clinical work prides itself.

Another human aspect which these pages attempt to exemplify involves the fact that people, particularly adolescents, are rarely, if ever, neatly self-consistent. Often we clinicians play down an individual's wide (and often wild) variety, so that a personality organization can more easily be fitted into a theoretically smoother, more immediately understandable and graspable, pattern. But one sees again and again that these young people are composed of a colorful variety of parts which seem to go off in different directions at the same time: behaviorally, characterologically, in terms of values, wishes, life goals and in a number of other ways. Just when the clinician may feel that he understands "all of" the personality of any adolescent, he finds some tendency which goes in a different, occasionally opposite, direction from the one he has come to expect (and, for reasons of theoretical neatness, from the one he might prefer). But few people, and even fewer adolescents, consistently go in one homogeneous set of directions. All a clinician can hope to accomplish in suggesting a diagnostic label is to indicate the person's dominant character and symptom trends. It may often be that the very direction which is not consistent with the others is the one that can effectively be exploited for treatment purposes. If one deals, for example, with a person who usually lacks external interests, but who is fascinated by some one area, then that area may be the entering wedge in instituting a useful treatment plan. The more one studies adolescents, as well as their elders, the more one realizes how multifaceted they are and how often they appear to be "inconsistent." The assigning of a diagnostic label, while often necessary, tends to obscure the rich variety present in each personality make-up. A "true" diagnosis (i.e., more than simply a label) takes much more account of the variety of personality tendencies which exist, of the wide spectrum of each person's dispositions, likes, values, wishes, needs and potentials, of his apparent inconsistencies, all of which contribute to the exquisitely varied, ever-changing spectrum of his personality.

The diagnosis of adolescents is complicated by the fact that they have not yet settled down to any sort of permanence in their personality organization. Probably their personalities are more integrated (although they may be quite different) than they were in childhood; probably they are *less* integrated (although, again, possibly quite different) than they later will be in adulthood. The personality hierarchization that will take place later on, which will involve certain characteristics being subsumed, or eliminated, or made less scratchy, or weakened, or modified in order to be integrated, is much less in evidence during adolescence. Inconsistency is much more characteristic during this period, when ways are being tried out to see how well they fit.

There are two reasons that the adolescents discussed in this book are presented by way of their reactions to psychological tests. First, the author is most familiar, and therefore most at home, with this form of personality investigation. Second, the various psychological tests offer an opportunity for tapping not only a *breadth* of behavior, but a hierarchical *depth* as well. Psychological tests seem to offer the possibility for discovering the personality multidimensionality which this book strives to emphasize.

Although psychological testing has established itself over the past years as a proper medium of exchange in the clinical marketplace, there is a question about how useful a supplement to a sensitive psychiatric investigation it often is. Except for an essential amount of basic (and relatively gross) information, how, even under the more auspicious circumstances, is additional subtle understanding useful for establishing or carrying out a treatment plan? The sensitive aide, or therapist, or nurse, or physician, or occupational therapist, or teacher takes his cues largely from some present interaction with the disturbed person.[1] On this more or less situational basis, the

[1] Although the psychotherapist will work with a person's internal relationships, he can work with them only as they emerge at any particular time. While there exists a strong point of view which holds that psychological tests can be helpful in psychotherapeutic planning, this view does not seem convincing to the author.

professional reacts in ways that are clinically appropriate. Using a less than recent diagnostic examination for current interventions carries with it the assumption that a person does not change basically: that any observed change can only be evanescent and superficial and that a personality organization, once developmentally established, remains immutable.

Psychological test findings tend frequently to be filled with the kinds of subtle personality nuances which, while they may be highly interesting, can probably be of no great use in the making of clinical decisions that involve initial disposition or later treatment planning. Clinicians are limited in the choices they have available to them in making their decisions. There are only so many things they can do—only so many ways that are available for clinical action.

It is not that psychological tests are of so little *potential* use; rather, we do not know *yet* how to apply the kinds of fine differentiations and distinctions which a sensitive diagnosis permits. Perhaps some day, once decisions based on diagnostic knowledge are more refined and differentiated, the kind of information that is derived from psychological tests can be more effective. As matters stand at the moment, however, the types of information derived from the psychological examination are primarily of training and research, rather than of applied, value. The information we derive from tests helps us to understand patients more thoroughly, even though we understand only a very small portion of that information well enough these days to do much with.

Regardless of the quality of the disorder which the adolescents in these pages manifest, they all share the problem of growing into adulthood, a problem they face in a variety of ways. The major picture, which appears over and over, involves the adolescents' confusion. They are confused about who they are, who they can become, what is important, where they are going at the moment, and where they will and can go in the future. Partly through their symptoms, they try to drown out the implicit and explicit demands to reach some sort of life decision, but this drowning out is usually only a moderately successful effort; it does not and cannot totally quiet the underlying affective restlessness, the impulse perturbation and the identity questioning. As an increasingly large portion of the total population falls into the adolescent category, it is necessary to find new methods to help the growth process of these young people. The ways that have served until now are no longer adequate (if they ever were). It is neither fair nor effective simply to patch up the old methods in order to adapt to the conditions of today. Possibly the old ways work less well now because mistakes are much more obvious when they are numerically so magnified. In any case, clinicians cannot be satisfied to enter the picture so late—to try to undo damage which has already had its disruptive effects. Although there has been a good deal of nonproductive talk about prevention, so that this concept is in danger of becoming a cliché, it nevertheless appears that a wholly new attitude and point of view will have to be developed to help young people across that complicated boundary, so difficult for many to step over, between the dependency of being a child and the autonomy of being an adult.

Bibliography

Babcock, H. (1930), An Experiment in the Measurement of Mental Deterioration. *Arch. Psychol.*, No. 117.

Bellak, L., & Bellak, S. S. (1949), *Children's Apperception Test.* New York: C. P. S.

Bender, L. (1946), *The Bender Gestalt Test.* New York: American Orthopsychiatric Association.

Bixler, H. H. et al. (1959), *The Metropolitan Achievement Test.* New York: Harcourt, Brace & World.

Blos, P. (1962), *On Adolescence.* New York: Free Press.

Erikson, E. (1956), The Problem of Ego Identity. *J. Amer. Psychoanal. Assn.*, 4:56-121.

Freud, A. (1958), Adolescence. *The Psychoanalytic Study of the Child,* 13:255-278. New York: International Universities Press.

Group for the Advancement of Psychiatry (1959), *Basic Considerations in Mental Retardation.* New York: Group for the Advancement of Psychiatry.

Machover, K. (1949), *Personality Projection in the Drawing of the Human Figure.* Springfield, Ill.: Charles C Thomas.

Menninger, K. A., Mayman, M., & Pruyser, P. (1963), *The Vital Balance.* New York: Viking Press.

Murray, H. A. (1943), *Thematic Apperception Test.* Cambridge: Harvard University Press.

Rapaport, D., Gill, M. M., & Schafer, R. (1945-1946), *Diagnostic Psychological Testing.* Chicago: Year Book Publishers. Revised edition, ed. R. R. Holt (1968). New York: International Universities Press.

Rorschach, H. (1921), *Psychodiagnostics.* Bern: Hans Huber, 1949. (Distributors for the United States, Grune & Stratton, New York.)

Schafer, R. (1948), *The Clinical Application of Psychological Tests.* New York: International Universities Press.

Strauss, A. A., & Lehtinen, L. E. (1947), *The Psychopathology and Education of the Brain Injured Child.* New York: Grune & Stratton.

644

Terman, L. M., & Merrill, M. A. (1916-1937), *Revised Stanford-Binet Intelligence Scale.* New York: Houghton-Mifflin.

―――― & ―――― (1937), *Measuring Intelligence.* New York: Houghton-Mifflin.

Wechsler, D. (1941), *The Measurement of Adult Intelligence* (2nd ed.). Baltimore: Williams & Wilkins.

―――― (1949), *Wechsler Intelligence Scale for Children.* New York: The Psychological Corporation.